Signals and Communication Technology

Series Editors

Emre Celebi, Department of Computer Science
University of Central Arkansas
Conway, AR, USA

Jingdong Chen, Northwestern Polytechnical University
Xi'an, China

E. S. Gopi, Department of Electronics and Communication Engineering
National Institute of Technology
Tiruchirappalli, Tamil Nadu, India

Amy Neustein, Linguistic Technology Systems
Fort Lee, NJ, USA

H. Vincent Poor, Department of Electrical Engineering
Princeton University
Princeton, NJ, USA

Antonio Liotta, University of Bolzano
Bolzano, Italy

Mario Di Mauro, University of Salerno
Salerno, Italy

This series is devoted to fundamentals and applications of modern methods of signal processing and cutting-edge communication technologies. The main topics are information and signal theory, acoustical signal processing, image processing and multimedia systems, mobile and wireless communications, and computer and communication networks. Volumes in the series address researchers in academia and industrial R&D departments. The series is application-oriented. The level of presentation of each individual volume, however, depends on the subject and can range from practical to scientific.

Indexing: All books in "Signals and Communication Technology" are indexed by Scopus and zbMATH

For general information about this book series, comments or suggestions, please contact Mary James at mary.james@springer.com or Ramesh Nath Premnath at ramesh.premnath@springer.com.

G. R. Kanagachidambaresan
Dinesh Bhatia • Dhilip Kumar • Animesh Mishra
Editors

System Design for Epidemics Using Machine Learning and Deep Learning

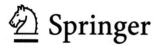

Editors
G. R. Kanagachidambaresan
Department of CSE
Vel Tech Rangarajan Dr Sagunthala R&D
Institute of Science and Technology
Chennai, India

Visiting Associate Professor
Department of Institute of
Intelligent Systems
University of Johannesburg
South Africa

Dhilip Kumar
Computer Science and Engineering
Vel Tech Rangarajan Dr. Sagunthala R&D,
Institute of Science and Technology
Chennai, TN, India

Dinesh Bhatia
Department of Biomedical Engineering
North Eastern Hill University
Shillong, Meghalaya, India

Animesh Mishra
North Eastern Indira Gandhi Regional
Institute
Shillong, India

ISSN 1860-4862 ISSN 1860-4870 (electronic)
Signals and Communication Technology
ISBN 978-3-031-19754-3 ISBN 978-3-031-19752-9 (eBook)
https://doi.org/10.1007/978-3-031-19752-9

© The Editor(s) (if applicable) and The Author(s), under exclusive license to Springer Nature Switzerland AG 2023

This work is subject to copyright. All rights are solely and exclusively licensed by the Publisher, whether the whole or part of the material is concerned, specifically the rights of translation, reprinting, reuse of illustrations, recitation, broadcasting, reproduction on microfilms or in any other physical way, and transmission or information storage and retrieval, electronic adaptation, computer software, or by similar or dissimilar methodology now known or hereafter developed.

The use of general descriptive names, registered names, trademarks, service marks, etc. in this publication does not imply, even in the absence of a specific statement, that such names are exempt from the relevant protective laws and regulations and therefore free for general use.

The publisher, the authors, and the editors are safe to assume that the advice and information in this book are believed to be true and accurate at the date of publication. Neither the publisher nor the authors or the editors give a warranty, expressed or implied, with respect to the material contained herein or for any errors or omissions that may have been made. The publisher remains neutral with regard to jurisdictional claims in published maps and institutional affiliations.

This Springer imprint is published by the registered company Springer Nature Switzerland AG
The registered company address is: Gewerbestrasse 11, 6330 Cham, Switzerland

To family, students, and friends.

Preface

The World Health Organization (WHO) proclaimed a COVID-19 pandemic in March 2020 (WHO 2020). COVID-19 is a multi-system disorder caused by the SARS-CoV-2 coronavirus. Vaccine development was prioritized for managing and controlling the pandemic due to concerns about the disease's spread and severity, as well as the effectiveness of available therapies. During epidemics or pandemics, such as the current Coronavirus Disease 2019 (COVID-19) crisis, healthcare practitioners (HCPs) face a variety of difficult situations. The stress of treating patients during an epidemic or pandemic may be detrimental to HCPs' mental health. Evidence-based recommendations on what would be useful in reducing this impact are lacking. Digital healthcare has been a hot topic among people for quite a while. The pre/post pandemic situations have led patients and subjects to be monitored outside the hospital environment with more digital equipment to avoid spreading of COVID. Tapping into the available data to extract useful information is a challenge that's starting to be met using the pattern matching abilities of machine learning (ML) – a subset of the field of artificial intelligence (AI). In order to provide smarter environments, machine learning needs to be implemented in the Internet of Things (IoT). Machine learning will allow these smart devices to become smarter in a literal sense. It can analyze the data generated by the connected devices and get an insight into the human's behavioral pattern. Without implementing ML, it would really be difficult for smart devices and the IoT-based digital healthcare to make smart decisions in real time, severely limiting their capabilities. This book provides the challenges and the possible solutions in these areas. Various image-based and data-based artificial intelligence approaches are discussed in this book to improve the healthcare services in hospital.

Chennai, India
Shillong, India
G. R. Kanagachidambaresan
Dinesh Bhatia
Dhilip Kumar
Animesh Mishra

Acknowledgments

We thank all authors, who have put a lot of time effort and their findings in this book project. We would like to thank our reviewers for providing timely reviews. The support from Vel Tech, North Eastern Hill University, and North Eastern Indira Gandhi Regional Institute of Health and Medical Sciences allowed editing and support of our projects. We hope this book will be a valuable material for all healthcare researchers.

Contents

Pandemic Effect of COVID-19: Identification, Present Scenario, and Preventive Measures Using Machine Learning Model... 1
A. Nazar Ali, Jai Ganesh, A. T. Sankara Subramanian, L. Nagarajan, and G. R. Subhashree

Introduction... 1
    Coronavirus First Case 2
    Corona Cases in India.. 2
Structure of Coronavirus... 4
    Growing Stages of Virus 4
Statistical Data of COVID-19 at Present Scenario 5
    COVID-19: Confirmed Cases and Causalities 5
    COVID-19: Transmission Rate and Statistics on Different Stages of Transmission 7
    COVID-19: Case Fatality Rate (CFR) 9
    COVID-19: Category-Wise Fatal Cases – Age Factor and Medical History 9
Machine Learning Model for COVID-19 Prediction 10
    Baseline Model... 10
    Training Using Unbiased Features 11
    Discussion... 11
    Development of the Model 12
    Evaluation of the Model 13
Transmission and Prevention of COVID-19 14
    Transmission of COVID-19 14
    Prevention and Control Measures 14
Conclusion 15
References 16

A Comprehensive Review of the Smart Health Records to Prevent Pandemic ... 19
Kirti Verma, Neeraj Chandnani, Adarsh Mangal, and M. Sundararajan

Introduction to a Smart Health Record ... 19
    Various Types of Records in Smart Health ... 21
    Development of EHR Standards for India ... 22
    Traditional Paper Records vs Smart Health Records ... 23
Comparison Between Paper-Based Records and Electronic Health Records ... 24
    Interoperability and Standards in the Smart Healthcare System ... 25
    Guidelines for Proposed Smart Health Records ... 26
    Introduction of Machine Learning in Healthcare ... 27
    Introduction to Vector Machine Techniques ... 28
    Introduction to OCR Techniques in Healthcare ... 30
    Flood of Paper Claims After the Arrival of Optical
        Character Recognition ... 30
    Electronic Exchange of Documents ... 32
    Advantages of OCR in Healthcare ... 32
    Privacy and Security in Smart Health Records ... 32
Conclusion ... 35
References ... 35

Automation of COVID-19 Disease Diagnosis from Radiograph ... 37
Keerthi Mangond, B. S. Divya, N. Siva Rama Lingham, and Thompson Stephan

Introduction ... 37
Materials and Methods ... 38
    Dataset ... 38
    Proposed Classification Model ... 39
Results and Discussion ... 41
    First Phase (Data Augmentation) ... 41
    Second Phase Pre-Trained VGG16 ... 42
    Performance Metrics ... 42
    COVID-19 Classification Results ... 42
    Confusion Matrix and Feature Maps ... 42
    Comparison with State-of-the-Art Methods ... 44
Results and Discussion ... 45
References ... 46

Applications of Artificial Intelligence in the Attainment of Sustainable Development Goals ... 49
Nisha Solanki, Archana Chaudhary, and Dinesh Bhatia

Introduction to Artificial Intelligence and Sustainable
    Developmental Goals (SDGs) ... 49
Artificial Intelligence and SDGs ... 51

Role of AI in Quantitative SDGs	51
Good Health and Well-Being	51
Quality Education	53
Affordable and Clean Energy	54
Decent Work and Economic Growth	54
Responsible Consumption and Production	55
Peace, Justice and Strong Institutions	56
Partnership for the Goals	56
Role of AI in Qualitative SDGs	57
No Poverty	57
Zero Hunger	58
Gender Equality	59
Clean Water and Sanitation	59
Industry, Innovation and Infrastructure	59
Reduced Inequalities	60
Sustainable Cities and Communities	60
Climate Action	60
Life Below Water	61
Life on Land	61
Conclusion	61
References	62

A Novel Model for IoT Blockchain Assurance-Based Compliance to COVID Quarantine 63
M. Shyamala Devi, M. J. Carmel Mary Belinda, R. Aruna, P. S. Ramesh, and B. Sundaravadivazhagan

Introduction to Blockchain	63
Blockchain	64
Blockchain Design Architecture	65
IoT Blockchain Assurance-Based Compliance to COVID Quarantine	66
IoT Design Architecture	67
Temperature Sensor Control Node	68
Respiration Sensor Control Node	72
Pulse Rate Sensor Control Node	73
Accelerometer Sensor Control Node	73
Blood Pressure Sensor Control Node	74
Motion Sensor Control Node	75
Glucometer Sensor Control Node	75
EMG and EEG Sensor Control Node	76
Patient Doctor Smartphone Sensor Control Node	77
Wi-Fi/Bluetooth Sensor Control Node	77
Health Authorization Sensor Control Node	78
Results and Efficiency Analysis	79
Conclusion	80
References	81

Deep Learning-Based Convolutional Neural Network with Random Forest Approach for MRI Brain Tumour Segmentation 83
B. Leena

Introduction. 83
Literature Review 86
System Design 89
    Convolutional Neural Network. 90
Result and Discussion. 92
Conclusion 94
References. 95

Expert Systems for Improving the Effectiveness of Remote Health Monitoring in COVID-19 Pandemic: A Critical Review 99
S. Umamaheswari, S. Arun Kumar, and S. Sasikala

Introduction. 99
    Internet of Things 101
    Artificial Intelligence (AI) and Robotics 101
    Wireless Body Area Networks 101
COVID-19 Pandemic 102
Remote Health Monitoring System 102
    Advantages of Remote Health Monitoring System for COVID-19 102
Wireless Body Area Network for Remote Monitoring of SARS-CoV-2 ... 104
    Workflow of WBAN Architecture. 106
    Security Constraints in Wireless Body Area Network 107
IoT in COVID-19 Remote Health Monitoring 108
    Remote Monitoring of Vitals 109
    Rapid Diagnosis 109
    Contact Tracking. 110
    Screening. 110
    Reducing the Workload of Healthcare Professionals 110
    Disease Containment and Tracking 110
Robotics and AI Technologies in COVID-19 Pandemic. 114
    COVID-19 Risk Assessment. 115
    Surveillance During COVID-19 116
    Telehealth Care Services During COVID-19 117
    Delivery and Supply Chain During COVID-19 117
    Disinfection. 119
    Research and Drug Development 119
Conclusion 119
References. 120

Artificial Intelligence-Based Predictive Tools for Life-Threatening Diseases ... 123
Vijay Jeyakumar, Prema Sundaram, and Nithiya Ramapathiran

Origin and Background of Diseases ... 125
   Classification ... 125
   Phases of Disease ... 126
   Transmission of Infection ... 127
   Routes of Transmission ... 128
Morbidity and Mortality Rates ... 129
Pathogens of Bacteria and Virus ... 130
   Plague or Black Death ... 130
   Cholera ... 132
   Influenza or Spanish Flu ... 132
   Smallpox ... 133
   HIV or AIDS ... 133
   Coronavirus ... 133
Disease Management System ... 134
Role of Expert Systems ... 135
   Mathematical Model for Predictive Modeling ... 136
   The Implication of Machine Learning Algorithms ... 137
   Deep Learning Model for Big Medical Data Analytics ... 141
Tools Used for Mass Screening ... 142
   Predictive Tool for Mass screening ... 142
COVID-19 Prediction Tools ... 143
   Machine Learning Algorithm-Based Predictive Tools ... 144
   Deep Learning-Based Predictive Tools ... 148
Summary ... 148
References ... 149

Deep Convolutional Generative Adversarial Network for Metastatic Tissue Diagnosis in Lymph Node Section ... 153
J. Arun Pandian, K. Kanchanadevi, Dhilip Kumar, and Oana Geman

Deep Convolutional Generative Adversarial Network ... 153
Data Augmentation on PatchCamelyon Dataset Using DCGAN ... 155
   PCam Dataset Preparation ... 155
   DCGAN Model Design and Parameter Optimization ... 155
   Training the DCGAN on PCam Dataset ... 157
   DCGAN Performance Testing Using Frechet Inception Distance ... 161
Development of Classification Models for Metastatic Tissue Detection ... 162
Results and Discussions ... 163
Conclusion ... 165
References ... 166

**Transformation in Health Sector During Pandemic
by Photonics Devices**... 167
Jyoti Ahlawat, Archana Chaudhary, and Dinesh Bhatia

Introduction.. 167
Existing Technologies for Healthcare Monitoring 168
Diagnostic Technologies on the Rise 174
Technologies for Disinfection...................................... 176
Future Outlook and Conclusion 179
Bibliography... 181

**Diagnosis of COVID-19 from CT Images and Respiratory
Sound Signals Using Deep Learning Strategies**...................... 185
S. Maheswaran, G. Sivapriya, P. Gowri, N. Indhumathi,
and R. D. Gomathi

Introduction... 185
   Economical Impact on the World 186
   Economical Impact of India 187
   Some Positives of COVID-19................................... 188
   Some Drawbacks of Covid 188
   Impact on Students 189
Dataset Description... 190
Proposed Methodology... 190
   Dataset Preprocessing... 192
   Data Augmentation... 192
   Feature Extraction... 193
   ResNet-50 Model 194
   Feature Selection.. 195
   LSTM 197
Classification.. 197
   Performance Metrics.. 198
   Random Forest 199
   XGBoost... 199
   Support Vector Machine 200
   LASSO, Ridge, and Elastic Net Regression...................... 200
Conclusion 203
References... 204

**The Role of Edge Computing in Pandemic and Epidemic
Situations with Its Solutions**..................................... 207
A. G. Balamurugan, R. Pushpakumar, S. Selvakumari, and
S. Pradeep Kumar

Introduction... 207
Related Works... 208
   Health Care in Affective Computing............................. 209

IIoMT Devices	209
Deep Learning Applications	210
Edge Computing	210
System Design	210
Edge Computing Applications	210
Selection of Edge IIoMT Device	213
Edge Deep Learning Stack Design	213
System Workflow	213
Implementation	214
Test Results	216
EEG Signal Classification	216
Drowsiness Analysis	216
ECG	217
Fever Detection	217
Face Mask Detection	218
Determination of Physiological State Using Excitement Analysis	218
Residential Cough Sound Analysis from Both Affected and Not Affected	218
Conclusion and Future Work	219
References	219

Advances and Application of Artificial Intelligence and Machine Learning in the Field of Cardiovascular Diseases and Its Role During the Pandemic Condition 221
Sohini Paul

Introduction	221
AI and Its Principles	222
Applications of AI in the Medical Field Settings	223
Application of AI in Cardiovascular Diseases	223
Precision Medicine	224
Clinical Prognosis	224
Cardiac Imaging Analysis	224
Intellectual Robots	225
Clinical Decision Support System and Preventive Cardiology: The Application of AI	225
Applications of AI During the COVID-19 Pandemic in the Domain of Cardiology	226
AI and Cardiology Treatment During the Pandemic Situation	227
COVID-19 Pandemic and Artificial Intelligence: The Challenges	227
The Future Scope of Artificial Intelligence	228
References	228

Effective Health Screening and Prompt Vaccination to Counter the Spread of COVID-19 and Minimize Its Adverse Effects.. 231
Sandip Bag and Swati Sikdar

Introduction... 231
Screening.. 233
COVID-19 Screening Tools and Procedure........................ 233
Vaccine... 239
COVID-19 Vaccine... 240
Working Mechanism of COVID-19 Vaccine..................... 243
Vaccination.. 244
Side Effects of COVID-19 Vaccine.................................. 250
Importance of COVID-19 Vaccination............................. 251
Conclusion.. 253
References... 253

Crowd Density Estimation Using Neural Network for COVID-19 and Future Pandemics... 257
S. U. Muthunagai, M. S. Girija, R. Iyswarya, S. Poorani, and R. Anitha

Introduction... 257
Tracking Framework for Objects...................................... 258
   Object Detection.. 258
   Object Modeling.. 259
   Object Tracking... 260
Proposed Model... 262
   Object Detection and Tracking Model........................... 264
   YOLO Object Detection... 264
   Pairwise Distance Calculation Using Manhattan Distance... 265
   Closeness Property... 266
   Possibility of the Breach in the Protocol and Transmission... 266
Object Detection and Distance Calculation Using Proposed Scheme...... 266
   Input Feed.. 266
   Object Detection.. 267
   Decision-Making and Output Formatting....................... 267
Performance Evaluation... 267
Conclusion and Future Work.. 269
References... 270

Role of Digital Healthcare in Rehabilitation During a Pandemic........ 271
Meena Gupta and Ruchika Kalra

Introduction... 271
   Different Digital Health Platforms in Rehabilitation......... 272
Discussion... 277
Conclusion.. 279
References... 279

**An Epidemic of Neurodegenerative Disease Analysis
Using Machine Learning Techniques** 285
M. Menagadevi, V. Vivekitha, D. Thiyagarajan, and G. Dhivyasri

Introduction. 285
Supervised Learning 287
Decision Tree 288
Linear Regression 289
Logistic Regression. 291
Naive Bayes 292
Support Vector Machine 293
Unsupervised Learning. 294
K-Means Algorithm 295
Mean-Shift Clustering Algorithm 295
Affinity Propagation and Hierarchical Clustering 296
Density-Based Spatial Clustering (DBSC). 298
Gaussian Mixture Modeling 299
Convolutional Neural Network (CNN). 299
    Convolutional Layer 300
    Activation Functions. 300
    Pooling Layer 301
    Fully Connected Layer 301
Conclusion 302
References. 302

**COVID-19 Growth Curve Forecasting for India Using
Deep Learning Techniques**. 305
V. Vanitha and P. Kumaran

Introduction. 305
Literature Review 306
Materials and Methods 308
    Description of Dataset. 308
    Forecasting COVID-19 with Recurrent Neural Network 308
    ADF (Augmented Dickey-Fuller) Test 310
    LSTM 311
    Stacked LSTM 312
    Bidirectional LSTM 313
    The Proposed Models 314
Results and Discussion. 315
Conclusion 319
References. 319

Index. 323

About the Editors

G. R. Kanagachidambaresan received his BE degree in electrical and electronics engineering from Anna University in 2010 and ME in pervasive computing technologies from Anna University in 2012. He has completed his PhD at Anna University, Chennai, in 2017. He is currently an associate professor in the Department of CSE, Vel Tech Rangarajan Dr. Sagunthala R&D Institute of Science and Technology. His main research interest includes body sensor network and fault-tolerant wireless sensor network. Kanagachidambaresan has published several reputed articles and undertaken several consultancy activities for leading MNC companies. He has also guest edited several special-issue volumes and books for Springer and serves as editorial review board member for peer-reviewed journals. He is presently working on several government-sponsored research projects by ISRO, DBT, and DST. He is an ASEM-DUO fellowship. Kanagachidambaresan has successfully edited several books in EAI Springer. He is presently editor-in-chief for Next Generation Computer and Communication Engineering series Wiley. He is a Visiting Associate Professor, Department of Institute of Intelligent Systems, University of Johannesburg, South Africa.

Dinesh Bhatia pursued his PhD in biomechanics and rehabilitation engineering from MNNIT, Allahabad, India, in 2010 with bachelor's (2002) and master's degree (2004) in biomedical engineering from Mumbai University. He completed his MBA (dual specialization) from IMT Ghaziabad in 2007. He is currently working as an associate professor in the Department of Biomedical Engineering, North Eastern Hill University (NEHU), Shillong, Meghalaya, India. Dinesh is the recipient of the "Young Scientist Award (BOYSCAST 2011–12)" by the Government of India to pursue research in osteoarthritis (OA) for 1 year at Adaptive Neural Systems Laboratory, Biomedical Engineering Department, Florida International University, Miami, Florida, USA, where he was leading a multidisciplinary team of researchers. He is also the recipient of "INAE fellowship award" in 2011 by the Indian National Academy of Engineering. Dinesh was selected as one of the 12 young biomedical scientists by the Indian Council of Medical Research (ICMR), Govt. of India, to pursue research fellowship (2014–15) in the field of sensory prosthetics at

University of Glasgow, Scotland, UK. He has attended biomechanics and human gait training at Munich, Germany, in March 2017, and training of use of neurodiagnostics equipment(s) at Ivanovo, Russia in September 2017. He delivered an Invited Talk on Gait and Osteoarthritis in Kaula Lumpur, Malaysia, in August 2018. Dinesh has several research papers in reputed journals, conference, seminars, and symposia with teaching and research experience of more than 17 years. He is invited panel member of several professional bodies, editorial boards, committees, societies, and forums. Dinesh has worked on various funded projects on physically challenged, disabled, and paralyzed persons, and few projects are still on-going. He has published 9 books and 21 books chapters till date and supervised several UG, PG, and doctoral students. His research focuses on understanding muscle mechanics, joint kinematics, and dynamics involved in performing locomotion and routine tasks and undermining it effects during an injury or disease. His areas of interest are medical instrumentation, biomechanics and rehabilitation engineering, medical informatics, signal and image processing, marketing, and international business.

Dhilip Kumar Associate Professor, Department of CSE, Vel Tech Rangarajan Dr. Sagunthala R&D Institute of Science and Technology, Avadi, dhilipkumarit@gmail.com. Dr. V. Dhilip Kumar, He was awarded PhD at North Eastern Hill University (A Central University of INDIA) in 2017. Presently, he is working as an associate professor in the Department of Computer Science and Engineering at Vel Tech Rangarajan Dr. Sagunthala R&D Institute of Science and Technology, Chennai. He has more than 10 years' experience in teaching as well as research. Dhilip did his BTech in information technology and ME computer science engineering under Anna University, Chennai. He has published in various international journals and international conferences in the field of vehicular communication and machine learning. Dhilip is an editorial board member and reviewer of various international journals and conferences by reputed publishers such as Springer, IEEE, Elsevier, and Wiley. His areas of interest are vehicular communication, soft computing techniques, Internet of Things, and machine learning. He is presently working on projects related to artificial intelligence for healthcare and automations.

Animesh Mishra Professor, Department of Cardiology, NEIGRIHMS (An autonomous institute, Under ministry of Health & Family Welfare, Government of India). Dr. Animesh Mishra has completed his DM in cardiology from MAMC Delhi University. He has completed his MD in internal medicine from the Institute of Medical Sciences, BHU Varanasi. Animesh has more than 25 years of professional experience. He has published his research in reputed publications.

Pandemic Effect of COVID-19: Identification, Present Scenario, and Preventive Measures Using Machine Learning Model

A. Nazar Ali, Jai Ganesh, A. T. Sankara Subramanian, L. Nagarajan, and G. R. Subhashree

Introduction

Coronaviruses are a category of viruses belonging to the *Coronaviridae* family. Coronaviruses produce enveloped virions with a diameter of around 120 nm. The envelope's club-shaped glycoprotein peaks give the infections a crown-like look. The viral nucleic acids are contained in a protein coat called a nucleocapsid that is either helical or spherical. One favorable strand of RNA makes up the entirety of the coronavirus DNA. Corona infections are wrapped, single-stranded, positive-sense RNA infections that are phenotypically and genotypically assorted. These components have not only prompted the occurrence of a variety of known coronaviruses but have also encouraged the rise of infections with new characteristics that permit the living being to adjust to new haven and ecologic specialties, in some cases causing zoonotic events. In humans, poultry, and cattle, coronaviruses are common causes of gastrointestinal illness. A kind of coronavirus known as SARS produces a highly contagious respiratory infection in humans that is characterized by

---

A. N. Ali (✉)
Department of Electrical and Electronics Engineering, Rajalakshmi Engineering College, Chennai, Tamil Nadu, India
e-mail: nazarali.a@rajalakshmi.edu.in

J. Ganesh · A. T. S. Subramanian
Department of Electrical and Electronics Engineering, K. Ramakrishnan College of Technology, Trichy, Tamil Nadu, India

L. Nagarajan
Department of Electrical and Electronics Engineering, Kathir College of Engineering, Coimbatore, Tamil Nadu, India

G. R. Subhashree
Kingston Engineering College, Vellor, Tamil Nadu, India

© The Author(s), under exclusive license to Springer Nature Switzerland AG 2023
G. R. Kanagachidambaresan et al. (eds.), *System Design for Epidemics Using Machine Learning and Deep Learning*, Signals and Communication Technology, https://doi.org/10.1007/978-3-031-19752-9_1

symptoms like fever, coughing, and muscle pain, frequently coupled with dynamic difficulty in relaxing. In 2002, more persons became infected; it likely infected humans from bats, i.e., horseshoe bats. Coronaviruses are not only found in bats, but they can also be found in numerous different species, including feathered creatures, felines, hounds, pigs, mice, ponies, whales, and people. Depending on the type of the organism, they may have varying degrees of severity; they may induce respiratory, intestinal, hepatic, or neurologic disorders. Without even a doubt, genetic alterations to the infection were necessary for the SARS coronavirus to be able to spread to humans. Since the SARS illness seen in horseshoe bats cannot legitimately infect people, it is believed that these progressions took place in the palm civet. Additionally, a SARS outbreak in humans was brought on by a heretofore unheard-of coronavirus in 2003. The RNA-subordinate RNA polymerase's dishonesty, the high frequency of RNA recombination, and the remarkably large genomes considering RNA infections all contribute to the coronaviruses' good diversity.

Coronavirus First Case

Some other coronavirus that was believed to cause the Middle East respiratory syndrome (MERS), a severe respiratory disorder, was discovered in people in 2012. The first case was discovered in Saudi Arabia, and since the identification of MERS, countries like United Arab Emirates, Germany, Qatar, Jordan, France, and the UK have also reported cases of MERS. Every case that was recorded had an indirect or direct connection to the Middle East respiratory syndrome. Roughly 33% of the alleged cases that were tallied as of 2019 ended in fatalities. The coronavirus that caused the Middle East respiratory syndrome was similar to other coronaviruses that were believed to have originated in bats and spread from bats to other species ultimately reaching humans. And the main reservoir of MERS was thought to be camels. An infection with clear links to the SARS coronavirus emerged in Wuhan, China, early in 2019. It was named COVID-19 disease which was caused by a virus named SARS-CoV-2 and has similar symptoms to SARS, i.e., fever and respiratory problems [10]. The disease is highly contagious and the infection is extremely difficult to prevent. By the middle of 2020, it had reached every part of China, as well as the USA and Europe, after being spread by travelers from the infected regions. The World Health Organization declared a pandemic to be in progress in March [2, 3].

Corona Cases in India

On January 30, 2020, the first case of COVID-19 infection in India was identified. A total of 1637 cases, 133 recoveries, and 38 deaths have been reported throughout the country as of April 1, 2020, according to the Ministry of Health and Family Welfare. Since India's sickness rates are some of the lowest in the world, experts believe there may be more ailments than we realize. The rate of COVID-19 exposure in India is taken into account; it is fundamentally lower than it is in the nations with the worst environmental conditions. Over 12 states and associate areas have declared the event to be a plague, and as a result, plans under the Epidemic Diseases Act of 1897 have indeed been made, leading to the closure of various corporate foundations as well as educational institutions. Due to the fact that the majority of the confirmed cases involved other nations, India has stopped all visitor visas. At the behest of Prime Minister Narendra Modi, India observed a 14-hour deliberate open limited time on March 22, 2020. In addition to every major city, the authorities planned lockdowns in 75 locations where COVID infections had occurred. Additionally, on March 24, the chief admin asked for a 21-day nationwide lockdown, affecting India's entire 1.3 billion people. As the second populous country, India would have a huge impact on the ability of the globe to control the coronavirus outbreak, according to World Health Organization official CEO Michael Ryan. Figure 1 displays the current COVID-19 cases in India. Those are the coronavirus introductions, which help us to understand how these viruses were created, how they spread around the world (e.g., in India), and how the countries around the world are combatting these viruses. In this paper, a machine learning method that can correctly predict the presence of SARS-CoV-2 illness by using RT-PCR testing is developed. It works by posing eight simple questions. The model has been trained

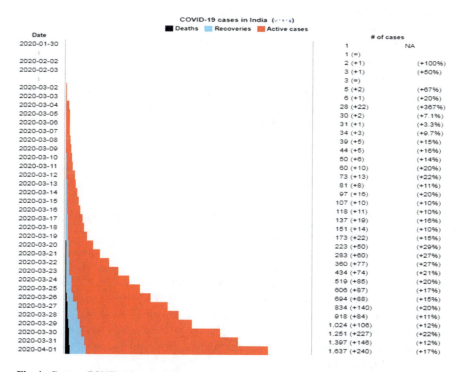

Fig. 1 Current COVID-19 cases in India

using information from each Israeli who had undergone a SARS-CoV-2 test during the initial months of the COVID-19 pandemic. Thus, for effective viral screening and prioritizing inhabitant testing, our approach may be used globally. The structure of coronaviruses is covered in Chap. 2, along with their developmental stages, and statistical data gathered from all around the world is covered in Chap. 3.

Structure of Coronavirus

The structure is characterized by spikes enveloped as crown-like on its exterior [1]. It is named after its spike structure that looks like a crown, which comes from the Latin term coronam, meaning crown. The coronavirus is composed of the following major components: spike protein, genome single-stranded +RNA (ss + RNA), nucleocapsid protein, membrane, and envelope. This coronavirus is nanometeric in size ranging between 65 and 125 nm. The spike protein is projected outside the envelope of the virus particle [3]. It is composed of glycoprotein. This glycoprotein helps in binding virus to the host cell surface especially to angiotensin-converting enzyme 2 (ACE2) receptor and facilitates entry into cytosol. This spike protein has more affinity to ACE2 than MERS and SARS that is why it is spreading widely. The genome (ss + RNA): The nuclei contain a single-stranded +RNA genome, with sizes ranging between 26 and 32kbs in length containing all information necessary for making viral component. Nucleocapsid protein: This ss + RNA contain a structured protein-forming complex known as nucleocapsid. This nucleocapsid again envelops the ss + RNA. Membrane and envelope: The nucleocapsid is enclosed by the membrane also composed of lipid protein; it forms the central organization of CoV assembly, which determines the shape of the virus [9]. Different from MERS and SARS, the sequence data and amino acid data of COVID replicate that is why this coronavirus spreads widely (Fig. 2).

Growing Stages of Virus

Stage 1: Binding of virus spike region to ACE2 of the host cell, which allows the entry of virus inside the cytoplasm.
Stage 2: Release of ss + RNA genome and its protein synthesis. In this stage, this ss + RNA is ready for translation.
Stage 3: Replication and transcription of complex substances. This is done by recognizing eukaryotic ribosome instantly as it has MRNA 5prime cap and a poly-A tail. Here replication of sub-genome also happens with all proteins.
Stage 4: Replication of RNA genome by the enzyme, which is RNA-dependent. Translation of sub-genome RNA forms nucleocapsid, spike protein, membrane, and envelop protein.

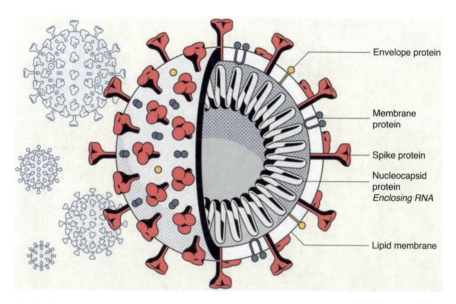

Fig. 2 Structure of coronavirus

Stage 5: Genome RNA is also released and it multiplies with the help of replication and genome is released into cytoplasm along with nucleocapsid.

Stage 6: Release of virion into the infected host cell and this multiplication goes on leading to pneumonia. Figure 3 shows the growth of coronavirus. Moreover, this virus replicates another virus called SARS [11–14].

Statistical Data of COVID-19 at Present Scenario

COVID-19: Confirmed Cases and Causalities

The coronavirus outbreak is said to have its first recorded case in a market in Wuhan, China, in the mid of December 2019 which rapidly becomes an epidemic infecting people with symptoms similar to a common cold or without symptoms. But if not addressed on time, it could become life-threatening to an infected individual. The sources of World Health Organization in its report clearly made a global warning and alerting all countries to make suitable arrangements for preventing their citizens from getting affected [4–8]. The total confirmed cases globally are around 750,890 with causalities of 36,405 as of the end of March. More cases with symptoms still need to be identified. The region-wise classification of confirmed cases is shown in Fig. 3. The WHO itself declares the situation is very crucial and the statistics available is changing from time to time. The data available from WHO is based on the

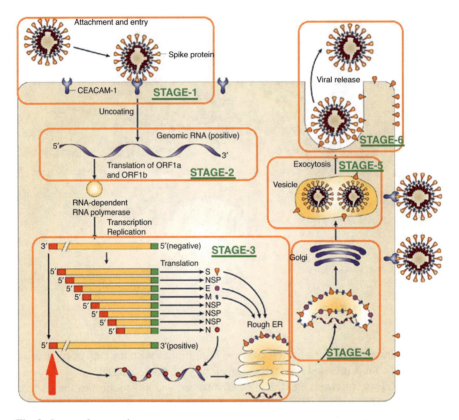

Fig. 3 Stages of coronavirus

hospitalized cases and one must be aware that there are even more cases with symptoms that still need to identified. From Fig. 4 it is observed that the European region is the most affected by sharing around 56% of the total confirmed cases followed by Region of Americas (22%), Western Pacific Region (14%), Eastern Mediterranean Region (7%), South-East Asian Region (1%), and finally African Region (0.5%).

Figure 5 shows the number of causalities among the confirmed cases. Though the Eastern Mediterranean Region has lower number of infections (50,349) when compared to Region of Americas (1,63,014) and Western Pacific Region(104,868), it has the second highest causalities with 5.8% of death among its confirmed cases. The most affected region is the European Region in terms of not only the number of confirmed cases but also the number of deaths, i.e., 6.2% of infected people so far lost their lives to this deadly disease.

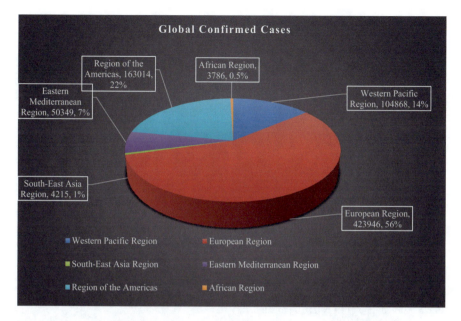

Fig. 4 Region-wise COVID-19 confirmed cases

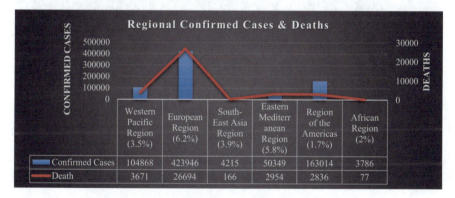

Fig. 5 Region-wise COVID-19 confirmed cases and causalities

COVID-19: Transmission Rate and Statistics on Different Stages of Transmission

With the global alert from the World Health Organization and the pandemic assessment sectors of individual countries, many countries started implementing self-quarantine procedures on their people. Since no vaccine has so far assured to cure the COVID-19 disease, there is no way other than preventing its spread further. But the statistical data presented in Fig. 6 is not encouraging as it clearly shows there is a tremendous growth in the spread of the disease starting from its first infection in

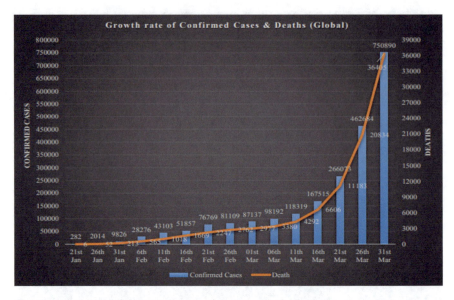

Fig. 6 Growth rate of COVID-19 globally

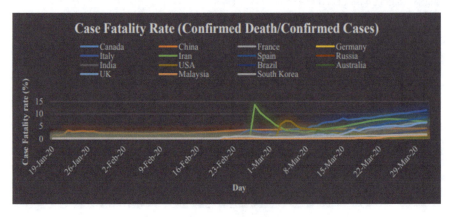

Fig. 7 Day-to-day changes in the CFR of different countries

Wuhan. It spreads throughout the world in a faster rate as an airborne or contact type viral spread. But still different countries or territories have different rates of transmission which depend on many factors such as climatic conditions, populations, sex ratio, age, etc. Everyday thousands of new cases are registered among millions of people who are tested globally [21, 22]. The scenario will become worse if the country enters into stage 3 of transmission, that is, the communal spread from unidentified infected people.

Figure 7 shows the stage of transmission of COVID-19 disease among different countries or territories among the six regions classified earlier. However, the statistics shows only two basic categories, namely, local transmission and imported cases.

There will be always many more combinations which cannot be accurate because of the complexity in identification and collection of data. As per the WHO report [23], it is clearly stated that the stages of transmissions are subjected to change based on the availability of detailed reports on root cause analysis. It is observed that many countries are already experiencing community transmission or at the verge of reaching that danger zone and it is not a good sign for human life. It is noticeable that there are more imported cases in American and African regions where infected people from other countries migrated to such countries resulting in more infections. However, local transmission is low in those two regions. Still more precautionary measures are needed as prescribed by WHO such as lockdown of infected areas or even countries.

COVID-19: Case Fatality Rate (CFR)

Case fatality rate is the ratio of confirmed deaths to confirmed cases. Figure 7 shows the day-to-day percentage of case fatality rate in a pool of 15 countries worldwide.

It is observed that China where the disease is first identified flattened its curve along with South Korea to some extent, whereas other countries such as Iran, Spain, Italy, the UK, and the USA are fighting hard to save their people. Germany, Malaysia, Australia, Brazil, and India are keeping their case fatality rate well within their control. The success of the countries purely depends on the concept of "flatten the curve" principle and it seems all the countries are working their best toward it [16–20].

COVID-19: Category-Wise Fatal Cases – Age Factor and Medical History

During outbreak of any worldwide pandemic, it is highly impossible to present the exact number of infections without testing all possible infected individuals, still from the available data and the best possible observations. Fatal cases of COVID-19 are categorized based on patients' age group and their medical history bringing out a clear idea about the worst result that this disease can give to a society. It is clearly observed that the elderly are more vulnerable compared to the young people to be infected with COVID-19 that targets the respiratory system of an individual. The data about the fatal cases in China, South Korea, Italy, and Spain is shown in Fig. 8. The elderly aged over 60 are more prone to be infected with COVID-19 and also children below 10 years of age but no casualties are observed under age 10. Still there are many other factors as discussed earlier apart from age that play an important role in transmitting and increasing the fatality rate of this disease. Italy and Spain are found to have more causalities as they have the most aged population

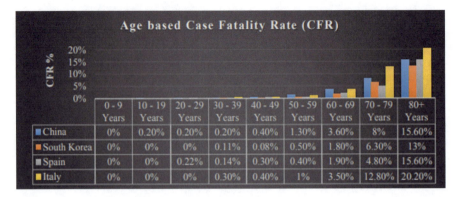

Fig. 8 Age-based case fatality rate in different countries

around the world, i.e., around 60% of their total population is more than 50 years of age. It replicates the data of CFR when it comes to age-wise diseased people [24, 26–29].

The case fatality rate in China is a sample-based analysis to predict what age groups of people are more vulnerable to COVID-19. There are also cases being confirmed without any major symptoms. But in general, based on the available data, healthy people with no medical history have less chance of being infected compared to people having long-term health issues such as allergic asthma, leukemia, cancer, hypertension, chronic respiratory diseases, diabetes, and cardiovascular diseases. It is observed that people with cardiovascular diseases have high mortality rate (10.50%) followed by people with diabetes (7.30%) and chronic respiratory diseases (6.30%). So it is advisable that people who already have the above health issues should be more cautious about the disease.

Machine Learning Model for COVID-19 Prediction

Baseline Model

The model made predictions based on the area under the receiver operating characteristic curve for the potential test set. The feasible working points based on test set predictions are 84.54% sensitivity and 78.20% specificity or 85.60% sensitivity and 70.68% specificity.

An additional spreadsheet file has all of the metrics from each ROC curve that was used in this study. Fever and cough were crucial indicators of the disease's impending onset. As predicted, close contact with a person who had been diagnosed with COVID-19 was also a significant factor, supporting the illness' high transmissibility and emphasizing the value of social isolation. Additionally, the model found that male gender was a predictive factor of a favorable outcome, correlating with the reported gender bias.

Training Using Unbiased Features

Limits and biases exist in the information that the Indian Ministry of Health reported. For example, symptom reports were more thorough for those who tested positive for COVID-19, and this finding was supported by a focused epidemiological investigation. Therefore, it is anticipated that people who tested negative for COVID-19 may mislabel their symptoms. The percentage of those who were COVID-19 positive compared to all of the people who were positive for each symptom reflects this. As a result, our approach distinguished between symptoms having balanced reporting and characteristics with biased reporting (headache, 95.1%; sore throat, 92.8%; shortness of breath, 92.6%; cough, 27.5%; and fever, 45.5%). Misclassification of sensations may also result from those who tested negative underestimating and underreporting their symptoms. Finally, it gets an auROC of 0.842 with a modest shift in the Shapley additive explanations summary plot if we train and test our model while pre-filtering out signs of strong bias (Figs. 9 and 10).

Discussion

Depending on straightforward clinical manifestations, the model offers first COVID-19 test screening. By enabling optimal administration of healthcare resources throughout upcoming waves of the SARS-Cov-2 pandemic, improving clinical priorities may lessen the strain now placed on health systems, which is particularly crucial in resource-constrained emerging nations. There are some issues with this study. For patients whose contact with a confirmed COVID-19 carrier was indicated, additional information such as the time and place of the encounter was not accessible. Previous research has found some symptoms as being highly indicative of a COVID-19 infection, but the Health Ministry did not document them. It demonstrated that a model may be trained and tested while having severe bias

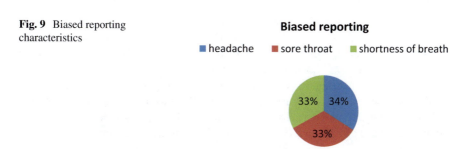

Fig. 9 Biased reporting characteristics

Fig. 10 Symptoms with balanced reporting characteristics

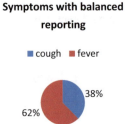

symptoms removed beforehand and yet attain very high accuracy. Additionally, keep in mind that all illnesses had been self-reported; hence, a negative result for a symptom may indicate that it was not recorded. Therefore, it's crucial to evaluate the performance of the model using absent or missing information rather than through negative ones. In the projected test set, researchers randomly picked negative reports for each of the five symptoms at a time and then deleted the negative values to create a less biased scenario. The model continued to produce encouraging results with regard to these generated test sets, boosting our faith in the approach. All the people tested had reasons for testing, notwithstanding the possibility that this model may have limitations due to variations in how symptoms are reported. This suggests that for the vast majority of the participants in this sample, there was no referral bias. Coughing and cold were listed as the primary symptoms in the Ministry of Public Health guidelines, and it is thought that even in people who tested negative for SARS-Cov-2, these indications are difficult to detect [15].

Furthermore, we assume that biases pertaining to the COVID-19-negative group were lessened by the comparatively large sample size. This emphasizes the need for more reliable data to supplement the concept and acknowledge the bias that always exists when symptoms are self-reported (Fig. 11).

As the COVID-19 epidemic spreads, it is essential that reliable data are continuously collected and shared between government agencies and the science process. Additional indications might be incorporated into future devices in addition to our awareness of how different symptoms affect the diagnosis of the disease.

Development of the Model

A gradient-boosting machine model created with selection base-learners was used to produce predictions. Many effective algorithms in the field of machine learning use gradient boosting, which is usually regarded as state-of-the-art for forecasting statistics. The gradient-boosting predictor treated missing data by default, as suggested by earlier investigations. We made use of the LightGBM Python package's gradient boosting predictor. Early halting was tested using the validation set, and auROC was utilized as the performance indicator. SHAP values were computed to determine the key characteristics influencing model prediction [40]. These

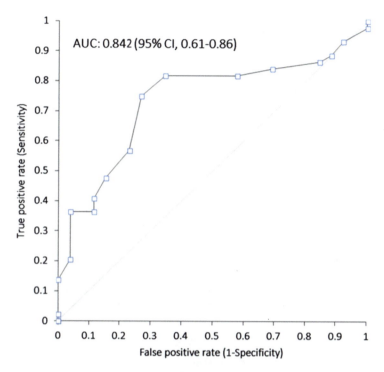

Fig. 11 Shapley Additive explanations summary plot – auROC

parameters are appropriate for sophisticated models like gradient-boosting machines and ANN [41]. The SHAP values, which have their roots in game theory, divide each sample's prediction performance into the contributions made by each individual feature value. This is accomplished by estimating model differences using subsets of the feature space. SHAP values calculate the relevance of each attribute to final predicted results by average across samples.

Evaluation of the Model

The auROC was used to evaluate the model on the test set. Plots of the PPV versus sensitivities were also created across several thresholds. Sensitive, specific, prognostic, and predictive values, false-positive and false-negative rates, false discovery rates, and accuracy rate were all determined for all the threshold values because of all the ROC curves. The bootstrap percentage approach with 1000 trials was used to derive confidence intervals (CI) for the different performance metrics [37–39].

Transmission and Prevention of COVID-19

Transmission of COVID-19

Exact mode of transmission cannot be predicted, but some modes of transmissions are discussed. Sneeze and Cough: When the infected person sneezes or coughs, then the infected droplets spread in the air for 1 meter and deposits on the nearby objects and cause aerosol. When the non-infected person touches the object, then he will become the host, and by this method, the transmission can be single or group depending upon the place [30].

Close Contact

When a person has a close contact with the infected person, then that person may also be infected [31, 32]. By this method, group of persons may have the chance being infected when they have contact with family members and healthcare workers. The shopkeeper who is infected may also spread this.

Prevention and Control Measures

The only method to avoid the transmission is quarantine, social distancing, wearing of face mask, frequent handwashing with soap and water, and alcohol sanitizing.

Self-quarantine: This is adopted by the infected person himself, in a room of his home, in order to avoid spreading of the virus [33, 34].

Quarantine ward (isolation ward): In this ward, persons who are severely infected are admitted. This ward is under the surveillance of NGO or government. These organizations are responsible of the infected persons. They provide all medicines and hygienic dieted food besides continuously monitoring the infection rate. If the person is cured from the disease, then he/she will be sent home [35, 36].

Social distancing: This is maintaining a distance of more than 1 meter from every person in the infected region. This will prevent the other person from inhaling the aerosols.

Wearing of face mask: Since the size of the COVID-19 is in nanometer, it will be filtered by mask during inhaling [28].

Hand washing and sanitizing: Hands should be frequently washed with soap and water for about 20 seconds with more foam, because the enveloped membrane of COVID-19 which is made of lipid can easily destroyed by soap and alcohol disinfectants.

Figure 12 shows COVID 19-transmission possibility and its preventive measures [25].

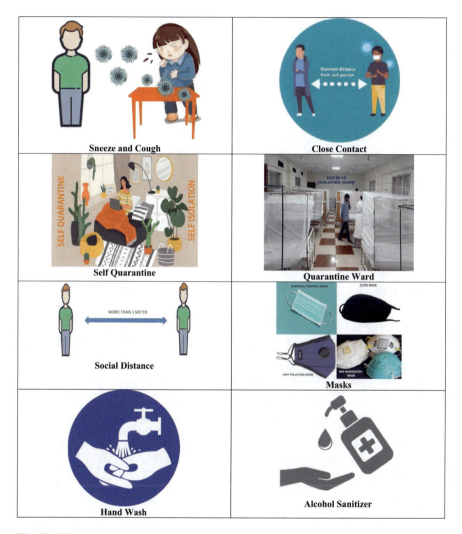

Fig. 12 COVID-19 transmission possibility and its preventive measures

Conclusion

With the analytical results of the current scenario of coronavirus outbreak based on the available subsets of data, the 2019-nCOV is found to have different growth pattern with different degree of casualties in different regions. It is observed that the changes in the structure of coronavirus are vital in creating this disgusting situation resulting in increased mortality rate throughout the affected areas. It is found that the elderly aged 70 and people with preexisting medical conditions such as cardiovascular problems, diabetes, and chronic respiratory diseases are more prone to get infected, and these factors play an important role in increasing the fatality rate. Now it has become an important responsibility of the individual to follow the proven preventive measures as discussed in this study. Moreover, there are also positive observations, i.e., more than 20% of infected people are treated in response to common antiflu microbial treatments, more than 70% of affected people are only experiencing mild symptoms, and only less than 15% of patients required intensive care treatment. "Flatten the curve" is the basic idea the countries are trying to achieve through continuous, tireless, well-planned, and disciplined medical and social measures to get away from the ruthless hands of COVID-19. In summary, this created a model that can predict COVID-19 diagnoses by posing eight fundamental questions based on data collected across the country and published by the Ministry of Health. When testing resources are limited, this methodology can be used, among several other things, i.e., to prioritize COVID-19 testing. The approach used in this study could also help the health system react to subsequent epidemic waves of this illness and of other respiratory pathogens in particular.

References

1. N. Wang, X. Shi, L. Jiang, S. Zhang, D. Wang, P. Tong, et al., Structure of MERS-CoV spike receptor-binding domain complexed with human receptor DPP4. Cell Res. **23**(8), 986 (2013)
2. C.-C. Lai, T.-P. Shih, W.-C. Ko, H.-J. Tang, P.-R. Hsueh, Severe acute respiratory syndrome coronavirus 2 (SARS-CoV-2) and corona virus disease-2019 (COVID-19): The epidemic and the challenges. Int. J. Antimicrob. Agents **105924** (2020)
3. Organization WH, *Laboratory Testing for Coronavirus Disease 2019 (COVID-19) in Suspected Human Cases: Interim Guidance, 2 March 2020* (World Health Organization, 2020)
4. C. Wang, P.W. Horby, F.G. Hayden, G.F. Gao, A novel coronavirus outbreak of global health concern. Lancet (2020)
5. L.T. Phan, T.V. Nguyen, Q.C. Luong, T.V. Nguyen, H.T. Nguyen, H.Q. Le, et al., Importation and human-to-human transmission of a novel coronavirus in Vietnam. N. Engl. J. Med. (2020)
6. J. Riou, C.L. Althaus, Pattern of early human-to-human transmission of Wuhan 2019 novel coronavirus (2019-nCoV), December 2019 to January 2020. Eur. Secur. **25**(4) (2020)
7. J. Parry, *China Coronavirus: Cases Surge as Official Admits Human to Human Transmission* (British Medical Journal Publishing Group, 2020)
8. Q. Li, X. Guan, P. Wu, X. Wang, L. Zhou, Y. Tong, et al., Early transmission dynamics in Wuhan, China, of novel coronavirus–infected pneumonia. N. Engl. J. Med. (2020)
9. J. Huynh, S. Li, B. Yount, A. Smith, L. Sturges, J.C. Olsen, et al., Evidence supporting a zoonotic origin of human coronavirus strain NL63. J. Virol. **86**(23), 12816–12825 (2012)
10. J.F.-W. Chan, K.-H. Kok, Z. Zhu, H. Chu, To KK-W, S. Yuan, et al., Genomic characterization of the 2019 novel human-pathogenic coronavirus isolated from a patient with atypical pneumonia after visiting Wuhan. Emerg. Microbes Infect. **9**(1), 221–236 (2020)
11. S. van Boheemen, M. de Graaf, C. Lauber, T.M. Bestebroer, V.S. Raj, A.M. Zaki, et al., Genomic characterization of a newly discovered coronavirus associated with acute respiratory distress syndrome in humans. MBio **3**(6), e00473–e00412 (2012)
12. X. Xu, P. Chen, J. Wang, J. Feng, H. Zhou, X. Li, et al., Evolution of the novel coronavirus from the ongoing Wuhan outbreak and modeling of its spike protein for risk of human transmission. Sci. China Life Sci. **63**, 457–460 (2020)
13. V.M. Corman, N.L. Ithete, L.R. Richards, M.C. Schoeman, W. Preiser, C. Drosten, et al., Rooting the phylogenetic tree of middle east respiratory syndrome coronavirus by characterization of a conspecific virus from an African bat. J. Virol. **88**(19), 11297–11303 (2014)

14. P. Richardson, I. Griffin, C. Tucker, D. Smith, O. Oechsle, A. Phelan, et al., Baricitinib as potential treatment for 2019-nCoV acute respiratory disease. Lancet (2020)
15. C.S. Ng, D.M. Kasumba, T. Fujita, H. Luo, Spatio-temporal characterization of the antiviral activity of the XRN1-DCP1/2 aggregation against cytoplasmic RNA viruses to prevent cell death. Cell Death Differ., 1–20 (2020)
16. M.L. Holshue, C. DeBolt, S. Lindquist, K.H. Lofy, J. Wiesman, H. Bruce, et al., First case of 2019 novel coronavirus in the United States. N. Engl. J. Med. (2020)
17. M. Wang, R. Cao, L. Zhang, X. Yang, J. Liu, M. Xu, et al., Remdesivir and chloroquine effectively inhibit the recently emerged novel coronavirus (2019-nCoV) in vitro. Cell Res., 269–271 (2020)
18. H. Bisht, A. Roberts, L. Vogel, K. Subbarao, B. Moss, Neutralizing antibody and protective immunity to SARS coronavirus infection of mice induced by a soluble recombinant polypeptide containing an N-terminal segment of the spike glycoprotein. Virology **334**(2), 160–165 (2005)
19. K. Stadler, A. Roberts, S. Becker, L. Vogel, M. Eickmann, L. Kolesnikova, et al., SARS vaccine protective in mice. Emerg. Infect. Dis. **11**(8), 1312 (2005)
20. U.J. Buchholz, A. Bukreyev, L. Yang, E.W. Lamirande, B.R. Murphy, K. Subbarao, et al., Contributions of the structural proteins of severe acute respiratory syndrome coronavirus to protective immunity. Proc. Natl. Acad. Sci. **101**(26), 9804–9809 (2004)
21. N. Takasuka, H. Fujii, Y. Takahashi, M. Kasai, S. Morikawa, S. Itamura, et al., A subcutaneously injected UV-inactivated SARS coronavirus vaccine elicits systemic humoral immunity in mice. Int. Immunol. **16**(10), 1423–1430 (2004)
22. K.V. Holmes, SARS coronavirus: A new challenge for prevention and therapy. J. Clin. Invest. **111**(11), 1605–1609 (2003)
23. C. Huang, Y. Wang, X. Li, L. Ren, J. Zhao, Y. Hu, et al., Clinical features of patients infected with 2019 novel coronavirus in Wuhan, China. Lancet (2020)
24. M. Bolles, E. Donaldson, R. Baric, SARS-CoV and emergent coronaviruses: Viral determinants of interspecies transmission. Curr. Opin. Virol. **1**(6), 624–634 (2011)
25. V. Vara, Coronavirus outbreak: The countries affected. 11 MARCH 2020.; Available from: https://www.pharmaceutical-technology.com/features/coronavirus-outbreak-the-countries-affected/
26. Q. Li, X. Guan, P. Wu, et al., Early transmission dynamics in Wuhan, China, of novel coronavirus infected pneumonia. N. Engl. J. Med. (2020)
27. A.E. Gorbalenya, Severe acute respiratory syndrome-related coronavirus e the species and its viruses, a statement of the coronavirus study group. bioRxiv (2020)
28. N. Zhu, D. Zhang, W. Wang, et al., A novel coronavirus from patients with pneumonia in China, 2019. N. Engl. J. Med. **382**, 727e33 (2020)
29. Y. Si, B. Tai, D. Hu, et al., Oral health status of Chinese residents and suggestions for prevention and treatment strategies. Glob Health J **3**, 50e4 (2019)
30. W.J. Guan, Z.Y. Ni, Y. Hu, W.H. Laing, C.Q. Ou, J.X. He et al., Clinical characteristics of 2019 novel coronavirus infection in China. medRxiv (2020)
31. N. Chen, M. Zhou, X. Dong, J. Qu, F. Gong, Y. Han, et al., Epidemiological and clinical characteristics of 99 cases of 2019 novel coronavirus pneumonia in Wuhan, China: A descriptive study. Lancet **395**, 507 (2020)
32. S. Ryu, B.C. Chun, An interim review of the epidemiological characteristics of 2019 novel coronavirus. Epidemiol Health **42**, e2020006 (2020)
33. P. Colson, J.M. Rolain, D. Raoult, Chloroquine for the 2019 novel coronavirus. Int. J. Antimicrob. Agents **55**, 105923 (2020)
34. H. Chen, J. Guo, C. Wang, F. Luo, X. Yu, W. Zhang, et al., Clinical characteristics and intrauterine vertical transmission potential of COVID-19 infection in nine pregnant women: A retrospective review of medical records. Lancet **395**, 809–815 (2020)
35. https://www.mohfw.gov.in/pdf/FAQ.pdf
36. https://en.wikipedia.org/wiki/2020_coronavirus_pandemic_in_India

37. B. Efron, R.J. Tibshirani, *An Introduction to the Bootstrap* (CRC Press, 1994)
38. S. Lundberg, S.-I. Lee, A unified approach to interpreting model predictions. arXiv:1705.07874 [cs, stat] (2017)
39. S.M. Lundberg et al., Explainable machine-learning predictions for the prevention of hypoxaemia during surgery. Nat. Biomed. Eng. **2**, 749–760 (2018)
40. J. Josse, N. Prost, E. Scornet, G. Varoquaux, On the consistency of supervised learning with missing values. arXiv:1902.06931 [cs, math, stat] (2019)
41. T. Chen, C. Guestrin, XGBoost: A scalable tree boosting system, in *Proceedings of the 22nd ACM SIGKDD International Conference on Knowledge Discovery and Data Mining* (Association for Computing Machinery, 2016), pp. 785–794

A Comprehensive Review of the Smart Health Records to Prevent Pandemic

Kirti Verma, Neeraj Chandnani, Adarsh Mangal, and M. Sundararajan

Introduction to a Smart Health Record

The meaning of smart is organized, precise, efficient, measurable, analytical, prosecutable, and technology-driven in all manner. We have to use the statistics of a patient in real time to store it on the cloud so that we can interpret the information through various mobile apps and smartphones and find out some patterns, images recognition techniques, and previous records of the patient, e.g., X-ray reports and ultrasound reports, to evaluate these records through machine learning model/techniques with maximum accuracy by accommodating advance health services that have never been existed before [1].

Technology is coming with conviction and zeal and the peoples are obtaining and grasping it openhandedly as it is a powerful and transformational technique to make millions of people's lives better and healthy. The intention behind the technology is to gather real-time data using wearable gadgets like a smartwatch, smart glasses, bio-patch, smart hearing aids, etc. to track the improvement or any implication through the day-to-day monitoring and to collect the real-time data at the

---

K. Verma (✉)
Department of Engineering Mathematics, Lakshmi Narain College of Technology, Jabalpur, Madhya Pradesh, India

N. Chandnani
Institute of Advance Computing, SAGE University, Indore, Madhya Pradesh, India

A. Mangal
Department of Mathematics, Engineering College Ajmer (An Autonomous Institute of Government of Rajasthan), Ajmer, Rajasthan, India

M. Sundararajan
Department of Mathematics & Computer Science, Mizoram University, Aizawl, Mizoram, India

© The Author(s), under exclusive license to Springer Nature Switzerland AG 2023
G. R. Kanagachidambaresan et al. (eds.), *System Design for Epidemics Using Machine Learning and Deep Learning*, Signals and Communication Technology, https://doi.org/10.1007/978-3-031-19752-9_2

centralized server and fetch these data through a mobile application in times of emergency [2].

This is the collective exercise between researchers, doctors, specialists, developers, and engineers to implement the machine learning algorithm by recognizing the patterns of previous images of organs and comparing them with a healthy one, so we can easily identify the ramifications with current health statistics of patients and start the treatments as early as possible [3].

Fig. 1 describes the various records smartly stored in any network device. Instead of managing a lot of documentation for a single patient, it is easier to have a single medical record. We are creating huge decentralized records through job cards, patient's admission forms, procedure sheets, evaluation sheet, medication sheets, recovery sheets, etc. as the day in and day out that are at present existing in almost every healthcare institution among health records of outpatient offices, ICUs, and treatments [4].

Physicians, healthcare experts, and medical professionals are spending a lot of time preparing the records of patients who have already been surrounded by chronic diseases or having such kind of history for a long time. They use to create the

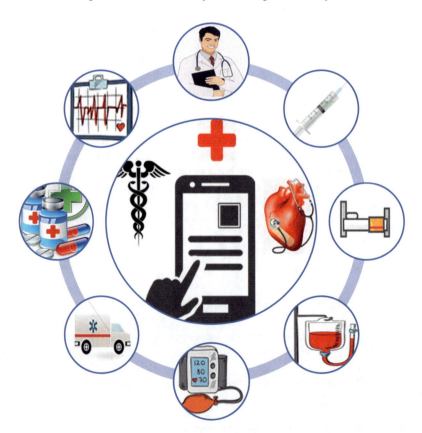

Fig. 1 Smart health management

documentation for a large number of patients as per day, week, and month by making files or manual diagnosis through huge previous medical records and repeating the tests to check the health implications of patients [5].

Various Types of Records in Smart Health

Health records are generally classified into four categories:

1. Clinical records: It is the awareness of various cases of patients' seizure, breakthroughs of their betterment, and various types of facilities provided by medical staff and higher authorities. Such kinds of records are having a few salient features like the following:

    (a) Experimental, objective, and authorized.
    (b) Records are prudently handled by medical personnel.
    (c) Proper documentation should be given to patients about their treatments.
    (d) Duplication should also be avoided as it enhances paperwork and a lot of documentation
    (e) Real data on research and other related modules have to be provided by the hospital.
    (f) Better service should be provided in the up-gradation of health.
    (g) Insurance and safety are also major concerns to the staff members, nurses, doctors, and physicians.
    (h) Proper sanitization of a building should be provided to disinfect the people near to patients.

      Some of the examples related to clinical records:

    - Physician's order form
    - Patient's procedure sheet
    - Nurse's admission appraisal form
    - Medical history of patients
    - Physician's annotations/impressions
    - Treatment records
    - Improvement statistics

2. Staff records: Independent set of records for each staff member. These individual records have to be maintained by producing the details of the particulars of their presence, their medical conditions, e.g., insurance, personal information, experience, etc., in the digital form [6].

    Some of the examples related to staff records:

    - An individual's appraisal form
    - The number of patients handled at a particular time
    - Daily attendance records
    - Medical history of an individual staff member

3. Department/ward records: It is the kind of records connected with an individual department or ward.
   Some of the examples related to ward records:
   - Circular of the ward to maintain the records daily.
   - Presence and absence record at a particular time or at the time of the round.
   - The ward duty of each individual should be checked on frequently.
   - The inventory of the ward should be kept in a digital form.
   - Patients about that particular ward record.
   - Billing of medicine records.
   - Records containing the ward's daily activities.
   - Numbers of patient's daily procedure records.
4. Administrative records: It is the kind of records in which the administration is responsible to make sure that every activity is under supervision electronically to achieve the goal of the better flow of everything in any organizations [7].
   Some of the examples related to ward records:
   - The daily basis treatment record
   - Discharge record with medications
   - Service records
   - Organization notice board records of various activities
   - The procedure of each manual frequently

Development of EHR Standards for India

The Ministry of Health, Government of India, proposed the EHR standards to recommend a system that is highly flexible in conserving and generating the health records of patients in the country in the long run by healthcare workers. So, in the coming generation of the twenty-first century, the government of India is focused on electronic health records with the mission of digital India. The vision of this new era would be implemented in such a way that in the case of emergency, a person does not need to take any documentation like the previous history of their health treatments, last visit summary reports, etc. So with these standards, a person can go to any hospital having the best medical facilities and physicians, specialists, or experts and start his treatments as early as possible without wasting a lot of time as a fully unified electronic record has already been there at the cloud and anyone can access it at the time of need through connecting devices like software and application-embedded laptops, tablets, etc. [8].

The Ministry of Health had planned to suggest the EHR standards for the country in 2013. Again it was revised in 2016 introducing information technology, machine learning, big data analytics, sensor-based live streaming of data by using the Internet of things, and other technologies to make healthcare system efficient and easy to access in the upcoming years throughout the country by hospitals, researchers, and development centers pertinent to healthcare, various organizations, and medical

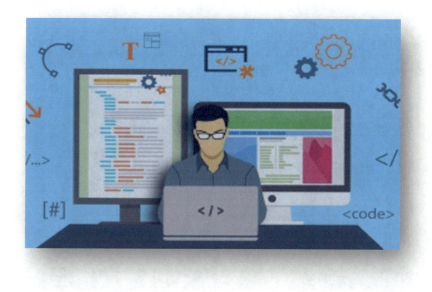

Fig. 2 The advancement of electronic health records through various devices with the help of web networks

institutions and advised them to update the system with new technology and implement the system in such a way that it would be within reach of a common man at the time of urgency with full transparency [9] (Fig. 2).

Traditional Paper Records vs Smart Health Records

Even in today's scenario, hospitals are still using traditional paper records to evaluate the files having the previous summary of their patients. A lot of documentation against the confidentiality of patients and the emphasis of being accessible to the records of patients delinquently the location from where they belong to take huge dominance to make the shift to EHRs. An electronic health record (EHR) is an electronic adaptation of a patient's admission form to any healthcare institution. EHRs belong to live data that proceeds as real-time information on the cloud; these records produce the data by using data analytics techniques which are easily accessible and steadily authorized [10].

Medical staff like nurses, practitioners, and trainers who are using electronic health records have seen a large attrition rate in paper work, patient's admission form, job cards, or other documentation by more than 40%. Electronic health records are one of the most impeccable approaches to get specific information on patients rapidly. Becoming paperless boosts our business. As we all know, in today's

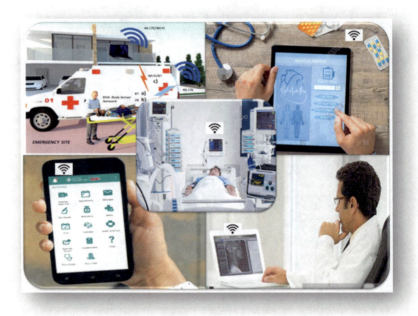

Fig. 3 Electronic health records

cut-throat competition, time is very crucial for all of us, and this has been proved that in various industries especially in the healthcare industry, electronic health records have become the buzzword as they help reduce a lot of time and efforts by using electronic gadgets, smartphones, etc. [11].

In electronic health records, we can get the data in real time by using telemedicine's techniques (Fig. 3).

Comparison Between Paper-Based Records and Electronic Health Records

Paper-based records	Electronic health records
Paper-based records dissipate among several hospitals and care centers and are inadequate as this piles up the records of patients as irrelevant and redundant	Electronic health records smartly curtail the redundant data by taking all information in mobile applications or software using smartphones, gadgets, tablets, etc.

Paper-based records	Electronic health records
Paper-based records are also disorganized as many physicians have to collect the records of the previous history of the patient from a lot of sources like documentation of the last admission submission forms, previous medications, procedures, as well as recovery rates	Electronic health records allow the accumulation of all previous records in one storage so that it can be easily accessible without viewing all previous documentation and a lot of files reducing the time and efforts of medical staff members, e.g., doctors, specialists, physicians, etc.
In paper-based records even if you are taking the records from various sources like email and fax, it will take a lot of time to proceed, and to start the treatment late would be fatal in case of emergency	In EHR, the system takes the complete records of the medical history of the patient, so there is no need to bring the data/information from any other resources and don't even need to fill the partial or full record in the system again
In this type of record, as you are not having the whole medical history of patients at one single location, this is very cumbersome to put all together with the previous medication and treatments	Due to real-time streaming of data/records application can be updated automatically as it can work 24/7 with the help of the internet like ATMs. Thus, we are not bothered about the current scenario of patient health because by wearing some connecting devices, these devices themselves fetch the real-time data and store it on a cloud
Physician's admittance is very less as he or she is only available within their job hours; thus, this can crunch the patient's health at the time of emergency or in any critical situations	In electronic health records, we can get the data live from any cloud platform and doctors can monitor this data from any location even from their home, and by using the telemedicine's techniques, they can prescribe any medicines at the time of any urgency

Interoperability and Standards in the Smart Healthcare System

The bundle of various standards circumscribed in this topic is introducing a cumulative approach:

1. Medical equipment and uses cases should be studied carefully.
2. Various wearables and connecting devices shall accept interoperability and standards.
3. Accepting standards and executing requirements for the flawless exchange of health information between various institutions and IT infrastructure.
4. Consolidate vendors around the domain with mutual medical issues and health-related challenges.
5. Establish various frequently used tools and gadgets and their related services.
6. Develop various phases of the requirement specification process by integrating attempts among public and private sector shareholders, in which vendors are collaborating to create willingness.
7. Various guidelines we should follow proposed by the government for health information networks throughout the country.

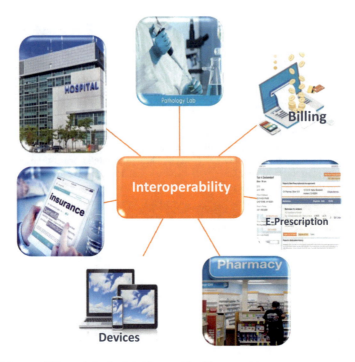

Fig. 4 Interoperability and standards in the smart healthcare system

8. Technology should be established to achieve the final goal of nationwide health measures so information technology, ICT, and machine learning will work together to fulfill the technical requirements (Fig. 4).

Guidelines for Proposed Smart Health Records

We all aware of the new technology named machine learning through which we are deliberately making our medical history on the server and with the help of RPC API and Google Cloud Vision using ML models to recognize the data with the pattern or recognition techniques and produce electronic health records in a digital form. Whole data would be stored on the cloud and we can access it through mobile apps by using smartphones, and these data or records can be easily accessed and controlled by our physicians, doctors, and pharmacists.

In recent times, many think tanks of the country in the health industry generate movable and "interoperable" electronic health records which means easy to access and understand by masses. Institutions of medical sciences, where a lot of information is participating against healthcare vendors, are amicably the most important domain; the deep-rooted EHR providers assured to intent their information exchange platforms instead of standards of the industry for partaking unprocessed information [12].

Electronic health records are less pricey to create and store and easy to move everywhere at the time of need. These are the reasons behind the picture of the new healthcare regime that the government is also taking interest to distribute and maintain the sharing regimen nationwide. Without the specialists and healthcare providers filling out the right information in the applications, electronic health records would become personal assets so that we can regulate it on our own at any time and send it to doctors to make urgent appointments or can take the help of telemedicine. Google Health and Microsoft's Health Vault online platforms are among the biggest IT giants in which consumers can accumulate and share their electronic health records.

Security and privacy specialists are concerned about the safeness and aegis of networked information of health records. Several experts, e.g., Center for Democracy and Technology, proposed guidelines that cannot be advocated, e.g., both buyers and consumers of the healthcare industry can share the common interest as their needs and requirements specifications are the same. According to the research, sources stated that the healthcare industry will see a 25% increase in IT jobs by 2022. In many hospitals that are having advanced medical facilities in almost every sector of the healthcare projects, there is a demand for productive smartphone applications and cloud servers for storing real-time data and computerized diagnosis.

Introduction of Machine Learning in Healthcare

Machine learning aggrandizes manual tasks without the intervention of humans. Electronic health records (EHR) are unregulated and enigmatic and opposing computerization so we can be muddled in fetching the information by taking the pricey time. Machine learning algorithms can forecast the data which is adjustable or fit according to patient's health specifications and is majorly on top priority so we can enlist the further steps to take appropriate actions as earlier as possible to save human lives and enhance the life expectancy of patients at the time of emergency. AI with machine learning algorithms work with generative adversarial networks (GANs) and anticipate the more precise shapes of molecules with high accuracy. Statistics uses R language to predict the chart for the remarkable representation of data so we can easily understand the graphs which gradually show the improvement measures of any individual to boost the capability and provide easy access.

Image recognition techniques, using machine learning classifying pathology e.g.: to find out tumors in healthcare modules by showing the images of different patterns showing in the human body so physicians can easily detect the body of having tumors with a healthy body which is showing a different image. Another pathway that is materializing is by using wearables with connecting devices like a smartwatch, Fitbit, etc. With the use of these wearables, we can store the real-time information of an individual, and with the machine learning model, we can conclude the data as a result, e.g., deterioration or wreckage. Wearables productively take the data while walking, running, and jogging. Because they are collecting data through live streaming module, when this data has reached to a particular danger point, it quickly informs a person or an individual to take appropriate actions before something worse can happen, e.g., a stroke risk, heartbeat enhancement, excessive sweating, etc.

Machine learning algorithms stimulate research in the field of healthcare with huge enthusiasm. Biologists, computer scientists, IT professionals, physicians, and faculties of applied science all are working together and practicing day and night in a collaborative environment to come up with all related technologies and to end up with some creative solutions like outbreak prediction and personalized medicines. And they often use the machine learning models to diagnose and identify the disease before happening. With the help of natural language processing, professionals related to this field can handle a lot of administrative tasks.

Introduction to Vector Machine Techniques

Machine learning (ML) has become the buzzword in almost every industry, and it has been acknowledged as an essential part of AI. Moreover, ML is a data analysis technique that computerizes the declarative structure. Algorithms used by machine learning are captivating all big IT giants in an industry collaborating with all major sectors, e.g., banking, transport, healthcare, etc. Support vector machines are one of the classification techniques that distribute pieces of information varying with patterns matching with supervised learning technique with hyperplanes provided by the machine learning technology. So SVM is well known as the ML technique for classification. SVM is a selective classifier. It generates the result as an outcome of the hyperplane, which organizes new data sets with examples that accept the technique of hyperplane called support vectors.

In the two-dimensional (2D) region, this technique is a straight line divided into two sectors wherein each sector is temporal on one side by taking two unique data sets or pieces of information shown in bullets or dots. This graphic representation proposes a confirmative interpretation as shown in the figure. Figure 5 shows various images differentiating sickly from healthy persons.

This visual representation comes up with an acquiescent interpretation (Fig. 5). The table below shows the various data set to analyze the data with the machine learning model.

Fig. 5 Various differentiation of the health categories

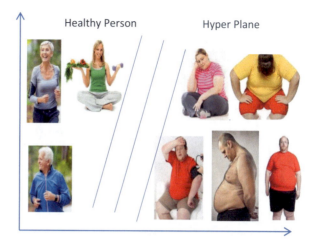

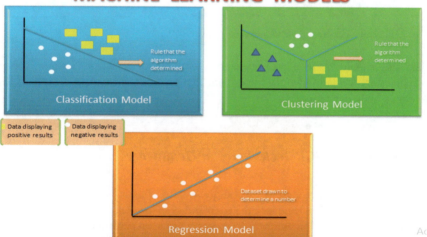

Fig. 6 Various types of machine learning models

Person suffering from obesity

	Fasting	Just after Eating	3 h after eating
Normal	80–100	170–200	120–140
Pre-diabetic	101–125	190–230	140–160
Diabetic	126+	220–300	200+

Data can be displayed through various models, e.g., classification model, clustering model, and regression Model (Fig. 6).

Sometimes we use to make mistakes while considering hyperplane as choosing an optimal one is a tedious job as noise sensitivity and rationalization of different

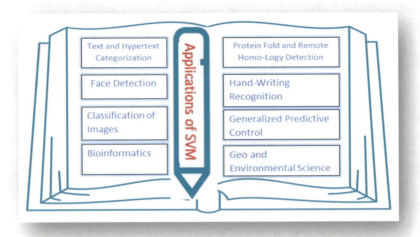

Fig. 7 Illustration of support vector machine

data sets should be in a proper manner with higher accuracy. Support vector machines are trying to upgrade hyperplane that provides substantially less distance to obtain skilled data set (Fig. 7).

Introduction to OCR Techniques in Healthcare

The optical character recognition technique we are using in healthcare is primarily helping us to process and enhance the adaptability of the plan you have taken related to your health status. The number of processes has been performed with the help of an image recognition technology which is used to remove the use of highly intensive data entry process on papers.

We are using the optical character recognition technique extensively in medical science which is based on the proficiency of an optical character recognition scanner. As the same suggests, it can scan alphanumeric characters present in files by recognizing the characters carefully and cache the data as e-files.

Flood of Paper Claims After the Arrival of Optical Character Recognition

In the insurance sector, a simple healthcare plan contains a huge number of individual paper claims which is used to be scanned by an OCR and translated into e-files which is based on the healthcare system's preference with a

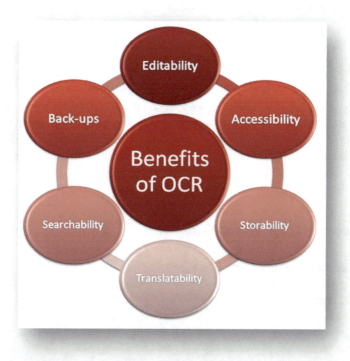

Fig. 8 Benefits of optical character recognition

predefined formatted model. We normally use the X.12 format to verify claims related to this technique. Like an electronic data exchange file, we can insert our file into the system. The images residing in the document are saved so that they can be used shortly by referencing the same images and comparing with future incoming data to understand patterns easily with the help of machine learning models. Machine learning models tend to be highly sophisticated so that in this interface our e-files having a lot of images can percolate and bring back quickly and comfortably. The whole process eliminates the use of papers and manual documentation.

The frequently incoming claims with manual documentation or in paper format per day are increasing at a fast speed. With the help of connecting devices like smartphones in a particular network having kiosks, cloud servers, and various apps, saving the electronic information, and transporting these e-files anywhere at the receiver end, has become an effortless system by the use of optical character recognition in healthcare.

Different modules have benefits of OCR using EDI (Fig. 8).

Electronic Exchange of Documents

Another application of optical character recognition in healthcare or medical sciences is that it composes the paper files or documents electronically exchangeable with the EDI module. By generating an on-screen paper module, all manual files that contain images are primarily stored in the system's forms. By doing this, we can easily accessed and simply transfer these files with efficiency. Later on, by using the EDI technique, images and pictures would be transformed into text format and be stored automatically into the databases in a cloud-based server worldwide so that we can retrieve this information easily for use at the time of need in a secure way [13].

Advantages of OCR in Healthcare

1. Tremendous speed to access and retrieve files.
2. Enhanced capacity of storing e-files, thus taking less space instead of storing very cumbersome paper files.
3. The accuracy rate is highly captivated even in a fraction of seconds.
4. Storage is less costly as compared to the storage of manual files for which we have to create a huge space to place the files.
5. Transportation is extremely easy as we are free to transfer the files from one location to another with a single click.
6. Many organizations are assisting with the problem of data loss and damage to unreliability. OCR has been extricating a lot of these problems to diminish errors.

Privacy and Security in Smart Health Records

With the invention of technology, the government of India has initiated a tremendous attempt to revolutionalize traditional health records by integrating them with information technology (IT). Electronic health records can produce huge profits and welfare by fixing responsibility and cutting costs. However, by computing and streamlining health records at the cloud, EHR systems have now become vulnerable to security threats as most of the vital information are made available not only in the hands of medical doctors or physicians but also on the cloud server, making them within the reach of hackers, crackers, and cybercriminals. Due to these privacy and security threats in health records, a new measure has emerged named cybersecurity because for policymakers this is an extreme affair for medical science in the era of the digital world. Many journals, articles, and papers have been issuing cyberbullying and security and privacy concerns in healthcare. A lot of research is still going on in recent times to amend the privacy and security in EHR systems [14].

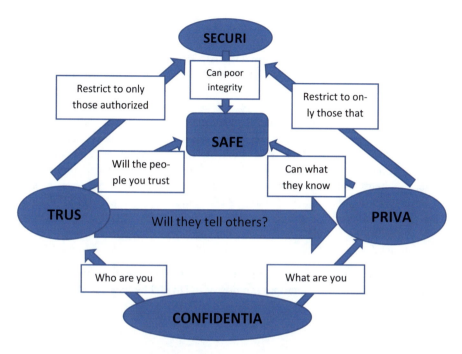

Fig. 9 Introduction to Google Cloud Vision API

Uncompromising security and privacy safeguards are now essential for the everlasting accomplishments of EHR systems. If the trust and belief of patients have evacuated that EHR systems are apprehensive, most probably they are not going to use it and feel hesitant to use it; thus, not a single piece of information should be available to unauthorized person. If a hacker is trying to access the record of any individual or trying to penetrate the medical history of any patient, then security is imposed (Fig. 9).

Google Cloud Vision endeavors the products that adopt machine learning concepts to understand our data as inputs by labeling the objects and after executing providing the result with a high level of accuracy interacting with the algorithms or pre-trained model in between our inputs and the final result. The following are the types of Google Cloud Vision:

1. AutoML Vision
2. Vision API

Let us explain each of them:

1. AutoML Vision: As the name suggests, personalizing our machine learning standard and developing a model, we can use AutoML Vision's technique which is easy to access with the feature of the API (application programming interface). With the help of code, which we use to perform different classification by using classes and objects concept, we can develop an application which is highly

optimized with the following features: low latency, small size, and maximum accuracy.

Later on, we can transport the complete structure to the application on the cloud and it can also be stored to an array of various connecting network devices at the end user and deploy the model to our apps and comprehend objects to make the difference from which we can easily compare right things to get the result with an optimized manner, e.g., prediction of diseases quickly, emotional intelligence patterns, buying behavior of customers, and business analysis.

2. Vision API: In this module, we can use the REST and Remote Procedure Call API, which is known as the elementary form of application programming interface. It helps us to deploy our block of code to another remote server through Remote Procedure call. If we have to take the code block into HTTP through HyperText Markup Language, it can be treated as Web API. By the REST and Remote Procedure Call API, we make our machine learning model as skilled and pre-trained.

Fig. 10 depicts the working of the training data set into optimal result by using AutoML Vision through the proper training of the model by flawless algorithms.

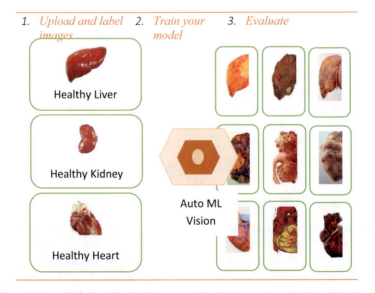

Fig. 10 Machine learning model in the healthcare system through the Google Cloud Vision API

Conclusion

From the above discussions, we have to conclude that as day in and day out, the healthcare system is now gripping into human's life without involving the absolute presence of patients as it has been diversified with a lot of devices and technologies to handle the data of any individual at various remote locations and prescribe them with any medicines with emerging techniques, e.g., telemedicine. As we all know that in the next decade, the number of older adults suffering from chronic diseases will increase, putting the health records and the previous history of their chronic diseases securely with the help of database servers and collecting them any time of urgent need will be of utmost importance so that doctors can give appropriate treatments in a limited time to save lives. The adoption of all the new technologies like smart health records, telemedicine, and virtual prescriptions of the treatments would improve well-being of patients.

References

1. L. Catarinucci et al., An IoT-aware architecture for smart healthcare systems. IEEE Internet Things J. **2**(6), 515–526 (2015). https://doi.org/10.1109/JIOT.2015.2417684
2. A. Kumar, G. Chattree, S. Periyasamy, Smart healthcare monitoring system. Wirel. Pers. Commun. **101**(1), 453–463 (2018). https://doi.org/10.1007/S11277-018-5699-0
3. R. Dautov, S. Distefano, R. Buyya, Hierarchical data fusion for smart healthcare. J Big Data **6**(1), 1–23 (2019). https://doi.org/10.1186/S40537-019-0183-6/FIGURES/5
4. N. Chandnani, C.N. Khairnar, A novel machine learning based secure protocol for data aggregation and efficient routing in IoT WSNs, in *Wireless Personal Communications, Springer*, Electronic ISSN: 1572-834X, Print ISSN: 0929-6212 (2019)
5. N. Chandnani, C.N. Khairnar, Bio-inspired multilevel security protocol for data aggregation and routing in IoT WSNs, in *Mobile Networks and Applications*, Springer, Electronic ISSN: 1572-8153, Print ISSN: 1383-469X (2022), doi: https://doi.org/10.1007/s11036-021-01859-6
6. K. Verma, N. Chandnani, G. Bhatt, A. Sinha, *Internet of Things and Smart Farming* (Springer, 2022), pp. 283–303. https://doi.org/10.1007/978-3-030-77528-5_15
7. N. Chandnani, C.N. Khairnar, A comprehensive review and performance evaluation of recent trends for data aggregation and routing techniques in IoT networks, in *Lecture Notes in Networks and Systems*, vol. 100 (Springer, 2020), pp. 467–484. doi: https://doi.org/10.1007/978-981-15-2071-6_37
8. N. Chandnani, C.N. Khairnar, Efficient data aggregation and routing algorithm for iot wireless sensor networks, in *IFIP International Conference on Wireless and Optical Communications Networks, WOCN, IEEE Conference*, vol. 2019 (2019), doi: https://doi.org/10.1109/WOCN45266.2019.8995074
9. N. Chandnani, C.N. Khairnar, A novel secure data aggregation in IoT using particle swarm optimization algorithm, in *2018 International Conference on Advanced Computation and Telecommunication, ICACAT 2018, IEEE Conference* (2018), doi: https://doi.org/10.1109/ICACAT.2018.8933784
10. N. Chandnani, A.M. Gupta, P. Fatnani, P. Jain, Development of distributed mains monitoring and switching system for indus complex, in *IOSR Journal of Electronics and Communication Engineering (IOSR-JECE)*, Electronic ISSN: 2278-2834, Print ISSN: 2278-8735, vol. 10, no. 6 (2015), pp. 01–09, doi: https://doi.org/10.9790/2834-10610109

11. N. Chandnani, K. Verma, S. Joshi, A. Mangal, M. Sundararajan, A. Mohan, Application of mathematics in research, education and medical science. Des. Eng., 13026–13037
12. M. Verma, K. Verma, Statistical analysis and effect of primary nutrient (N, P, K) in coal ash admixed wasteland soil through vesicular–arbuscular mycorrhizae invasion, in *Nveo-Natural Volatiles & Essential Oils Journal Nveo* (2021), pp. 6816–6824
13. P. Vijayashanthi, K. Verma, S. Dixit, S. K. Pandey, E. Sathya, M. Arunkumar, An overview on sequentially g-quotient maps, in *Materials Today: Proceedings* (2021)
14. R. JatinKikani, K. Verma, R. Navalakhe, G. Shrivastava, V. Shrivastava, Cryptography: Recent research trends of encrypting mathematics, in *Materials Today: Proceedings* (2021)

Automation of COVID-19 Disease Diagnosis from Radiograph

Keerthi Mangond, B. S. Divya, N. Siva Rama Lingham, and Thompson Stephan

Introduction

Coronavirus is indeed a highly infectious disease, known as COVID-19. It doesn't have a specific treatment and can also be lethal with a 2% mortality rate. Because of extensive lung damage and respiratory failure, this severe illness can result in death [1]. The COVID-19 virus, which started on December 31, 2019, by the unawareness of the reasons for lung fever in Wuhan, Hubei province of China, turned out to be a pandemic. Many recent articles [2–4] have discussed the impact of COVID-19 on people's livelihoods and their health. COVID-19 is caused by the virus SARS-CoV-2. In a short period of 1 month, this virus has spread from Wuhan to most of the world [5, 6]. Severe acute respiratory syndrome coronavirus (SARS-CoV) and Middle East respiratory syndrome coronavirus (MERS-CoV) have caused severe acute respiratory syndrome and many deaths [10].

To that end, we have explored the possibility of using technology to help detect patients who are infected with the virus. Furthermore, unlike laboratory procedures that require the patient's respiratory system to be controlled, X-rays may be performed without an increased risk of pathogen aerosolisation [7]. X-rays can also allow patients to be categorised as having COVID-19 positive or negative. The purpose of this research work is to automate the identification of the COVID-19 virus in the patient's respiratory system using their chest X-ray images. Society will benefit from early identification of COVID-19 as it facilitates quarantining the patients

K. Mangond · B. S. Divya · T. Stephan (✉)
Department of Computer Science & Engineering, M. S. Ramaiah University of Applied University, Bengaluru, Karnataka, India

N. Siva Rama Lingham
Department of Computer Science and Engineering, Vel Tech Rangarajan Dr. Sagunthala R&D Institute of Science and Technology, Chennai, Tamil Nadu, India

promptly. Using lung X-ray radiograph images, the automated identification of COVID-19 has life-saving value for both patients and physicians. The automated diagnosis of COVID-19 will decrease the diagnosis's price and result in a fast report. This cost reduction will be a boon to the governments of the countries that pay for the healthcare services.

A doctor may conveniently and precisely diagnose a chest X-ray for pneumonia with a computer-aided diagnostic (CAD) [5]. Due to their ability to perform beyond human capacity in the medical field, the use of artificial intelligence techniques is rapidly growing in medical services [8]. Implementing CAD methods into radiologists' diagnostic systems significantly decreases doctors' workload and increases performance and quantitative analysis [9]. Machine learning and medical imaging CAD systems are more popular fields of study [10]. Many researchers [22] have recently developed various automated diagnostic algorithms based on machine learning techniques. This research aims to build an automated system with the capacity to detect coronavirus diseases by using computer vision and medical image processing techniques. There are also differences in the volume of data used in studies. This research aims to present the use of machine learning over lung X-ray images for high-precision diagnosis of coronavirus with a limited dataset. The state-of-the-art coronavirus analysis solution using lung X-rays can be implemented by applying the latest deep learning techniques and computer vision techniques. One of the efficient architectures for analysing visual imagery is the convolutional neural network (CNN), a deep learning method. CNN is formulated to mimic the brain in analysing visual data [11, 12]. Alex designed a CNN with Ilya Sutskever and Geoffrey Hinton and submitted the design in the completion of the ImageNet Large Scale Visual Recognition Challenge (ILSVRC-2012) and showed a surprising result of 15.3%, followed by the runner-up with 26.2%. From then on, CNN opened a new era for computer vision. K. Simonyan and A. Zisserman proposed the VGG16 model again at ILSVRC-2014, which obtained an error rate of 7.3%. VGG16 improves over AlexNet by reducing the kernel size from 11 to 5 to 3.

Materials and Methods

Dataset

We have collected the lung X-ray radiographs of normal and COVID-19 lung X-ray radiograph images. The COVID-19 patient dataset was taken from Dr. Joseph Paul's account and the normal patient dataset was taken from the Kaggle website [13]. And the collected dataset was split into two categories: COVID-19 and normal. These two categories were provided for both the training and testing phases. For this purpose, two separate training and testing folders are created. For training normal, 70 images, and COVID-19, 60 images, and for testing normal, 25 images, and COVID-19, 25 images, were used.

Proposed Classification Model

The proposed image automatic classification architecture is as depicted in Fig. 1. It follows majorly two phases:

1. Data preprocessing.
2. A pre-trained VGG16 model.

Data Preprocessing

The number of images in the present dataset was too small for a deep learning algorithm. So the number of images in the dataset was increased. ImageDataGenerator class was called to increase the size of the dataset. The images were resized to 224, 224.

The number of images was increased in only the training set, not the validation or test data. This data augmentation is different from the preparation of data, such as resizing of images and pixel scaling. The data augmentation methods used are as follows:

1. Image shifting was done by the width shift range and height shift range.
2. Image flipping was obtained by the horizontal flip and vertical flip.
3. Rotation of the image was done by the rotation range.
4. Zooming of the images was also done by the zoom range.

The proposed X-ray radiograph classification model is as shown in Fig. 1. As the dataset was too small to train the CNN, data augmentation techniques were used to increase the size of the dataset. The CNN architecture for VGG16 [7], shown in Fig. 1, was used for feature representation, as it has several convolutional layers, max-pooling layers, and fully connected layers for classification. The convolutional layers detect the discriminative features from the image regions by identifying pixel

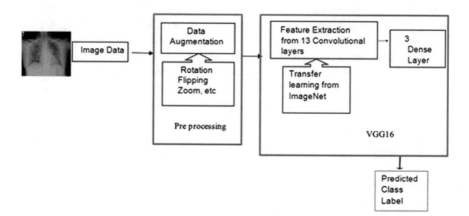

Fig. 1 Proposed classification model architecture

patterns. The max-pooling layers scale back computational complexity by only choosing the utmost output value of the output of the convolutional layers. The resulted output from the convolution and max-pooling layers will be flattened, which will then be provided as input to the 512-d dense layer, and finally to the output layer, which is a softmax activation function for getting the classification result [14].

The Pre-Trained VGG16 Architecture

VGG framework was introduced by Simonyan. The two main VGG16 CNN architecture blocks are as follows:

The First Block The VGG16 framework had 13 convolutional layers in the order Cn1, Cn 2, Max pool 1, Cn 3, Cn 4, Max pool 2, Cn 5, Cn 6, Cn 7, Max pool 3, Cn 8, Cn 9, Cn 10, Max pool 4, Cn 11, Cn12, Cn13. Three dense layers follow this with softmax as transfer function for the classification. Cn 1 and Cn 2 have 64 feature maps resulting from 64 filters of size 3×3. Cn 3 and Cn 4 have 128 maps resulting from 128 of size 3×3. Cn 5, Cn 6, and Cn 7 have 256 feature maps resulting from 256 masks of size 3×3. Cn 8, Cn9, and Cn10 have 512 maps resulting from 512 masks of size 3×3. Cn 11, Cn 12, and Cn 13 have 512 maps resulting from 512 filters of size 3×3.

The convolutional layers were calculated by a one-pixel stride and one pixel of zero padding. All four Max pools were done on a 2×2 pixel window and with stride 2. Every convolutional layer will follow a ReLU layer. The convolutional layers and pooling layers are considered the first blocks, so the first block will do the feature extraction. For this, it will do the template matching by applying filter operations, and in this block, the first layer will filter the image with kernels and then give back feature maps, and then these feature maps are resized with a max-pooling layer. This process is repeated, and at the end, the values of the last feature maps are combined into a vector. This obtained vector is the output of the first block, and at the same time, it will be the input for the next block.

The Second Block This block has three dense layers for the classification, of which two serve as hidden layers and the last one will be the classification layer. This block is mainly helpful for classification, so it is used at the end of the CNN networks. The input vector values are transformed to give back another new vector to the output along with many activation functions and linear combinations. And the final vector holds many elements in which each element i represents the image probability that belongs to a class. Therefore, every element resides between 0 and 1. For the calculation of these probabilities, the last layer of the second block is used. Finally, logistic activation is used for binary categorisation in the final layer, and the softmax transfer function is used for multiclass classification [6, 15].

Transfer Learning Algorithm Transfer learning uses previously learned knowledge from one dataset to solve similar problems on another dataset with less information and fewer data points. The network may use these learned features instead of training the model from the beginning.

Results and Discussion

The required system specifications are the Intel Core i5 processor, a graphics card of 2 GB, the 64-bit operating system at 1.80 GHz, and RAM that should be 4 GB. For this work, we needed a considerable number of radiographs of COVID-19-positive cases for better classification, but due to a small dataset, we applied data augmentation techniques and transfer learning techniques. Further, the model will mine the attributes from the training images and use those attributes to detect class labels (COVID-19 and normal).

First Phase (Data Augmentation)

Data augmentation was used to increase the size of the dataset. And this data increment will also help to succeed in dealing with the overfitting problem in transfer learning. The dataset contains 60 COVID-19-positive images and 70 images of normal patients, as tabulated in Table 2. Figure 2 will represent the sample chest radiographs of normal and COVID-19 cases from the dataset. X-ray radiograph images were used in this. At the first stage of the detection, the images given as input data had varied resolutions. So, in the prepossessing, the images were processed to have a resolution of 224x224x3 to maintain uniformity. The types of augmentation applied are shown in Table 1. Augmentation was applied only to the training images, not to test images.

Table 1 Types of data augmentation

Data augmentation technique	Parameters
Flip	Vertical/horizontal (true)
Rotation	Rotate (50)
Zoom	Zoom range (0.1)
Split	Validation split (0.2)
Shift	Width/height (0.2)
	Channel shift (20)

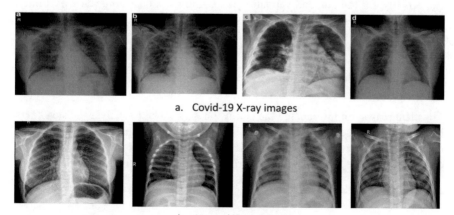

a. Covid-19 X-ray images

b. Normal X-ray images

Fig. 2 Sample chest X-ray images of COVID-19 and normal patients. (**a**) COVID-19 X-ray images (**b**) Normal X-ray images

Table 2 Dataset details used in the work

Category	Training data	Testing data
COVID-19	60	25
Normal	70	25

Second Phase Pre-Trained VGG16

The required image size for the transfer learning model is VGG16 (224x224x3). Only the last three dense layers were trained to classify the chest radiograph images based on the class labels of the training images that were normal and COVID-19. Furthermore, if we need to classify other different images, we can retrain the model by updating the layers based on the new input images. In the training phase, the parameters given to the developed model were as follows:

Performance Metrics

The model's performance was calculated based on the following parameters: accuracy, precision, sensitivity, F1-score, and specificity. A confusion matrix is a table that provides us with a summary of the model's performance. The format of the confusion matrix for a binary categorisation is shown in Table 3.

COVID-19 Classification Results

The data was split into training and validation to avoid overfitting during the training phase. Figures 3 and 4 present categorical entropy loss and model accuracy, respectively, for training and validation data. And the model achieved a maximum score of 98% on the validation data, as shown in Fig. 5.

Confusion Matrix and Feature Maps

The main reason for introducing the confusion matrix was to analyse the steadiness between the guessed result produced by the proposed technique and the actual results. And the confusion matrix is one of the best methods for classifying multi-class objects. Here, each column will represent the predicted class, and each row

Table 3 Confusion matrix

Predicted values	Actual values	
	T P	F P
	T N	F N

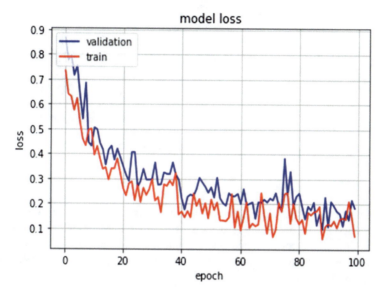

Fig. 3 Training and validation loss

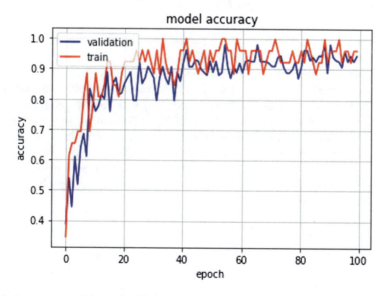

Fig. 4 Accuracy on training and validation set

Fig. 5 Confusion matrix

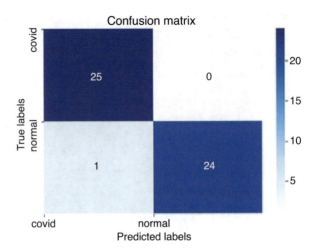

will represent the actual class. The confusion matrix for COVID-19 categorisation is represented in Fig. 5, and the feature maps for the trained model layers are represented in Fig. 6. The performance was evaluated and tabulated as shown in Table 4. Table 4 shows the score of the performance metrics of the X-ray classification VGG16-based model.

Comparison with State-of-the-Art Methods

In the automatic classification of images, deep learning methods can be helpful in the very first diagnosis of a disease. As shown in Table 5, using the methods of deep learning techniques, we can easily achieve faster and better results in comparison with other classification techniques. In this work, an efficient COVID-19 detection technique is proposed. The methodology will classify chest radiographs into different classes such as normal and COVID. The comparison of the performance in this work with the state-of-the-art methods is given here to assess the proposed CNN model. While Table 5 shows the performance values of the listed studies [9, 16–21] but using different datasets, our design outperformed almost all the previous studies, except Khan et al., who used a comparatively large dataset and complex network.

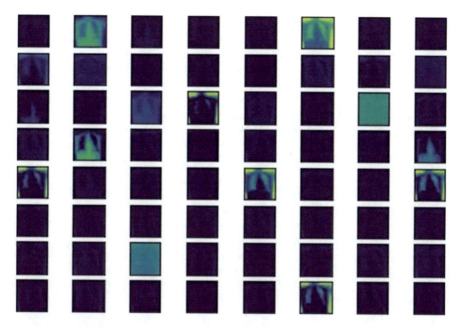

Fig. 6 Feature maps from second CNN layer

Table 4 Performance measures

Accuracy	98%
Precision	0.961
Recall	1
F1-score	0.97

Results and Discussion

In the present research work, the detection of COVID-19 from radiograph was done by the VGG16 convolutional neural network architecture. The experiment was conducted to evaluate the pre-trained VGG16 convolutional neural network's performance on the publicly available COVID-19 dataset. As the dataset was small, the data augmentation method was adapted to increase the number of images in the dataset. T, the data augmentation method, was adapted. To achieve an effective result, the transfer learning-based model was used. This work proposes a two-phase methodology to identify the considered radiograph into COVID-19 and normal classes. In phase 1 data, augmentation was implemented. In phase 2 classification, the operation was performed using a transfer learning-based architecture known as VGG16. The proposed framework will support the fast and precise detection of COVID-19 from X-ray radiograph images.

Table 5 Comparison with state-of-the-art methods

Author	Model	Dataset used	Accuracy	F1-score
Sethy and Behera (2020)	ResNet50 + SVM	Dr. Joseph Cohen+ open-i repository	95.38	
Narin et al. (2020)	ResNet50	Dr. Joseph Cohen	98	0.98
Apostolopoulos and Mpesiana (2020)	VGG19	Public medical repositories- Cohen+ Radiological Society of North America, Radiopaedia, and Italian Society of Medical and Interventional Radiology	98.75	
Hemdan et al. (2020)	VGG19	Dr. Joseph Cohen1 + Dr. Adrian Rosebrock	90	0.91
Ozturk et al. (2020)	DarkCOVIDNet	Cohen JP+ Wang	98.08	0.96
Khan et al. (2020)	CoroNet	Joseph+ (Radiological Society of North America (RSNA)	99	0.98
Toraman et al. (2020)	CoroNet	Cohen JP+ Wang	97.24	0.97
This study	VGG16	Dr. Joseph +Cohen JP	98%	0.97

References

1. Z. Xu, L. Shi, Y. Wang, J. Zhang, L. Huang, C. Zhang, S. Liu, P. Zhao, H. Liu, L. Zhu, et al., Pathological findings of covid-19 associated with acute respiratory distress syndrome. Lancet Respir. Med. **8**(4), 420–422 (2020)
2. S. Kumar, R. Viral, V. Deep, P. Sharma, M. Kumar, M. Mahmud, T. Stephan, Forecasting major impacts of COVID-19 pandemic on country-driven sectors: Challenges, lessons, and future roadmap. Pers. Ubiquit. Comput (2021)
3. M.S. Kaiser, M. Mahmud, M.B. Noor, N.Z. Zenia, S. Al Mamun, K.M.A. Mahmud, S. Azad, V.N.M. Aradhya, S. Punitha, T. Stephan, R. Kannan, M. Hanif, T. Sharmeen, T. Chen, A. Hussain, iworksafe: Towards healthy workplaces during COVID-19 with an intelligent pHealth app for industrial settings. (2021). https://doi.org/10.20944/preprints202101.0092.v1
4. A. Aggarwal, M. Chakradar, M.S. Bhatia, M. Kumar, T. Stephan, S.K. Gupta, S.H. Alsamhi, H. AL-Dois, Covid-19 risk prediction for diabetic patients using fuzzy inference system and machine learning approaches. J. Healthcare Eng. **2022**, 1–10 (2022). https://doi.org/10.1155/2022/4096950
5. Z. Wu, J.M. McGoogan, Characteristics of and important lessons from the coronavirus disease 2019 (covid-19) outbreak in China: Summary of a report of 72 314 cases from the chinese center for disease control and prevention. JAMA **323**(13), 1239–1242 (2020)
6. M.L. Holshue, C. DeBolt, S. Lindquist, K.H. Lofy, J. Wiesman, H. Bruce, C. Spitters, K. Ericson, S. Wilkerson, A. Tural, et al., First case of 2019 novel coronavirus in the United States. N. Engl. J. Med. (2020)
7. T. Singhal, A review of coronavirus disease-2019 (covid-19). Indian J. Pediatr. **87**(4), 281–286 (2020)

8. P. Stephan, T. Stephan, R. Kannan, A. Abraham, A hybrid artificial bee colony with whale optimization algorithm for improved breast cancer diagnosis. Neural Comput. & Applic. **33**(20), 13667–13691 (2021)
9. G. Ga'al, B. Maga, A. Luk'acs, Attention u-net based adversarial architectures for chest x-ray lung segmentation. arXiv preprint arXiv **2003**, 10304 (2020)
10. A. Jaiswal, N. Gianchandani, D. Singh, V. Kumar, M. Kaur, Classification of the covid-19 infected patients using densenet201 based deep transfer learning. J. Biomol. Struct. Dyn. **39**, 1–8 (2020)
11. H. Greenspan, B. Van Ginneken, R.M. Summers, Guest editorial deep learning in medical imaging: Overview and future promise of an exciting new technique. IEEE Trans. Med. Imaging **35**(5), 1153–1159 (2016)
12. L. Deng, D. Yu, Deep learning: Methods and applications, foundations and trends in signal processing. **7**(3–4), 197–387 (2014)
13. Cohen JP (2020) COVID-19 image data collection.. https://github.com/ieee8023/covid-chestxray-dataset
14. P. Lei, Z. Huang, G. Liu, P. Wang, W. Song, J. Mao, G. Shen, S. Zhou, W. Qian, J. Jiao, Clinical and computed tomographic (ct) images characteristics in the patients with covid-19 infection: What should radiologists need to know? J. Xray Sci. Technol. **28**(3), 369–381 (2020)
15. W. Kong, P.P. Agarwal, Chest imaging appearance of covid-19 infection. Radiol. Cardiothor. Imag. **2**(1), e200028 (2020)
16. P. K. Sethy, S. K. Behera, Detection of Coronavirus Disease (Covid-19) based on deep features (2020)
17. I.D. Apostolopoulos, T.A. Mpesiana, Covid-19: Automatic detection from x-ray images utilizing transfer learning with convolutional neural networks. Phys. Eng. Sci. Med. **43**(2), 635–640 (2020)
18. E.E.-D. Hemdan, M.A. Shouman, M.E. Karar, Covidx-net: A framework of deep learning classifiers to diagnose covid-19 in x-ray images. arXiv preprint arXiv **2003**, 11055 (2020)
19. T. Ozturk, M. Talo, E.A. Yildirim, U.B. Baloglu, O. Yildirim, U.R. Acharya, Automated detection of covid-19 cases using deep neural net- works with x-ray images. Comput. Biol. Med. **121**, 103792 (2020)
20. A.I. Khan, J.L. Shah, M.M. Bhat, Coronet: A deep neural network for detection and diagnosis of covid-19 from chest x-ray images. Comput. Methods Prog. Biomed. **196**, 105581 (2020)
21. S. Toraman, T.B. Alakus, I. Turkoglu, Convolutional capsnet: A novel artificial neural network approach to detect covid-19 disease from x-ray images using capsule networks, chaos. Solitons & Fractals **140**, 110122 (2020)
22. S. Punitha, T. Stephan, A.H. Gandomi, A novel breast cancer diagnosis scheme with intelligent feature and parameter selections. Comput. Methods Prog. Biomed. **214**, 106432 (2022)

Applications of Artificial Intelligence in the Attainment of Sustainable Development Goals

Nisha Solanki, Archana Chaudhary, and Dinesh Bhatia

Introduction to Artificial Intelligence and Sustainable Developmental Goals (SDGs)

In its basic form, artificial intelligence is a multidisciplinary strategy that combines computer science with substantial datasets to solve problems. AI not only is confined to systems that think and act like humans but also provides rationalised thinking to act accordingly. With the emergence of new technologies in the nineteenth century, lots of progress is made in computer sciences which has influenced society Hanson III and Marshall [7]. The majority of technologies were beneficial; however, some have a detrimental impact on society which needs to be criticised rationally and needs to be worked on so that loopholes may be overcome. Artificial intelligence has attained breakneck speed and made progress in every aspect of life and has supercharged humanity. The AI makes further benchmark by incorporating more data computing and other applied areas such as image progressing, artificial neural network (ANN) and Internet of things (IoT). This multiplier effect of AI can accelerate the achievement of objectives and goals of SD Hanson III and Marshall [7]. The application of AI having multiplying effect allows the achievement of the SD goals. This plays an extremely important and a decisive role in the evolution of

---

N. Solanki
Maharaja Surajmal Institute, GGSIP University, Delhi, India

A. Chaudhary (✉)
Department of Environmental Science, Faculty of Science, SGT University Gurugram, Delhi, India

D. Bhatia
Department of Biomedical Engineering, North Eastern Hill University, Shillong, Meghalaya, India

© The Author(s), under exclusive license to Springer Nature Switzerland AG 2023
G. R. Kanagachidambaresan et al. (eds.), *System Design for Epidemics Using Machine Learning and Deep Learning*, Signals and Communication Technology, https://doi.org/10.1007/978-3-031-19752-9_4

changes towards a new model that involves improving development and accelerating the achievement of objectives and goals of SDs [3].

The entire world is synergising combined efforts to achieve the Sustainable Development Goals (SDGs) for anticipating the future needs of upcoming generations in the developed economy. 'Circular economy' and 'smart cities' are considered as common concepts to boost sustainable development for a nation [3]. Artificial intelligence (AI) has been proved as an efficient and effective tool for developing the economy by contributing to various sectors. According to the latest report published by *Nature*, AI has contributed to the achievement of a major portion of SDGs (79%) [10]. This contribution of AI is the sum of all contributions from various sectors such as agriculture, transportation, manufacturing, construction, etc. AI helps transportation with traffic management and conservative mobility by sharing vehicles that not only save energy and effort but also benefit the environment. It also helps farmers in agriculture for better surveillance and pest control through drones and microscopes that help in enhancing the crop quality by efficient manuring and also stops the damage by effective control [10]. AI helps to overcome major errors which could be ignored by human oversight and helps in improving the overall supply chain management of any industry and manufacturing unit. AI also helps in ensuring the safety of millions of people through quality checks in buildings, dams and other infrastructural units. Hence, the contribution of AI is immense in several fields, and it could help in the near future to the fulfilment of the SDGs through various dimensions [4].

The Sustainable Development Goals (SDGs) are a worldwide plan to end poverty, protect the environment and ensure the prosperity of all people. They consist of 17 goals totalling 169 targets. While the United Nations Sustainable Development Goals (SDGs), which were established as part of the 2030 Agenda for Sustainable Development, do not need a long explanation, their effective implementation certainly requires a thorough assessment of investment and corporate strategies [4]. Fortunately, it was in 2015 that the SDGs had a significant impact on the worldwide investment climate. Their inherent granularity offered the necessary flexibility and universality, enabling investors and private sector players to identify and solve key sustainability issues linked to their business models while staying consistent with their fiduciary obligations. International cooperation's development efforts through 2030 will be guided by these benchmarks and indicators [4]. In order to achieve sustainable development, the 17 goals need to be treated as a whole, and AI aids in giving answers for the difficulties encountered. Our future behaviours will be greatly influenced by AI, which is one of the most rising technologies. AI is anticipated to expand at a compound annual growth rate (CAGR) of 42.2% between 2020 and 2027, according to Grand View Research. Because of its rapid development, technology will be used in many aspects of society, including ensuring sustainability. Though there is no denying that AI is still in its infancy and has the potential to make game-changing advancements, there is a constant need to improve by combining advanced and customised technology [4]. Human interactions, on the other hand, are always vital and must be embraced properly as the need of the hour, particularly in building a sustainable society.

Applications of Artificial Intelligence in the Attainment of Sustainable Development...

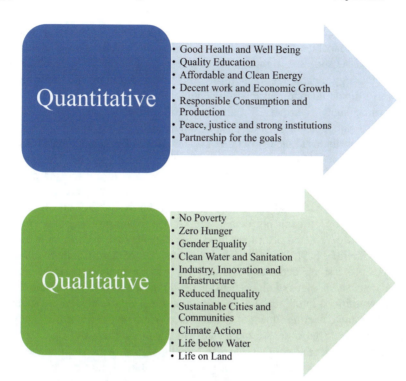

Fig. 1 Categorisation of SD goals as quantitative and qualitative goals

Artificial Intelligence and SDGs

Although United Nations SDGs were well elaborated with basic targets and indicators so that the progress can be calculated and tracked still out of 17 SDGs, some goals are qualitative and some are quantitative in nature if we compare with each other based on the extent of quantification of indicators for each SDG. The different SD goals require customised AI technologies and skills for achieving targets [12]. For better understanding, the SDGs can be classified into two categories of quantitative and qualitative (Fig. 1) for proper understanding the concept behind them.

Role of AI in Quantitative SDGs

Good Health and Well-Being

The 2030 agenda recognises the interdependence between good health and sustainable development. We've made tremendous strides against many major killers with the help of AI and have raised life expectancy significantly by attaining good health and well-being [12]. This is further achieved by significant decrease in mortality rates of newborn babies and maternal cases, along with halved malaria fatalities. On the one hand, AI addresses fight against hunger through successful implementation of biotechnology techniques to multiply crop yields, while on the other hand, it addresses climate change and environmental concerns, giving earlier predictions and warning sign to farmers for growing crop varieties resistant to inclement weather and pathogens to grow crops accordingly [12].

AI also contributes to the resolution of issues such as no communicable diseases by eradicating poverty and reducing inequality through the successful implementation of universal health coverage [15]. AI open the way to customised precision medicines and treatments for diseases and epidemics. Now it is possible to make projections on diseases and outbreaks, favouring the availability and forecast of health services by utilising big data. With AI, healthcare professionals are more prepared for illnesses and health practices, and patients have more access to treatments and facilities [15]. The artificial intelligence-based identification method outperformed professional dermatologists, according to the findings. Wearable gadgets that can detect early signs of diabetes using heart rate sensor data are another example of how artificial intelligence is being used in the health sector. AI is capable of anticipating and detecting illness at a faster rate than the majority of medical practitioners. In one study, an AI model combining algorithms and deep learning detected breast cancer at a higher rate than 11 pathologists, demonstrating the power of artificial intelligence [13]. Another aspect of healthcare that can be improved through artificial intelligence is drug development. It is possible that the application of deep learning algorithms to whole-slide pathology images would increase the accuracy and efficiency of diagnostic evaluations [15].

According to Mara Geller (2020), one of AI's possible advantages is keeping people healthy so they don't need doctors as frequently. As AI and the Internet of Medical Things (IoMT) are already benefiting patients, apps and technology promote better behaviour and assist in maintaining a healthy lifestyle to give customers control over their health [13]. Also, AI helps healthcare practitioners better understand their patients' daily routines and requirements, allowing them to offer greater feedback, advice and support for remaining healthy. It helps healthcare companies use cognitive technologies to better diagnose patients and examine and retain more medical data than any person, including every medical publication, symptom and case study of therapy and reaction worldwide [13].

It is also solving real-world healthcare issues alongside doctors, researchers and patients. The technique blends machine learning and systems neuroscience to create neural networks that resemble the human brain. Beyond scanning health data to detect chronically sick patients at risk of adverse events, AI can assist doctors in better controlling illness, coordinating care plans and helping patients better manage and adhere to long-term treatment regimens. Medical robots have been around for almost 30 years. In addition, they may assist a human surgeon or do surgeries on their own. They are also utilised in hospitals and laboratories for repeated activities, rehabilitation, physical therapy and long-term diseases [13]. It is finding widespread use in the assistive and wearable devices market which has huge growth potential.

Quality Education

Certain rising nations' growth has been hampered by poverty, conflict and other difficulties. More youngsters are not attending school as a result of the ongoing armed conflict in Western Asia and North Africa [1]. The gravity of the situation is now becoming apparent. The primary school enrolment rate in Sub-Saharan Africa increased from 52% in 1990 to 78% in 2012, the largest increase of any rising region. As many as four times as many children from destitute homes skip school as those from rich ones. Disparities between rural and urban areas persist.

Quality education for all students is an important part of ensuring a more prosperous future for everybody [1]. There will be free elementary and secondary education for all children of all sexes by the year 2030. Equal access to high-quality education for all students is also a goal of the programme. As per the changing role of AI technology in education, many shifts have been seen especially in distance education where VR emerged as a subtheme to bring vivid experiences to classrooms, big data for student profiling models and learning analytics [1]. It has brought a boom in the field of education and made changes in acquiring education.

AI-based systems can assist students with their learning experience, especially in changing the form and nature of content to suit the student. 'Smart content' is generated to ensure that learning takes place through frequent testing which can be used as feedback to alter the course content and trajectory [1]. AI cannot entirely replace the human teacher, but an AI system can play an intermediate role by providing timely feedback to students and teachers.

While educators, psychologists and parents argue how much screen time is acceptable for children, another new technology, artificial intelligence, and machine learning, is starting to change education tools and institutions, and altering the future of education [5]. According to the study, artificial intelligence market in the US education sector would increase by 47.5% from 2017 to 2021. Even while most experts think teachers' essential presence is irreplaceable, the work and educational best practices will change.

Artificial intelligence (AI) is a strong technology that has a wide range of applications. Globally, the education sector is no exception. Various schools throughout the nation are using AI in education [5]. The application of AI in education has offered instructors, students, parents and educational institutions a fresh viewpoint on education.

Here are some facts about AI in education:

- It will be worth $1 billion by 2020. Between 2021 and 2027, it is projected to expand at a 40% CAGR (GMI).
- It is projected to generate 25.7 billion USD by 2030 (strategic intelligence).
- It is projected to reach USD 3.68 billion by 2023 (markets).

Affordable and Clean Energy

To promote the use of clean and reasonably priced renewable energy by using artificial intelligence (AI), it is possible to coordinate the use of electricity against a wide range of renewable energy sources using smart power grids, for example. However, we must be cautious here as well [5]. The need for ICT solutions is increasing as digital technology advances. As a result, electricity consumption is increasing as a result of the expanding manufacturing of ICT solutions.

As more renewable energy is sent into the system, anticipating capacity levels is critical to maintaining a stable and efficient grid [5]. Because renewables are taking up more grid space, sources like coal, which supply grid inertia through heavy rotating equipment like steam and gas turbines, are losing out. Power grids will be unstable and prone to blackouts without grid inertia [14]. Sensor technology now allows solar and wind production to give massive amounts of real-time data, enabling AI to forecast capacity levels. Before AI, most forecasting depended on specific weather models that only looked at a few factors that influence renewable energy supply [14]. New AI algorithms integrate self-learning weather models, historical data, real-time weather station measurements, sensor networks and satellite and sky camera cloud data.

The outcome is a 30% increase in solar forecasting accuracy, leading to numerous benefits. According to IBM Distinguished Researcher and Chief Scientist for Geoinformatics Hendrik Hamann, better solar predictions lowered operating energy production costs and reduced start-up and shutdown costs of conventional generators [14]. It is possible to forecast the basic factors, such as wind speed and global horizontal irradiance, together with the resultant power production, minutes to hours ahead (for grid stability and resource dispatching), days ahead (for plant availability) and even weeks ahead (scheduling maintenance). With bigger datasets available, computers may now be trained to anticipate more spectacular events [14], e.g. the extra electricity consumed during a vacation or large-scale international event, or how altitude affects a community's energy use. It also enables generators and dealers to better plan their production and bid in the wholesale and balance markets – all while avoiding fines.

Decent Work and Economic Growth

Employees living in extreme poverty have reduced by a third in the last 25 years, according to a news report. In developing countries, the middle class rose almost thrice between 1991 and 2015. The global economy is rebounding at a slower rate because of a growing workforce. The International Labour Organization (ILO) estimated that 204 million people were looking for work in 2015. Aiming towards the SDGs helps to boost economic growth, worker efficiency and technological advancement. This can only be accomplished via the promotion of commerce and the creation of jobs, as well as the elimination of slavery and other forms of human trafficking. These targets must be accomplished if we are to have full and productive employment for all women and men by 2030. Experimentation is no longer an option for established businesses. Large corporations are pouring money into AI technology and applications. Since 2010, the number of patents registered on AI technology in G20 nations has grown at a compound annual growth rate of more than 26%. The amount of money invested in AI companies has increased at a compound annual growth rate of almost 60%. Governments in the G20's most powerful nations are embracing AI for the greater benefit.

With the exponential increase, invaluable data and computer power are being used by both public and commercial entities all around the globe [2]. With the recent convergence of a revolutionary collection of technologies, economies are entering a new age in which artificial intelligence (AI) has the potential to transcend the physical constraints of capital and labour, opening up new sources of value and development. In India, the stakes for AI are enormous. The country is still the most competitive in South Asia, although it lags behind several other G20 nations in terms of AIQ. Despite Indian businesses embracing AI on a wider scale, the country's expenditures in digital infrastructure and its people's increasing computer abilities, this remains the case [2]. To fully exploit AI's potential, India's policymakers, universities, businesses, entrepreneurs and workers must work together and accomplish much more. Indeed, India must leverage both an inventive private sector and a supportive governmental and regulatory environment to increase its AIQ, adopting a balanced approach to AIQ improvement across stakeholders.

Responsible Consumption and Production

To accomplish this objective, proper management of natural resources and the disposal of hazardous waste and pollutants are both responsibilities we all share. By 2030, we should assist developing countries adopt more environmentally friendly consumption patterns by encouraging businesses and individuals alike to recycle and reduce their own personal trash [2]. More than half of the world's population does not consume enough food. Global food waste per capita must be reduced in order to improve production and supply chain efficiency. Food safety and resource conservation may be improved as a result. With vertical green farms, artificial intelligence is achieving optimum consumption and output levels while reducing waste and increasing yields and resource efficiency [2]. Individuals may interact with others and monitor personal progress on daily habits via the United Nations Campaign for Individual Action Act Now, which enables them to make a difference and have an effect for the better. On a global scale, 79 nations and the European Union stated that they have implemented at least one strategy to encourage sustainable consumption and production. In addition, 93% of the world's 250 biggest corporations are now required to report on their environmental and social performance [6]. The United Nations Development Programme (UNDP) collaborates with governments and organisations to develop carbon-neutral economic models. Individual towns and nations across the globe, including Bhutan, Chile, Costa Rica, Norway and Morocco, have made commitments to achieve carbon neutrality by 2050.

Peace, Justice and Strong Institutions

Armed conflict and instability impede the expansion of a country's economy and breed resentment across generations. Governments must protect people who are most at risk from crimes such as sexual assault, crime, exploitation and torture that are frequent under conflict and lawlessness [6]. The SDGs work with governments and communities to eliminate conflict and insecurity by partnering with them. Rule of law and human rights, as well as reducing illegal arms transfers and increasing the participation of poor countries in global governance organisations, are critical. One of the most interesting applications of artificial intelligence is in the criminal justice system [6]. AI may assess the danger posed by a criminal and assist courts in making sentence choices. Understandably, the application of artificial intelligence in criminal justice is raising concerns about the technology's inherent bias.

Criminal activity like money laundering and terrorist financing can be detected by using artificial intelligence to help law enforcement agencies better prosecute these crimes. This includes more mundane offences like employee theft or cyber-fraud or fake invoices, which can also be detected using artificial intelligence [6]. The use of artificial intelligence technologies may aid in the monitoring of content. Content monitoring may aid in the prediction process. And, in the long run, anticipating crimes will assist in their prevention. Artificial intelligence can assist in monitoring a person's digital traces and identifying any odd behaviours.

Partnership for the Goals

It's simpler than ever before. Improving access to technology and knowledge encourages people to share their ideas and be more creative. It is vital to coordinate strategies to assist rising countries in controlling their debt in order to achieve long-term growth and development. Through the support of national plans, the goals seek to strengthen North-South and South-South cooperation. Promoting international commerce results in a global, rules-based and equitable economic system that is fair and open to everyone.

Despite the fact that the Sustainable Development Goals (SDGs) did not enter the global lexicon until 2015, investors have been known to direct their focus and concerted efforts towards 'socially responsible investments', which were essentially designed on an early premise of 'social screening', which had enabled them to weed out companies with detrimental business models and/or obvious exacting environmental impact. Investors were better able to match their interests and tactics with

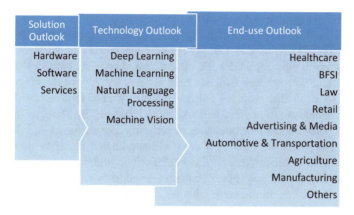

Fig. 2 Categorisation of global intelligence market (revenue, USD billion, 2017–2028)

broader societal aims once the UN Principles of Responsible Investing embraced ESG (environmental, social and governance) issues in 2006. This paved the way for ESG investing to gain traction. Surprisingly, the global movement now has over 1600 participants managing over USD 70 trillion in assets, indicating rapid global expansion. Despite this positive market response, corporate participation and activities frequently fall short of both commitment and output, which is often attributed to their inability to integrate sustainable business practices into their overall business plan. Investors and enterprises, it is claimed, have challenges in terms of thinking and direction in order to maximise capital utilisation for social and environmental development. While ESG investing has paved the path for more rapid and meaningful market reforms, there has always been a considerable disconnect between possible investment opportunities and their execution. Unfortunately, chronic hunger and malnutrition continue to obstruct many countries' progress. In 2017, it was estimated that 821 million people were chronically hungry, owing to environmental deterioration, drought and biodiversity loss. Obesity affects around 90 million children under the age of 5. Undernutrition and severe food insecurity seem to be rising in virtually all African and Latin American areas. For this study, Grand View Research has segmented the global artificial intelligence market report based on solution, technology, end-use and region (Fig. 2).

Role of AI in Qualitative SDGs

No Poverty

Getting rid of poverty is one of the most serious challenges in the world at the moment. People in severe poverty reduced by half between 1990 and 2014, yet far too many still lack even the most basic necessities in their homes. 738 million people were living on less than $1.91 a day in 2016. Food, clean water and sanitation are all in short supply for many people [9]. Millions have been lifted out of poverty as a result of globalisation, yet development has been uneven. Poor women have less opportunities for paid work, education and property than wealthy women. South Asia and Sub-Saharan Africa, which account for 80% of the world's impoverished, have made little progress. Climate change, war and food insecurity all mean that lifting people out of poverty will take more effort [9]. By 2030, the SDGs indicate a firm commitment to eradicating poverty in all of its forms and dimensions. Aiding communities affected by war or climate-related disasters necessitates a focus on the most vulnerable. People, particularly in underprivileged communities and remote or resource-poor places, can receive education, thanks to online access and 5G reach. We can mimic scenes that we conceive in fiction using virtual reality.

Zero Hunger

In order to feed the world's population by 2050, the United Nations estimates that we would need to increase the global food supply by 70%. AI systems may be used to speed up the discovery of possible answers when time is of the essence [8]. As a result of rapid economic growth and increased agricultural output, undernutrition has dropped by about half in the previous two decades. There are no longer any famines in many developing countries. In Central and East Asia, Latin America and the Caribbean, extreme hunger has been considerably decreased. The progress of a child's cognitive growth and physical health may be tracked using AI-based solutions [8]. The early detection of diseases, such as stunted development and epidemics, may be helped by image recognition systems. Using this information, the programme officers may then propose remedial measures. The AI systems may help with the identification of issues such as drought, poor sanitation and insufficient supply by integrating information from various sources [8].

'Precision farming' can be developed with the assistance of AI. *Scientific American* reports that techniques have resulted to more efficient use of inputs and greater harvests. Sensors measure the moisture content of the soil and the condition and colour of the leaf. The system uses this data to calculate how much water and fertiliser are needed. It also identifies which section of the plant requires these resources. Higher yields and lower agricultural inputs have also been reported for these systems. It's important to keep in mind that under Indian circumstances, farmers have far smaller land holdings and are less well-off.

Around half of the food produced today is thrown away, a shocking statistic. When it comes to food, AI can classify it as either 'good' or 'bad'. This is terrible. The use of big data and machine learning may help identify areas that are particularly vulnerable to food shortages, droughts and floods, as well as to increasing food prices and the deterioration of agricultural land. One example of how AI may be used is to better predict the spread of illnesses and viruses by integrating many types of alternative data, such as geolocation information (such as social media data), telecommunications data (such as Internet search data) and vaccination data.

Gender Equality

A growing body of research shows that empowering young women and girls has a positive impact on the nation's economy. This commitment to gender equality is a 20-year-old UNDP priority. Since 1990, the number of girls attending school has increased, and gender parity has been attained in most regions of primary education. Land, property, sexual and reproductive health and technology must all be accessible to women on an equal basis. Gender equality will be achieved if more women are given the opportunity to serve in high-ranking positions in the public sector. Algorithms and artificial intelligence (AI) provide enormous potential for human advancement, but they also represent significant dangers. But technology frequently absorbs and reproduces restrictive conceptions of gender and race that are then perpetually re-enforced. Consequently, the use of AI technology necessitates a highly advanced and well-planned infrastructure. When bias is present in AI systems, gender preconceptions and prejudices are reflected in the outputs, leading to discriminatory behaviours and choices.

Policymakers seem to have fallen short of adequately addressing the issues of an algorithmic society, according to this analysis. Research on how to include human rights into AI is still lacking, despite all the reports and plans about AI's role in reaching sustainable objectives. There is a significant issue with the lack of gender diversity in the AI industry, which is exacerbated by language processing and biassed ML algorithms in several sectors. Some of the Sustainable Development Goals' social objectives are hampered by these issues.

Clean Water and Sanitation

As temperatures rise, the number of individuals affected by water shortages is expected to climb as well. Despite gains in sanitation for 2.1 billion people, there is still not enough water on every continent. Several countries are already experiencing worsening conditions due to drought and desertification. At least one in four individuals will be affected by water shortages by 2050.

For the year 2030 to be a reality, we must put money into infrastructure, sanitisation and personal cleanliness. Protecting and restoring aquatic environments is essential.

Industry, Innovation and Infrastructure

Eco-economic development is fuelled by investments in infrastructure and innovation. There is a pressing need for public transportation, renewable energy and new businesses, as well as the use of ICT in cities. Technology aids in the creation of new jobs as well as the promotion of greater efficiency in the use of energy. One of the most effective ways to encourage long-term progress is to provide resources to scientific research and development.

People in developing nations account for 90% of those without Internet access, according to a recent report from the World Bank. Access to information, knowledge and entrepreneurship is critical if the digital divide is to be closed.

Reduced Inequalities

The richest 10% of the population earns up to 40% of global income, while the poorest 10% only get 2–7% of world income. When population growth is taken into account, inequality has increased by 11%. Inequality has increased over the world over the last several decades, although at different rates. The lowest and highest points may be found in Europe. There must be policies that empower low-income earners in order to achieve economic equality for everybody.

It is critical to address global wealth disparities, control the financial system, and promote foreign direct investment in regions with the highest need. The importance of ensuring the safety and mobility of people cannot be overstated.

Sustainable Cities and Communities

For the most part, our lives are spent in cities. More than 6.5 billion people will live in cities by the year 2050. Cities must undergo significant shifts in their design and management in order to expand sustainably. A result of population growth and migration, especially in developing countries, are the proliferation of megacities and slums. Creating employment, affordable housing and resilient communities and economies are essential to making cities sustainable. There is an emphasis on public transportation, the creation of green public spaces and the improvement of equitable urban planning and management. AI might also be used to keep tabs on the health of public transportation networks like trains and bridges. Traffic light systems, for example, may be modified using real-time traffic camera data and Internet of things sensors in order to enhance vehicle throughput.

Climate Action

Goal 13 and other SDGs are directly supporting underprivileged regions. Catastrophe risk reduction, sustainable resource management and human security must also be included in national development plans in order to keep global average temperatures from rising by more than 2 °C above preindustrial levels. Moreover, we also need strong political will, more investment and the best available technology.

Life Below Water

Oceans also take up around 30% of the CO_2 that is created by humans, and since the Industrial Revolution, there has been a 26% rise in the acidity of oceans. There is a concerningly high level of pollution in the ocean; around 13,000 pieces of plastic rubbish are found in every square kilometre of water. One of the Sustainable Development Goals (SDGs) that takes into consideration ocean acidification is included in this list. The improvement of ocean conservation and the usage of resources in a sustainable manner via international legislation would be beneficial to our waters as well.

Life on Land

Each year, 13 million hectares of forest are cut down, and 3.6 billion hectares of dry land are turned into desert. This has a disproportionately negative effect on individuals who are already living in poverty. On the other hand, just 15% of the land is protected in some way. The illicit trade of animals and plants involves around 7000 different species. The illegal trade in wildlife leads to the loss of biodiversity, exacerbates existing conflicts and fosters corrupt practices. The conservation of natural ecosystems and biological diversity is an immediate need for achieving global food and water security, mitigating and adapting to the effects of climate change and maintaining peace and security. Technologies that are driven by AI may be utilised to construct automated processes that gather data about biodiversity via the use of remote sensing. This data may assist stakeholders in recognising trends in the behaviour of the species and acting appropriately when they see anything that is not typical.

Therefore, technologies that are based on AI have the potential to play a significant role in the preservation of the environment. A more in-depth comprehension of the particular behavioural patterns of the inhabitants of protected areas allows for more efficient administration of such regions.

Conclusion

The advent of modern technology such as artificial intelligence and machine learning has led to their massive applications in almost all known fields. They have led to opening up of new areas having immense potential for sustainable development and growth. This would allow efficient, quality-based task accomplishment and ease of doing business. It would also help in achievement of the sustainable goals as decided by member UN nations, thereby improving human life and opening new avenues.

References

1. R. Abduljabbar, H. Dia, S. Liyanage, S.A. Bagloee, Applications of artificial intelligence in transport: An overview. Sustainability **11**(1), 189 (2019)
2. S. Alonso, R. Montes, D. Molina, I. Palomares, E. Martínez-Cámara, M. Chiachio, et al., Ordering artificial intelligence based recommendations to tackle the SDGs with a decision-making model based on surveys. Sustainability **13**(11), 6038 (2021)
3. A. Bahrammirzaee, A comparative survey of artificial intelligence applications in finance: Artificial neural networks, expert system, and hybrid intelligent systems. Neural Comput. & Applic. **19**(8), 1165–1195 (2010)
4. J. Bullock, A. Luccioni, K.H. Pham, C.S.N. Lam, M. Luengo-Oroz, Mapping the landscape of artificial intelligence applications against COVID-19. J. Artif. Intell. Res. **69**, 807–845 (2020)
5. A. Di Vaio, R. Palladino, R. Hassan, O. Escobar, Artificial intelligence and business models in the sustainable development goals perspective: A systematic literature review. J. Bus. Res. **121**, 283–314 (2020)
6. N. Efremova, D. West, D. Zausaev, AI-based evaluation of the SDGs: The case of crop detection with earth observation data. **1907**, arXiv preprint arXiv, 02813 (2019)
7. C.W. Hanson III, B.E. Marshall, Artificial intelligence applications in the intensive care unit. Crit. Care Med. **29**(2), 427–435 (2001)
8. A. E. Hassanien, R. Bhatnagar, A. Darwish (eds.), *Artificial intelligence for sustainable development: Theory, practice and future applications*, vol 912 (Springer, 2020)
9. A. Holzinger, E. Weippl, A.M. Tjoa, P. Kieseberg, Digital transformation for sustainable development goals (SDGs)-a security, safety and privacy perspective on AI, in *International cross-domain conference for machine learning and knowledge extraction*, (Springer, Cham, 2021, August), pp. 1–20
10. J. Korbicz, J. M. Koscielny, Z. Kowalczuk, W. Cholewa (eds.), *Fault diagnosis: models, artificial intelligence, applications* (Springer, 2012)
11. I. Palomares, E. Martínez-Cámara, R. Montes, P. García-Moral, M. Chiachio, J. Chiachio, F. Herrera, A panoramic view and swot analysis of artificial intelligence for achieving the sustainable development goals by 2030: Progress and prospects. Appl. Intell., 1–31 (2021)
12. W. R. Reitman (ed.), *Artificial Intelligence Applications for Business: Proceedings of the NYU Symposium, May 1983* (Intellect Books, 1984)
13. A.W. Sadek, Artificial intelligence applications in transportation. Transport. Res. Circ., 1–7 (2007)
14. R. Vinuesa, H. Azizpour, I. Leite, M. Balaam, V. Dignum, S. Domisch, et al., The role of artificial intelligence in achieving the sustainable development goals. Nat. Commun. 11(1), 1–10 (2020)
15. O. Zawacki-Richter, V.I. Marín, M. Bond, F. Gouverneur, A systematic review of research on artificial intelligence applications in higher education–where are the educators? Int. J. Educ. Technol. High. Educ. **16**(1), 1–27 (2019)

A Novel Model for IoT Blockchain Assurance-Based Compliance to COVID Quarantine

M. Shyamala Devi, M. J. Carmel Mary Belinda, R. Aruna, P. S. Ramesh, and B. Sundaravadivazhagan

Introduction to Blockchain

Blockchains are made up of any number of nodes, each of which has its own distributed ledger that allows numerous system nodes to contact and manipulate a single edition of a ledger while maintaining mutual contact regulation [1]. The blockchain nodes contain a disseminated ledger which could securely and permanently saves the action among the system devices. By connecting databases among nodes, blockchain expertise eradicates the requirement for third-party mediators to turn as reliable representatives to verify, detect, stock, and organize connections [2]. Blockchain effectively released statistics from the record that was previously reserved in a secure manner by succeeding the field from traditional integrated to decentralized [3] and then to distributed grid systems and is shown in Fig. 1 and Fig. 2.

M. S. Devi (✉) · M. J. Carmel Mary Belinda · R. Aruna · P. S. Ramesh
Computer Science and Engineering, Vel Tech Rangarajan Dr. Sagunthala R&D Institute of Science and Technology, Chennai, Tamilnadu, India
e-mail: carmelbelinda@veltech.edu.in; drraruna@veltech.edu.in; drpsramesh@veltech.edu.in

B. Sundaravadivazhagan
Faculty of IT, Department of IT, UTAS-AL Mussanah, Mussanah, Oman
e-mail: sundaravadi@act.edu.om

© The Author(s), under exclusive license to Springer Nature Switzerland AG 2023
G. R. Kanagachidambaresan et al. (eds.), *System Design for Epidemics Using Machine Learning and Deep Learning*, Signals and Communication Technology, https://doi.org/10.1007/978-3-031-19752-9_5

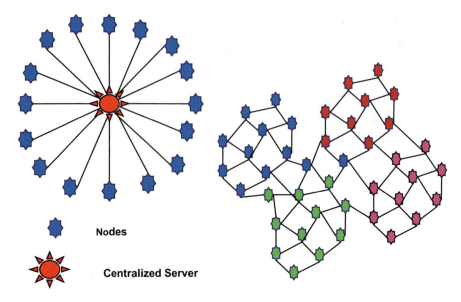

Fig. 1 (Left) centralized system framework, (right) distributed system framework

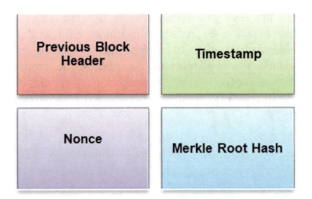

Fig. 2 Blockchain data structure

Blockchain

The blockchain data structure [4] is depicted in Fig. 2 and comprises the following apparatus:

- Former header block.
- Merkle root hash.
- Timestamp.
- Nonce.

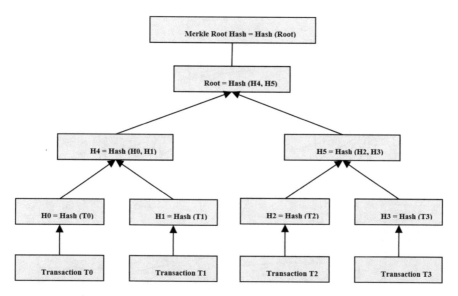

Fig. 3 Blockchain header Merkle hash root

A blockchain is an organized information assembly that is being utilized to generate a cardinal register of connections and is pooled among nodes in a distributed network [5]. Using cryptographic techniques, each network node user needs to perform secure manipulation on the distributed ledger without the need for a central authority [6]. The Merkle root hash of the blockchain is exposed in Fig. 3.

It is not necessary to alter or remove data from the blockchain after it has been updated on the blockchain distributed ledger [7]. Miners are contributors in the blockchain network. The blockchain miners have duplicates of the prevailing blockchain. When a fresh contestant node wishes to supplement a fresh action [8], network's miners use procedures to estimate and authenticate the projected contract [9].

Blockchain Design Architecture

Blockchain system is a promising application [10] that allows businesses to generate and authenticate economic businesses on an Internet in real time without the need for a dominant expert [11]. The blockchain architecture enables dispersed network of systems to achieve agreement deprived of relying on centralized authentication [12], and the design architecture of blockchain is shown in Fig. 4. The implementation steps involved in the blockchain network are depicted in Fig. 5.

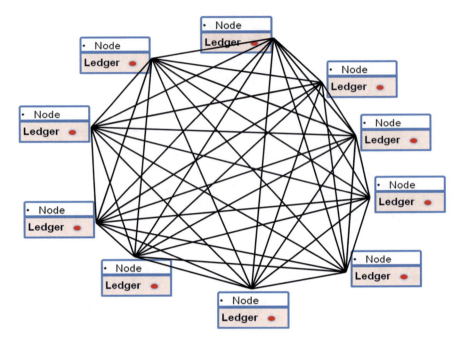

Fig. 4 Blockchain design architecture

IoT Blockchain Assurance-Based Compliance to COVID Quarantine

This paper presents a proposed model for IoT Blockchain Assurance-Based Compliance to COVID Quarantine. In COVID Quarantine blockchain network, the system in the blockchain gets the input data from the sensors that are integrated to sensor nodes in the COVID Quarantine process. The overall framework is modeled for IoT Blockchain Assurance-Based Compliance to COVID Quarantine and is shown in Fig. 6.

The systems that are integrated with the IoT Blockchain Assurance-Based Compliance to COVID Quarantine are as follows and are shown in Fig. 7:

1. Temperature sensor node.
2. Respiration sensor node.
3. Pulse rate sensor node.
4. Accelerometer sensor node.
5. Blood pressure sensor node.
6. Motion sensor node.
7. Glucometer sensor node.
8. EMG and EEG sensor node.
9. Patient doctor smartphone node.
10. Wi-Fi/Bluetooth node.
11. Health authorization node.

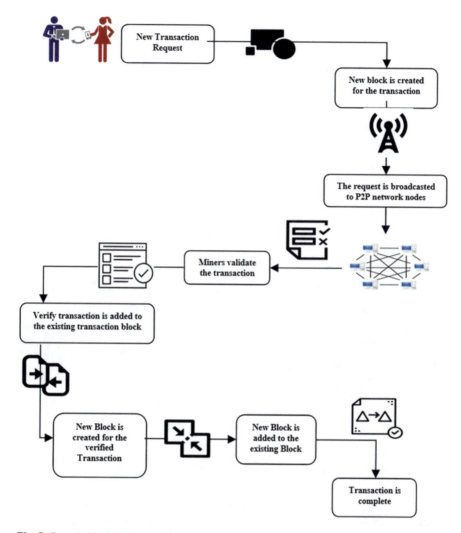

Fig. 5 Steps in blockchain technology

IoT Design Architecture

The IoT allows system nodes to be organized by end-user procedures such as computers or portable phones. The Internet of Things network can communicate an infinite number of devices. The sensors collect information about the things, which is then retrieved by mobile terminals that are linked to the devices via Internet entries. The end system nodes participate in the IoT system with absence of mortal interference. The design framework of IoT is depicted in Fig. 8 and it has high degree of scalability.

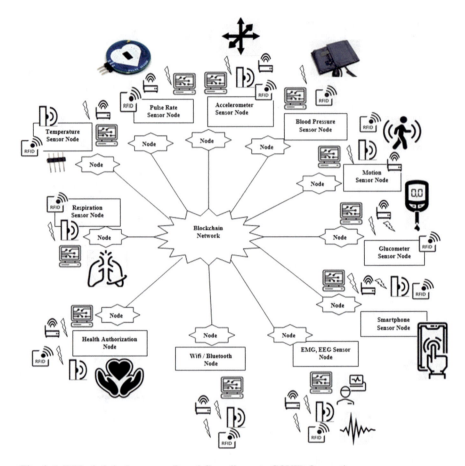

Fig. 6 IoT Blockchain Assurance-Based Compliance to COVID Quarantine

In this paper, we attempt to integrate blockchain with IoT technology in order to improve security, overcome data loss, and increase data transparency. Let us begin by discussing the blockchain development process [13, 14]. The steps involved in the blockchain development process are depicted in Fig. 9.

Temperature Sensor Control Node

All the nodes in the blockchain grid are depicted as a miner. Every system point contains the current replicate of the blockchain with the entire sanctioned transactions. Accessing, storing, and monitoring sensor data are the transactions involved in each node. The updating of information occurs concurrently with the storage process. The operations of the temperature sensor node in IoT Blockchain Assurance-Based Compliance to COVID Quarantine are as follows:

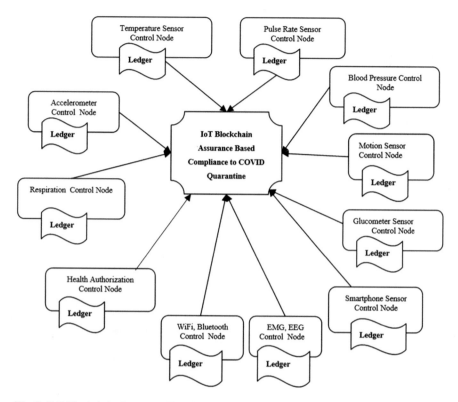

Fig. 7 IoT Blockchain Assurance-Based Compliance to COVID Quarantine

1. Temperature initial process.
2. Store and access temperature details transaction.
3. Monitor temperature status transaction.

The global policy-checking consensus and link embedding sensor for blockchain algorithm are shown below.

Blockstructure = hash[Previous block], timestamp, Nonce, Merkle Root, hash[current block].

Algorithm 1: Policy-Consensus-Checking (IncomingDetails[ ])

1. *Policy checking of the smart contract operation is done.*
2. *Raising the consensus for storing Incomingdetails[ ] from other blockchain nodes*
3. *Permit the temperature range information to enter in blockchain.*
4. *Store {Blockstructure, Incomingdetails[ ] }.*
5. *Combine this fresh node block along with the earlier one.*
6. *Refresh the disseminated ledger with the most recent blockchain.*
7. *Distribute updated blockchain distributed ledger to all blockchain nodes.*

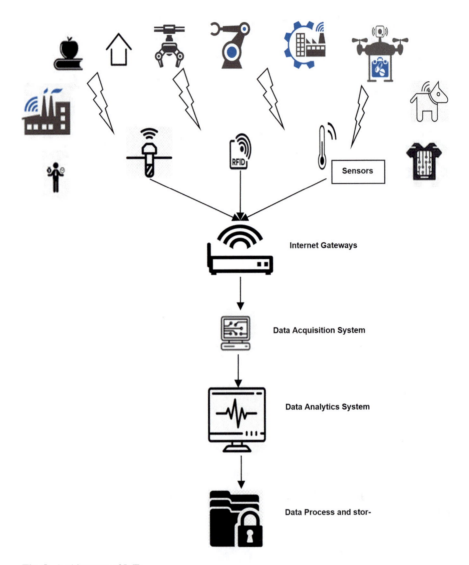

Fig. 8 Architecture of IoT

Algorithm 2: Link-Embedding-Sensor (IncomingSensorNode, IncomingDetails[ ])

1. *Embed the IncomingSensorNode based on smart contract to patient.*
2. *Link the IncomingSensorNode with RFID sensors.*
3. *Assign IncomingSensorNode identifier.*
4. *Receive the IncomingDetails from RFID sensors through Internet gateways.*
5. *IncomingDetails is stored for data analysis in the cloud storage.*
6. *IncomingDetails is retrieved by IncomingSensorNode.*

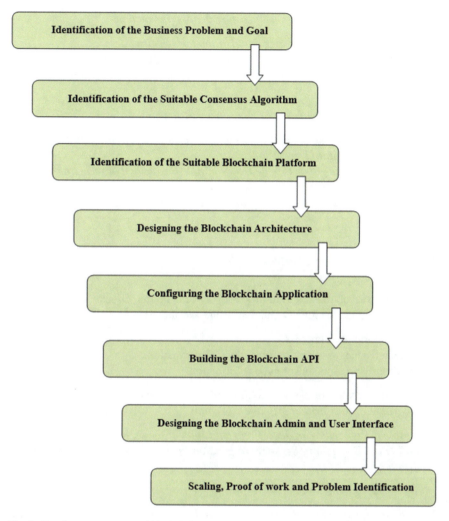

Fig. 9 Development process of blockchain

The algorithms for all the transactions of the temperature sensor control node are explored here.

Algorithm 3: Temperature primary procedure

1. *Initiate the procedure of accessing the temperature of the patient.*
2. *Call Link-Embedding-Sensor (temperature sensor node, temperature range details)*

Algorithm 4: Store and access temperature details transaction

1. *Get patient temperature range details from the sensor node.*
2. *Call Policy-Consensus-Checking (temperature range details).*
3. *Acquire and extract patient's temperature range details from temperature sensor node.*

Algorithm 5: Monitor temperature status transaction

1. *Monitor the continuous fluctuations of temperature range information of patient from the temperature sensor node.*
2. *If the needed time gap is expelled, then initiate the method of receiving temperature range information from the sensor node.*
3. *Call Policy-Consensus-Checking (temperature range details).*

Respiration Sensor Control Node

The procedures of the respiration sensor system in IoT Blockchain Assurance-Based Compliance to COVID Quarantine are as follows:

1. Respiration initial process.
2. Store and access respiration sensor node information.
3. Monitor respiration sensor node Information.

The processes for all the transactions are explored below.
Algorithm 6: Respiration primary procedure

1. *Initiate the procedure of accessing respiration of the patient.*
2. *Call Link-Embedding-Sensor (respiration sensor node, respiration range details).*

Algorithm 7: Store and access respiration sensor node information

1. *Get patient movement of the chest wall and abdomen circumference during respiration to compute the respiration rate and volume details from the sensor node.*
2. *Call Policy-Consensus-Checking (respiration rate, volume details).*
3. *Acquire and extract patient's respiration rate and volume details from respiration sensor node.*

Algorithm 8: Monitor respiration sensor node information

1. *Track the frequent motion of the chest wall and abdomen circumference during respiration to obtain the respiration rate and volume information of patient from the respiration sensor node.*
2. *If the needed time gap is expelled, then initiate the method of receiving respiration rate and volume details from the sensor node.*
3. *Call Policy-Consensus-Checking (respiration rate, volume details).*

Pulse Rate Sensor Control Node

The procedures of the pulse rate sensor node in IoT Blockchain Assurance-Based Compliance to COVID Quarantine are as follows:

1. Pulse rate initial process.
2. Store and access pulse rate sensor node information.
3. Monitor pulse rate sensor node information.

   The processes for all the transactions are explored below.
   Algorithm 9: Pulse rate primary procedure

1. *Start the process of accessing the pulse rate of the patient.*
2. *Call Link-Embedding-Sensor (pulse rate sensor node, pulse wave signal details).*

   Algorithm 10: Store and access pulse rate sensor node information

1. *Monitor the change in blood vessel volume which is the blood flow rate of the person that changes following heart contractions over time to calculate the pulse wave signal from the pulse rate sensor node.*
2. *Call Policy-Consensus-Checking (pulse wave signal details).*
3. *Acquire and extract patient's pulse wave signal details from pulse rate sensor node.*

   Algorithm 11: Monitor pulse rate sensor node information

1. *Track the blood flow rate (change in blood vessel volume) that changes following heart contractions over time to obtain the pulse wave signal details of patient from the pulse rate sensor node.*
2. *If the needed time gap is expelled, then initiate the method of receiving pulse wave signal details from the sensor node.*
3. *Call Policy-Consensus-Checking (pulse wave signal details).*

Accelerometer Sensor Control Node

The procedures of the accelerometer sensor node in IoT Blockchain Assurance-Based Compliance to COVID Quarantine are as follows:

1. Accelerometer initial process.
2. Store and access accelerometer sensor node information.
3. Monitor accelerometer sensor node information.

   The processes for all the transactions are explored below.
   Algorithm 12: Accelerometer primary procedure

1. *Initiate the procedure of accessing the vibration details of the patient.*
2. *Call Link-Embedding-Sensor (accelerometer sensor node, vibration details).*

Algorithm 13: Store and access accelerometer sensor node information

1. *Get patient activity count and vibration rate details from the accelerometer sensor node.*
2. *Call Policy-Consensus-Checking (activity count, vibration rate).*
3. *Acquire and extract patient's activity count and vibration rate details from accelerometer sensor node.*

Algorithm 14: Monitor accelerometer sensor node information

1. *Track the activity count and vibration rate details from the accelerometer sensor node.*
2. *If the needed time gap is expelled, then initiate the method of receiving vibration rate details from the sensor node.*
3. *Call Policy-Consensus-Checking (activity count, vibration rate).*

Blood Pressure Sensor Control Node

The methodologies of the blood pressure sensor node in IoT Blockchain Assurance-Based Compliance to COVID Quarantine are as follows:

1. Blood pressure initial process.
2. Store and access blood pressure sensor node information.
3. Monitor blood pressure sensor node information.

The processes for all the transactions are explored below.
Algorithm 15: Blood pressure primary procedure

1. *Initiate the method of accessing the blood pressure of the patient.*
2. *Call Link-Embedding-Sensor (blood pressure sensor node, blood pressure details).*

Algorithm 16: Store and access blood pressure sensor node information

1. *Get patient systolic, diastolic, and mean arterial pressure details from the accelerometer sensor node.*
2. *Call Policy-Consensus-Checking (systolic pressure, diastolic pressure, mean arterial pressure).*
3. *Acquire and extract the patient's systolic, diastolic, and mean arterial pressure details from blood pressure sensor node.*

Algorithm 17: Monitor blood pressure sensor node information

1. *Track the systolic, diastolic, and mean arterial pressure details from the blood pressure sensor node.*
2. *If the needed time gap is expelled, then initiate the method of receiving systolic, diastolic, and mean arterial pressure details from the sensor node.*

3. *Call Policy-Consensus-Checking (systolic pressure, diastolic pressure, mean arterial pressure).*

Motion Sensor Control Node

The methodologies of the motion sensor node in IoT Blockchain Assurance-Based Compliance to COVID Quarantine are as follows:

1. Motion initial process.
2. Store and access motion sensor node information.
3. Monitor motion sensor node information.

The processes for all the transactions are explored below.
Algorithm 18: Motion primary procedure

1. *Initiate the method of accessing the motion details of the patient.*
2. *Call Link-Embedding-Sensor (motion sensor node, motion details).*

Algorithm 19: Store and access motion sensor node information

1. *Get patient step count, motion rate, and movement range details from the motion sensor node.*
2. *Call Policy-Consensus-Checking (step count, motion rate, movement range details).*
3. *Acquire and extract patient's step count, motion rate, and movement range details from motion sensor node.*

Algorithm 20: Monitor accelerometer sensor node information

1. *Track the patient's step count, motion rate, and movement range details from the motion sensor node.*
2. *If the needed time gap is expelled, then initiate the method of receiving patient's step count, motion rate, and movement range details from the sensor node.*
3. *Call Policy-Consensus-Checking (step count, motion rate, movement range details).*

Glucometer Sensor Control Node

The methodologies of the glucometer sensor node in IoT Blockchain Assurance-Based Compliance to COVID Quarantine are as follows:

1. Glucometer initial process.
2. Store and access glucometer sensor node information.
3. Monitor glucometer sensor node information.

The processes for all the transactions are explored below.

Algorithm 21: Glucometer primary procedure

1. Initiate the method of accessing the glucose level of the patient.
2. Call Link-Embedding-Sensor (glucometer sensor node, glucose level).

Algorithm 22: Store and access glucometer sensor node information

1. Get patient glucose level details from the glucometer sensor node.
2. Call Policy-Consensus-Checking (glucose level).
3. Acquire and extract patient's glucose level details from the glucometer sensor node.

Algorithm 23: Monitor glucometer sensor node information

1. Track the patient's glucose level details from glucometer sensor node.
2. If the needed time gap is expelled, then initiate the method of receiving patient's glucose level details from the sensor node.
3. Call Policy-Consensus-Checking (glucose level).

EMG and EEG Sensor Control Node

The methodologies of the EMG and EEG sensor node in IoT Blockchain Assurance-Based Compliance to COVID Quarantine are as follows:

1. EMG and EEG initial process.
2. Store and access EMG and EEG details transaction.
3. Monitor EMG and EEG status transaction.

The processes for all the transactions are explored below.

Algorithm 24: EMG and EEG primary procedure

1. Initiate the method of accessing the EMG and EEG of the patient.
2. Call Link-Embedding-Sensor (EMG and EEG sensor control node, glucose level).

Algorithm 25: Store and access EMG and EEG transaction

1. Get patient EMG and EEG details from the sensor node.
2. Call Policy-Consensus-Checking (EMG and EEG details).
3. Acquire and extract patient's EMG and EEG details from EMG and EEG sensor node.

Algorithm 26: Monitor EMG and EEG

1. Monitor the continuous updation and fluctuation of EMG and EEG details of patient from the EMG and EEG sensor node.
2. If the needed time gap is expelled, then initiate the method of receiving EMG and EEG details from the sensor node.
3. Call Policy-Consensus-Checking (EMG and EEG details).

Patient Doctor Smartphone Sensor Control Node

The methodologies of the patient doctor smartphone sensor node in IoT Blockchain Assurance-Based Compliance to COVID Quarantine are as follows:

1. Patient doctor smartphone initial process.
2. Store and access patient details transaction.
3. Monitor patient details transaction.

   The processes for all the transactions are explored below.
   Algorithm 27: Patient doctor primary procedure

1. *Initiate the method of accessing the patient details to doctor's smartphone.*
2. *Call Link-Embedding-Sensor (patient doctor smartphone sensor node, patient health details).*

Algorithm 28: Store and access patient details transaction

1. *Get patient details from all the sensors from the sensor node.*
2. *Call Policy-Consensus-Checking (patient health details).*
3. *Acquire and extract patient's details from all the sensor node.*

Algorithm 29: Monitor patient details

1. *Monitor the continuous fluctuation of patient details from all the sensors.*
2. *If the needed time gap is expelled, then initiate the method of receiving patient's details from the sensor node.*
3. *Call Policy-Consensus-Checking (patient health details).*

Wi-Fi/Bluetooth Sensor Control Node

The methodologies of the Wi-Fi/Bluetooth sensor node in IoT Blockchain Assurance-Based Compliance to COVID Quarantine are as follows:

1. Wi-Fi/Bluetooth initial process.
2. Store and access Wi-Fi/Bluetooth details transaction.
3. Monitor Wi-Fi/Bluetooth details transaction.

   The processes for all the transactions are explored below.
   Algorithm 30: Wi-Fi/Bluetooth initial process

1. *Initiate the method of accessing the smartphone of the patient and doctor through Wi-Fi/Bluetooth.*
2. *Call Link-Embedding-Sensor (Wi-Fi/Bluetooth sensor node, Wi-Fi/Bluetooth connection details).*

Algorithm 31: Store Wi-Fi/Bluetooth connection details transaction

1. *Get Wi-Fi/Bluetooth connection details between the patient and doctor smartphone.*
2. *Call Policy-Consensus-Checking (Wi-Fi/Bluetooth connection details).*
3. *Acquire and extract patient's details from all the sensor node.*

Algorithm 32: Monitor Wi-Fi/Bluetooth connection

1. *Monitor the continuous fluctuation of Wi-Fi/Bluetooth connection details between the doctor and patient smartphone.*
2. *If the needed time gap is expelled, then initiate the method of receiving Wi-Fi/Bluetooth connection details from the sensor node.*
3. *Call Policy-Consensus-Checking (Wi-Fi/Bluetooth connection details).*

Health Authorization Sensor Control Node

The methodologies of the health authorization sensor node in IoT Blockchain Assurance-Based Compliance to COVID Quarantine are as follows:

1. Health authorization initial process.
2. Store and access health authorization details transaction.
3. Monitor health authorization details transaction.

The processes for all the transactions are explored below:
Algorithm 33: Health authorization initial process

1. *Initiate the method of health authorization of the patient through doctor's smartphone.*
2. *Call Link-Embedding-Sensor (health authorization sensor node, health authorization details).*

Algorithm 34: Store and access health authorization details transaction

1. *Get health authorization details from the doctor smartphone.*
2. *Call Policy-Consensus-Checking (health authorization details).*
3. *Acquire and extract health authorization details from all sensor node.*

Algorithm 35: Monitor health authorization details

1. *Monitor the continuous fluctuation of health authorization details between the doctor and patient smartphone.*
2. *If the needed time gap is expelled, then initiate the method of receiving health authorization connection details from the sensor node.*
3. *Call Policy-Consensus-Checking (health authorization details).*

Results and Efficiency Analysis

This paper proposes a proof of concept for the proposed IoT Blockchain Assurance-Based Compliance to COVID Quarantine System using the Ethereum Private Blockchain network as a genesis block. The throughput of the management hub is assessed, which influences the latency of blockchain methods and is shown in Table 1 and Fig. 10.

IoT devices are built using the LibCoAP library, which is a C procedure of the built-in CoAP framework. The LibCoAP framework was altered to produce a public key and private key for each system node, which uniquely authorizes the IoT systems. In this paper, the benchmark tool CoAPBench is used to validate the effectiveness of the proposed model. The latency timeout analysis of the management hub and IoT device is shown in Table 2 and Fig. 11.

Table 1 Management hub throughput analysis

Number of concurrent users	IoT device throughput	Management hub throughput
1	5	900
2	10	945
3	15	960
4	20	980
5	25	1000
6	30	975
7	35	950
8	40	920
9	45	900

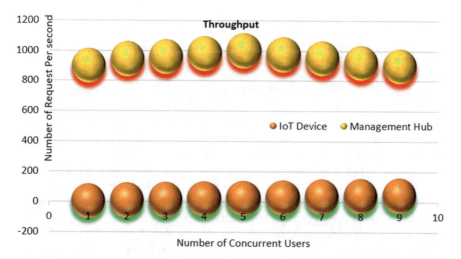

Fig. 10 Management hub throughput

Table 2 Management hub timeout analysis

Number of concurrent users	IoT device latency timeout	Management hub latency timeout
1	5	20
2	10	40
3	15	50
4	20	60
5	25	70
6	30	80
7	35	90
8	40	100
9	45	120

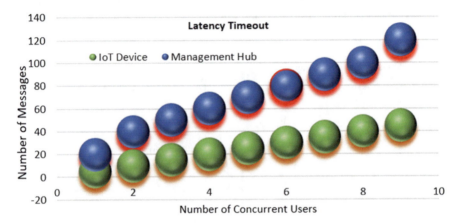

Fig. 11 Timeout latency of management hub

Conclusion

This work is explored to investigate the characteristics of blockchain and the Internet of Things. The theoretical verification of this proposed model, namely, IoT Blockchain Assurance-Based Compliance to COVID Quarantine, remains to be assessed. This work ended up with the model called IoT Blockchain Assurance-Based Compliance to COVID Quarantine System, as well as a framework of working process model that improves data safety and transparency. The systems that are integrated with the IoT Blockchain Assurance-Based Compliance to COVID Quarantine System are depicted clearly, and the blockchain algorithm for all the nodes is elaborated. The throughput and the latency timeout of the management hub and IoT device are assessed and the results are discussed. Furthermore, the proposed model can be upgraded by employing several consensus procedures to forecast efficiency indices. This paper's future work will include adding and upgrading the devices that are utilized to estimate the clinical attributes of patients. The security of the sensor devices is also developed to be implemented with respect to context-based clinical data.

References

1. I.F. Akyildiz, W. Su, Y. Sankarasubramaniam, E. Cayirci, Wireless sensor networks: A survey. Comm. ACM **38**(4), 393–422 (2002)
2. D.A. Anisi, *Optimal motion control of a ground vehicle*, Master's thesis (Royal Institute of Technology (KTH), Stockholm, 2003)
3. P. Bahl, R. Chancre, J. Dungeon, SSCH: Slo.Ed Seeded Channel hopping for capacity improvement in IEEE 802.11 ad-hoc wireless networks, in *Proceeding of the 10th International Conference on Mobile Computing and Networking (MobiCom'04)*, (ACM, New York, 2004), pp. 112–117
4. K.L. Clarkson, *Algorithms for Closest-Point Problems (Computational Geometry)*, Ph.D. Dissertation (Stanford University, Palo Alto, CA, 1985) UMI Order Number: AAT 8506171
5. Jacques Cohen (Ed.)., Special Issue: Digital Libraries. Commun. ACM **39**, 11 (1996)
6. B.P. Douglass, Statecarts in use: Structured analysis and object-orientation, in *Lectures on embedded systems*, Lecture notes in computer science, ed. by G. Rozenberg, F. W. Vaandrager, vol. 1494, (Springer, London, 1998), pp. 368–394. https://doi.org/10.1145/3-540-65193-429
7. I. Editor (ed.), *The title of book two*, 2nd edn. (University of Chicago Press, Chicago, Chapter 100, 2008). https://doi.org/10.1145/3-540-09237-4
8. C. Qu, M. Tao, J. Zhang, X. Hong, R. Yuan, Blockchain based credibility verification method for IoT entities. Secur. Commun. Netw. **2018**, 1 (2018)
9. A. Iftekhar, X. Cui, M. Hassan, W. Afzal, Application of Blockchain and internet of things to ensure tamper-proof data availability for food safety. J. Food Qual. **2020**, 1–14 (2020). https://doi.org/10.1155/2020/5385207
10. O. Cheikhrouhou, A. Koubaa, BlockLoc: Secure Localization in the Internet of Things using Blockchain, in *15th International Wireless Communications & Mobile Computing Conference (IWCMC), Tangier, Morocco*, (2019), pp. 629–634. https://doi.org/10.1109/IWCMC.2019.8766440
11. O. Novo, Blockchain Meets IoT: An architecture for Scalable Access Management in IoT. IEEE Internet of Things J. **5**, 2 (2018)
12. M.T. Hammi, B. Hammi, P. Bellot, A. Serrhouchni, Bubbles of trust: A decentralized blockchain-based authentication system for IoT. Comput. Secur. **78**, 126–142 (2018). https://doi.org/10.1016/j.cose.2018.06.004
13. M.J. Fischer, N.A. Lynch, M.S. Paterson, Impossibility of distributed consensus with one faulty process. J. ACM **32**(2), 374–382 (1985)
14. G.-T. Nguyen, K. Kim, A survey about consensus algorithms used in blockchain. J Inf Process Syst **14**(1), 101–128 (2018)

Deep Learning-Based Convolutional Neural Network with Random Forest Approach for MRI Brain Tumour Segmentation

B. Leena

Introduction

The medical business has profited in recent years from the advancement of information technology and e-healthcare systems, which have enabled clinical professionals to provide better healthcare to patients. Pereira et al. [26] define tumour as an abnormal rise of cancerous cells in several areas of the body, whereas a brain tumour is an abnormal proliferation of cancerous cells in the brain. A benign brain tumour does not harm the surrounding normal and healthy tissue, whereas a malignant tumour can harm the brain's surrounding tissues, perhaps leading to death. Accurate brain tumour segmentation is essential to locate the tumour, as well as to give the appropriate treatment for a patient and to provide the key to the surgeon who will do the surgery. Tumours are produced from the tissues of the brain itself and are known as primary brain tumours. The cancer tumour from another place in the body will extend to the brain part and it is called as metastasis. The options of treatment can be differed according to the tumour form, range and place [4].

The aims of treatment are therapeutic or focus to lessen the symptoms. The tumour symptoms can be repeated headache and migraines. It can still direct to vision failure. By this time, science can be insufficient about the beginning and the factor directing to this unusual expansion of tumour. In common, the tumours can be categorised depending on the two bases such as their source place and whether they can be cancer tumour or not [25]. The noncancerous tumour is called as benign tumour because it does not affect other parts of the human body. It can be simply noticeable and it contains a slow rate of expansion. Cancer-based brain tumour also known as malignant tumour can affect other parts of the brain, and it can be very

B. Leena (✉)
KGiSL Institute of Technology, Coimbatore, India

Fig. 1 MRI image of the brain

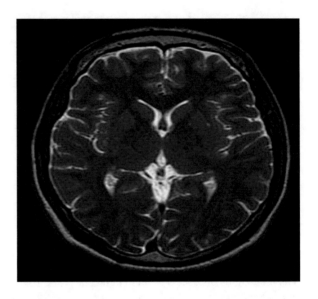

life-threatening as it can be difficult to identify. The doctors will select either a magnetic resonance imaging (MRI) or X-ray in identifying a tumour. If every examination fails to give adequate information, then MRI scan can be suitable. The magnetism properties and radio waves are utilised by the MRI scan to make perfect images [28]. The images of the brain parts are more clearly seen in the MRI scan than in CT, X-ray and ultrasound scans, which produces detailed two- or three-dimensional images of the brain stem and pituitary gland. The MRI image of the brain has been illustrated in Fig. 1.

Basically, MRI scan is a high-quality imaging technique used to image the brain's activity, and this kind of scanning technique is the most reliable in identifying the tumours in the brain area. However, it cannot take images of skull bones, and consequently CT scans they will not demonstrate the tumour effects on the skull part of the human body. The radio waves and strong magnets have been exploited by the MRI scans to take the images of the brain. Contrast objects, e.g., gadolinium, can be injected into a vein before the examination to aid in observing the details. MRI scan of the brain can give a secure and painless experiment that will utilise the radio waves and magnetic area to make comprehensive images of the brain parts of the human body. An MRI scan has been varied from a computed tomography (CT) since it will not utilise radiation waves [3].

In general, the MRI scanner has a huge doughnut-shaped magnet field that frequently contains a channel in the middle. In this testing process, the patients will be located on a table that slides into the channel. The various of centres can be opened in MRI machines that contains superior opening and it can be supportive to patients with claustrophobia. In hospitals and radiology centres, MRI machine is available to test the brain. The radio waves are direct the magnetic location of the human body atoms while the testing process that can be selected by an influential antenna and be sent to a computer. The computer can execute millions of estimations, resulting in the body's obvious white images [12]. These kinds of images have been transformed into three-dimensional (3-D) image of the scanned region of the body [2]. This type of scanning process will assist in finding out the disorders in the brain, while the test focuses on those locations. On the medical side, radiologists may face the challenge of differentiating brain cells and their nuclei from the content of an MRI image. Nowadays, segmenting brain tumours from MRI images might be problematic due to the shape and location of tumours in the human brain when using multimodal imaging data. As a result, picture segmentation may be the most difficult component of brain MRI image tumour identification. However, in order to distinguish the cancer tumour and provide an accurate diagnosis, the task of tumour segmentation and separation must be prioritised. The correct segmentation process can provide quantitative and qualitative data about a benign or cancerous tumour, which can be utilised to select the best treatments for the patient and assist the treating physician in developing a better plan [16].

The medical image processing is the most important method to examine the people's health position and sentimental analysis [18]. The mass is discovered by using the image processing methods with some enhancements, whether it is present in the inner organs or not. Methods that can execute this process are known as CAD methods. CAD methods can be used as a tool to augment the effectiveness of medical imaging procedure. The principles of the CAD methods are to enhance diagnostic accurateness; to identify abnormal structures, e.g. tumour in the brain or breast or any part of the body; and to assist radiologists by applying the computer methods. Pre-processing, image segmentation, feature analysis, feature extraction [17, 31], collection of feature and confirmation of feature, and finally, the classification phase that has been established in Fig. 2 are some of the phases in the CAD approach. The high-quality images can be utilised in the recognition methods.

This is an important concept that speaks directly to the success rate in the field of medical image processing. The pre-processing phase's main purpose is to increase the image quality of the brain MRI. Histogram equalisation is now the most commonly used method for improving image quality in MRI brain images. Two key histogram-based strategies that can be used to improve the MRI image quality are histogram equalisation and histogram equalisation of an image's dynamic set of values. The following method is offered to overcome the aforementioned challenges with brain **tumour** segmentation and to efficiently segment the brain tumour from an MRI image at an early stage in order to save the patient's life. The Convolutional neural network (CNN) with RF (Random Forest) algorithm for brain tumour segmentation are proposed.

The remainder of this chapter is organised as follows: Section "Literature review" discussed about brain tumour prediction and its related work, Section "System

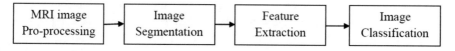

Fig. 2 Image processing of MRI image

design" discussed about proposed algorithm and implementation process, Section "Result and discussion" compares the experimental findings of the proposed and current systems, and Section "Conclusion" concludes with some closing remarks and a discussion of the work's future scope.

Literature Review

In this chapter, computer vision-based and image processing methods for brain tumour detection can be surveyed. The importance of accuracy and tumour classification has been extensively discussed in this literature. Different research works are obtainable on brain tumour detection utilising an effective image classifier in this survey.

Demirhan et al. [6] developed a new brain MR imaging tissue segmentation method that separated tumour, WM, GM, CSF, and oedema. Since the emergence of tumours on healthy brain tissues, the identification of healthy brain tissues has been done in tandem with the identification of malignant tissues. It has the potential to be the most crucial when it comes to treatment planning. In this investigation, T1, T2, and fluid-attenuated inversion recovery MR images of 20 people with glial tumours were employed. Before the segmentation phase, an algorithm for striped skull was improved. A self-organising map was created utilising a learning vector quantisation technique and an unsupervised learning algorithm to accomplish picture segmentation. In this way, an algorithm for clustering the SOM replacement of an additional network was enhanced. The input feature vector was measured using the features generated from the coefficients of the stationary wavelet transform.

The brain tissues' automatic segmentation from MRI image is more significant for the scientific research and the clinical purpose. In supervoxel-level examination, new development has enabled the robust segmentation of brain tissues by discovering the intrinsic data amongst multiple extracted features on the supervoxel process. The complexities are occurring within this common structure in clustering reservations compulsory by the redundancy of the MRI features and the heterogeneity of tissues. Kong and Hong [20] have presented a robust discriminative segmentation technique from the vision of information theoretic examination. The famous objective of the technique was to concurrently choose the useful feature and to decrease the supervoxel assignment's uncertainties for the process of discriminative brain tissue segmentation.

Meiyan Huang et al. proposed a new automatic tumour segmentation technique for MRI brain images [13]. In the therapy of tumour segmentation, this method has been proven to be highly effective. In addition, using the LIPC technique, each voxel was classified into several classes. To create this categorisation framework, the LIP was incorporated into the standard classification approach. The computation of local independent projections for LIPC required a high level of locality. Locality has also been investigated to see if local fix embedding is better than other coding approaches for resolving linear projection weights. Furthermore, LIPC looked into a softmax regression method that produced classification performance in order to assess data sharing between different classes.

El-Melegy and Mokhtar [8] developed a novel fuzzy method for segmenting standard and volumetric datasets of sick brain MRI. The well-known FCM technique has been altered in this way to extract information about the image's class centre. These data have also been simulated to account for uncertainty. This type of information helped to standardise the FCM algorithm's clusters, improving their presentation in unexpected data collection and noisy settings. In addition, the convergence process of the approach has been improved. This method was compared to other well-known fuzzy and non-fuzzy methods on simulated and real MRI volumes of the human brain, both normal and pathological, and it was discovered that this method had much greater segmentation accuracy, noise resistance and response time [10].

Atiq Islam et al. [15] proposed a new multiFD feature extraction and supervised classifiers for improved brain tumour segmentation and identification, as well as a modified AdaBoost algorithm to account for the extensive unpredictability in surface features of hundreds of multiple patients' MRI slices for expanded tumour and non-tumour tissue. The process of separating distinct brain tumour tissues from normal brain tissues is known as brain tumour segmentation. In most cases, the survival of abnormal tissues may be easily measured during a brain tumour examination. On the other hand, consistent and exact abnormality segmentation and categorisation has been proven difficult. A review of the brain tumour segmentation procedure was published by several researchers in the fields of MRI imaging and soft computing. The semiautomated and fully automated methods were presented at this time. Medical segmentation approaches were chosen based on the ease of segmentation and the degree of user management. Semiautomated or interactive procedures were used to keep the performer in charge for an extended period of time, especially in situations when erroneous understandings are unacceptably dangerous. After obtaining the image, Nelly Gordillo et al. [11] gave a basic overview of the most commonly used brain tumour segmentation techniques. Because of the benefits that MRI has over other types of diagnostic imaging, the focus of this review was on MRI brain tumour segmentation approaches. The semiautomated and fully automated methods have been highlighted in this survey.

This segmentation method was utilised by Friedrich et al. [9] to investigate simple scenarios such as fitting a circle, line, cubic spline contour, or ellipse. In phase-contrast magnetic resonance (PC-MR) pictures, the cross-section shaving the CSF wherever the object of interest was indicated by applying the deformed ellipse was utilised to discover subarachnoid gaps. The findings were used to segment a CSF structure utilising a s–t graph cut in this technique. The arithmetical contour method and force area were successfully configured using this way. This approach has the potential to effectively eliminate noise and defects in MRI images. This method does not require huge training datasets and does not require physical labelling of the training images when employing point sharing methods because it uses an arithmetical contour method.

D. Divyamary et al. [7] proposed a quick and forceful useful approach for solid tumour segmentation with the least amount of user intervention to aid researchers and clinicians in radio-surgery planning and treatment response evaluation. On contrast-enhanced T1-weighted MR images, a CA-based kernel tumour segmentation technique was utilised, which normalised the kernel selection and volume of interest (VOI). Initially, the CA-based segmentation connection was demonstrated to the graph-theoretic techniques to demonstrate that the iterative CA structure has solved the shortest path difficulty. In this method, the CA's state transition function has been modified in order to compute the accurate solution of shortest path problem. In addition, a parameter of sensitivity was presented to adjust to the heterogeneous tumour segmentation difficulty. An implied level set outside was progressed on a tumour likelihood map built from states of CA to inflict spatial softness. From the user, adequate data to initialise the method has been gathered by using the line drawn on the utmost tumour size. In addition, CA was introduced to distinguish the necrotic and improving the tumour tissue content that has obtained significance for a comprehensive evaluation of radiation therapy reaction [21].

Jason J Corso et al. [5] proposed a novel approach for automatically segmenting heterogeneous picture data that bridges the gap between top-down generative model-based methods and bottom-up affinity-based segmentation techniques. By introducing a Bayesian formulation into the computation of similarities, this method made a substantial contribution to the integration of soft model assignments. The model-aware affinities were incorporated into the multilevel segmentation process using the weighted aggregation methodology, and the method was applied to the process of finding and segmenting brain tumours using MRI. The solution was implemented faster than current state-of-the-art methods that can produce equivalent or superior results.

Heba Mohsen et al. [24] suggested a method for classifying brain MRI images into normal, metastatic, sarcoma and glioblastoma using the DWT and DNN. For brain tumour segmentation, fully convolutional networks (FCNs) were the most often employed convolutional neural networks. FCNs are voxels that have a direct spatial relationship between units in FMs and comparable classified voxels at a specific place. Because the FMs were combined in a convolutional layer to create novel FMs, channel mixing may be required. On the other hand, not all FMs are equally applicable to each class. The Squeeze-and-Excitation (SE) blocks were presented in classification concerns to recalibrate FMs as a whole and reduce the less beneficial ones. On the other hand, during the spatial association of voxels and units in FCN, this cannot be the best [29].

Sergio Pereira et al. [27] demonstrated feature recombination for semantic segmentation using linear extension and compression to generate more complex features as a consequence. In addition, a segmentation SE (SegSE) block for feature recalibration that has collected contextual data while keeping spatial meaning has been constructed. Finally, these techniques were approximated in brain tumour segmentation utilising the given data. CNNs have become the state-of-the-art presentation for automatic medical picture segmentation techniques [30]. They were, on the other hand, insufficiently precise and effective for medical use. They were also limited by the need for image-specific edition and the need for generalisability to previous concealed object classes.

Guotai Wang et al. [33] proposed a new deep learning-based interactive segmentation method by merging CNNs into a scribble-based segmentation pipeline and bounding box methodology. Image-specific fine-tuning was employed to create a CNN model that could adapt to either a supervised or unsupervised detailed examination image in this work. For fine-tuning, a weighted loss function was created that took interaction-based uncertainty and the network into consideration. This framework was used for two purposes: 2-D multiple organ segmentation from foetal MR slices and 2-D multiple organ segmentation from foetal MR slices with only two types of these organs explained for the training process. More than half of cancer patients were treated with radiotherapy. If artificial intelligence techniques aren't used to assist with the preparation and release of radiotherapy treatment, it can be a difficult task. Deep learning is the hottest issue in artificial intelligence right now, and it's being applied successfully in a variety of medical applications.

Philippe Meyer et al. [23] were the first to propose the concept of deep learning, which they came upon while researching machine learning. The typical architectures were available, but with a focus on CNNs [14]. Following that, a study of various studies on deep learning methods employed in radiation was undertaken, and they were categorised into seven divisions linked to patient workflow, as well as a number of future application ideas. This research used radiotherapy and deep learning communities, which was motivated by a unique collaboration between these two domains to increase enthusiastic radiotherapy applications.

Using the CNN deep learning technique, Wang Mengqiao et al. [22] proposed architecture for segmenting brain tumours. This method incorporates both global and local aspects as structure, which could be significant in the development of brain tumour segmentation in brain MRI images. Zeynettin Akkus et al. [1] deep learning architectures for anatomical brain lesions and brain structure segmentation were examined and contrasted in terms of speed, implementation and advantages.

System Design

In general, deep learning algorithms can pass data through several neural network layers, each of which transmits a compressed data representation to the next layer of the neural network approach. Deep learning algorithms will examine the MRI picture more closely as it passes through each NN layer. Initial layers can learn to recognise low-level aspects such as edges, while following layers have combined the properties of previous layers to create a more holistic depiction. Convolutional neural networks, deep auto-encoders and deep belief networks are examples of common deep learning approaches. These methods are described in detail and demonstrated in Fig. 3.

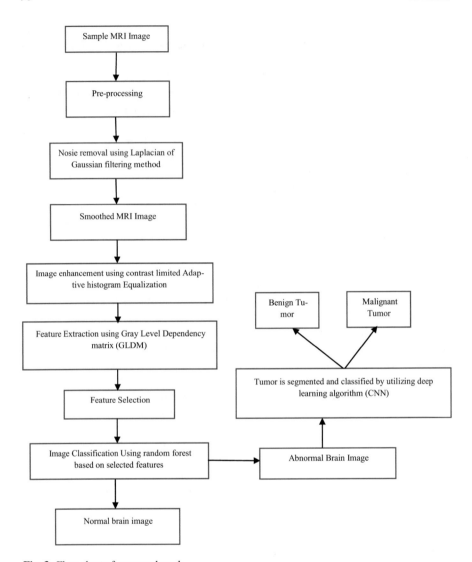

Fig. 3 Flow chart of proposed work

Convolutional Neural Network

CNNs are created through stimulating design of a visual system, and they are most wealthy literature approach for multilayer network training structures. This strategy combines spatial linkages with a smaller number of factors to investigate in order to increase training performance. CNN can be acted as a multilayer sensor neural network, in which every n-plane is described by a plurality of individual neurons and each layer contains plurality of two-dimensional plane. In handwritten character detection, the CNN has been used [19].

In most cases, CNN may be used to identify dislocation in two-dimensional images, as well as other types of deformation invariance and scaling. This strategy, which examines the training data without reservation, prevents the explicit feature sampling type. This can result in a CNN that is notably different from other neural network-based classifiers, and the network is a separate study, and it can be a big advantage of the convolutional neural network over neurons that are connected to each other. A convolutional neural network features a hierarchical local connection structure and a relatively tiny input for each neuron, which can help biological neural network's CNNs become more definite. It offers particular benefits in image processing and picture segmentation, with good feature extraction outcomes. This method will be utilised to handle medical photographs directly based on the classification process, and it will also deal with grey level images.

DBN is a DAG that can have any number of variables. The subsequent layer has linked a top-down directly from the previous layer, the bottom unit condition may be seen as an input data vector, and therefore this model has been defined as a bias probability technique generation since the CNN and DAE layers lack symmetry. In order to build a DBN from the bottom-up, the DBN unit joins different restricted Boltzmann machines (RBM).

The greedy unsupervised learning technique works by splitting a DBN network into numerous layers and doing unsupervised learning on each layer. Finally, the complete network is fine-tuned using the supervised learning method. The training process can map visible vector values to hidden units, which then reconstruct picture components in the hidden layer unit. Finally, the novel hidden unit is created by mapping the hidden unit to the new image component. If the random forest classifier classified the MRI image as abnormal, then there's the technology of deep learning. With a lower error rate and less time, CNN might be utilised to efficiently separate tumour cells from a brain MRI picture based on kernels. In this approach, CNN is combined with a random forest classifier. A CNN can be used to segment the tumour, and a random forest classifier can be used to classify it as benign or malignant. A CNN is a multilayer neural network with a general architecture. The popular RBF kernel is currently being used as a smart basic kernel choice. This chapter introduces spectrum mixing to the fundamental kernel in order to boost the tumour segmentation procedure's versatility.

When image analysis is simple to grasp and segment, effective tumour identification can be achieved. As a result of the difficult tumour segmentation process in MRI images, several algorithms and methods for manual, semiautomatic and fully automated tumour segmentation have been developed. Many of them were only performed on limited datasets. As a result, deep learning-based approaches and algorithms are now being used to improve tumour segmentation and tumour recognition in the brain. Deep convolutional neural networks have already been used to tackle tumour segmentation difficulties, and this methodology has produced significant performance improvements over earlier algorithms or methodologies. This chapter demonstrates an automated system kernel-based CNN with RF M for brain tumour segmentation with minimal time complexity, high accuracy and low error rate.

Result and Discussion

This section discusses the proposed hybrid for brain tumour segmentation utilising CNN with random forest, which efficiently deals with MRI brain image datasets (https://www.kaggle.com/datasets/sartajbhuvaji/brain-tumor-classification-mri) in the tool of matlab2013a and classed outcomes. The image matrix is created after extracting the pixel intensities from the test MR brain image and assigning a window with a certain number of rows and columns. This pixel's value is compared to the value of the neighbouring pixel, and if the deviation is large, the mean value of the pixels is calculated, or a Gaussian value is determined. Throughout the image, the window is also moved. As a result, as illustrated in Fig. 4, the filtered output is free of image acquisition noise and artefacts.

Adoptive histogram removes the skull from the test image with two separate thresholds that attempt to detect the strong and weak edges, respectively, as well as

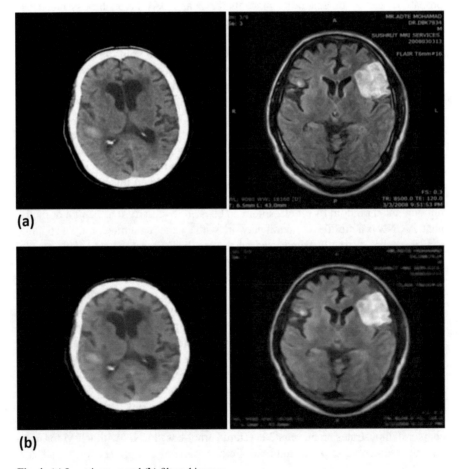

Fig. 4 (a) Input images and (b) filtered images

noise removal using the Laplacian filtering technique stated earlier. Figs. 5 and 6 demonstrate the extraction of the skull's output image.

The filtered image is now transformed to its binary counterpart, and each pixel in the image is labelled. The test image after deleting all the unnecessary pixels in the edges is shown in Fig. 7 and Table 1. The skull is eliminated from the given input image using morphological processes, which compare the intensities of each pixel with the intensities of the surrounding pixels. Fig. 8 shows the MR test image after the skull has been removed.

Table 1 MRI brain image segmentation: normal and abnormal image result

	Description	Normal image	Abnormal image
Figure 5	Adoptive histogram process of normal image and abnormal images		
Figure 6	Pixels of zero value adaptive histogram of normal image and abnormal images		
Figure 7	Removal of unnecessary pixels from normal image and abnormal images		
Figure 8	MRI brain image after skull elimination of normal image and abnormal images		

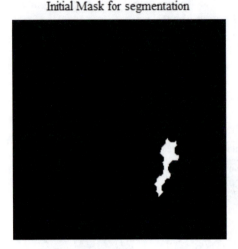
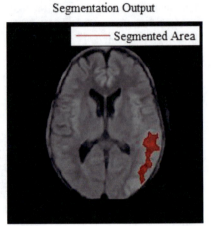

Fig. 9 Segmented output of MR brain image with astrocytoma

As a result, a proper segmentation algorithm is necessary to solve the constraints of combinational segmentation. The combinational segmentation methodology based on CNN with random forest method and other segmentation techniques are limited by the limits of the textural pixel connection-based technology. Figure 9 depicts an example of MR image segmentation.

Sensitivity, specificity and accuracy are the metrics used to evaluate the performance. This approach was put to the test using a variety of datasets from various data bases. The results are given in Table 2 and Fig. 10, respectively.

This section shows that proposed CNN with random forest method can be applied to MRI brain image datasets and compared to different existing methods: SVM [32], decision tree and random forest. Typically, only below 90% conventional accuracy could be achieved which even proposed system exceeded in 95.4% of the cases.

This shows that deep learning approach has better potential in CVD diagnosis. Comparatively, other conventional methods proposed systems that have more efficiency and time consumption for predicting the final result with better classification result.

Conclusion

When compared to prior studies, the provided CNN with random forest algorithm produces better results. The purpose of MRI image segmentation is to find questionable spots in an MRI image. It's a lengthy procedure. The detection of suspicious areas must be done with greater precision. A CNN with a random forest algorithm is used to detect brain cancers by identifying questionable spots in an MRI brain

Table 2 Performance analysis of proposed and existing system

Parameters	Proposed method	SVM	Decision tree	Random forest
Sensitivity	94.6	84	81.55	84.65
Specificity	95.8	86.4	79.84	88
Accuracy	95.4	83.22	83.14	84.22

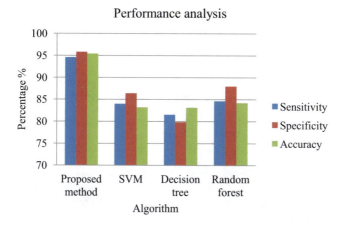

Fig. 10 Performance analysis of proposed and existing system

image. These methods are then integrated with a deep learning methodology to adaptively calculate the threshold value. The results of the experiments showed that the proposed strategies outperformed standard algorithms and delivered very accurate segmentation results. In the future, the research could be expanded to address issues with detecting various types of tumours and predicting the development direction in cases of grade I and II tumours, allowing for simple cell elimination in the early stages.

References

1. Z. Akkus, A. Galimzianova, A. Hoogi, D.L. Rubin, B.J. Erickson, Deep learning for brain MRI segmentation: State of the art and future directions. J. Digit. Imaging **30**(4), 449–459 (2017)
2. M. Amian, M. Soltaninejad, Multi-resolution 3D CNN for MRI brain tumor segmentation and survival prediction, in *International MICCAI Brainlesion workshop*, (Springer, Cham, 2019, October), pp. 221–230
3. J. Amin, M. Sharif, M. Yasmin, S.L. Fernandes, A distinctive approach in brain tumor detection and classification using MRI. Pattern Recogn. Lett. **139**, 118–127 (2020)
4. S. Bauer, R. Wiest, L.P. Nolte, M. Reyes, A survey of MRI-based medical image analysis for brain tumor studies. Phys. Med. Biol. **58**(13), R97 (2013)
5. J.J. Corso, E. Sharon, S. Dube, S. El-Saden, U. Sinha, A. Yuille, Efficient multilevel brain tumor segmentation with integrated bayesian model classification. IEEE Trans. Med. Imaging **27**(5), 629–640 (2008)

6. A. Demirhan, M. Törü, I. Güler, Segmentation of tumor and edema along with healthy tissues of brain using wavelets and neural networks. IEEE J. Biomed. Health Inform. **19**(4), 1451–1458 (2014)
7. D. Divyamary, S. Gopika, S. Pradeeba, M. Bhuvaneswari, Brain tumor detection from MRI images using naive classifier, in *2020 6th international conference on advanced computing and communication systems (ICACCS)*, (IEEE, 2020, March), pp. 620–622
8. M.T. El-Melegy, H.M. Mokhtar, Tumor segmentation in brain MRI using a fuzzy approach with class center priors. EURASIP J. Imag. Video Process. **2014**(1), 1–14 (2014)
9. F. Friedrich, J. Hörner-Rieber, C.K. Renkamp, S. Klüter, P. Bachert, M.E. Ladd, B.R. Knowles, Stability of conventional and machine learning-based tumor auto-segmentation techniques using undersampled dynamic radial bSSFP acquisitions on a 0.35 T hybrid MR-linac system. Med. Phys. **48**(2), 587–596 (2021)
10. N.N. Gopal, M. Karnan, Diagnose brain tumor through MRI using image processing clustering algorithms such as fuzzy C means along with intelligent optimization techniques, in *2010 IEEE international conference on computational intelligence and computing research*, (IEEE, 2010, December), pp. 1–4
11. N. Gordillo, E. Montseny, P. Sobrevilla, State of the art survey on MRI brain tumor segmentation. Magn. Reson. Imaging **31**(8), 1426–1438 (2013)
12. A. Harshavardhan, S. Babu, T. Venugopal, An improved brain tumor segmentation method from MRI brain images, in *2017 2nd international conference on emerging computation and information technologies (ICECIT)*, (IEEE, 2017, December), pp. 1–7
13. M. Huang, W. Yang, Y. Wu, J. Jiang, W. Chen, Q. Feng, Brain tumor segmentation based on local independent projection-based classification. IEEE Trans. Biomed. Eng. **61**(10), 2633–2645 (2014)
14. S. Iqbal, M.U. Ghani, T. Saba, A. Rehman, Brain tumor segmentation in multi-spectral MRI using convolutional neural networks (CNN). Microsc. Res. Tech. **81**(4), 419–427 (2018)
15. A. Islam, S.M. Reza, K.M. Iftekharuddin, Multifractal texture estimation for detection and segmentation of brain tumors. IEEE Trans. Biomed. Eng. **60**(11), 3204–3215 (2013)
16. G. Jothi, Hybrid tolerance rough set–firefly based supervised feature selection for MRI brain tumor image classification. Appl. Soft Comput. **46**, 639–651 (2016)
17. S. Kalimuthu, Sentiment analysis on social Media for Emotional Prediction during COVID-19 pandemic using efficient machine learning approach. Comput. Intell. Healthcare Inform. **215** (2021)
18. S. Kalimuthu, F. Naït-Abdesselam, B. Jaishankar, Multimedia data protection using hybridized crystal payload algorithm with chicken swarm optimization, in *Multidisciplinary approach to modern digital steganography*, (IGI Global, 2021), pp. 235–257
19. P.Y. Kao, S. Shailja, J. Jiang, A. Zhang, A. Khan, J.W. Chen, B.S. Manjunath, Improving patch-based convolutional neural networks for MRI brain tumor segmentation by leveraging location information. Front. Neurosci. **13**, 1449 (2020)
20. M. Kong, S.E. Hong, Tumor regression patterns based on follow-up duration in patients with head and neck squamous cell carcinoma treated with radiotherapy or chemoradiotherapy. Clin. Exp. Otorhinolaryngol. **8**(4), 416 (2015)
21. G.P. Mazzara, R.P. Velthuizen, J.L. Pearlman, H.M. Greenberg, H. Wagner, Brain tumor target volume determination for radiation treatment planning through automated MRI segmentation. Int. J. Radiat. Oncol. Biol. Phys. **59**(1), 300–312 (2004)
22. W. Mengqiao, Y. Jie, C. Yilei, W. Hao, The multimodal brain tumor image segmentation based on convolutional neural networks, in *2017 2nd IEEE international conference on computational intelligence and applications (ICCIA)*, (IEEE, 2017, September), pp. 336–339
23. P. Meyer, V. Noblet, C. Mazzara, A. Lallement, Survey on deep learning for radiotherapy. Comput. Biol. Med. **98**, 126–146 (2018)
24. H. Mohsen, E.S.A. El-Dahshan, E.S.M. El-Horbaty, A.B.M. Salem, Classification using deep learning neural networks for brain tumors. Future Comput. Inform. J. **3**(1), 68–71 (2018)

25. A. Myronenko, 3D MRI brain tumor segmentation using autoencoder regularization, in *International MICCAI Brainlesion workshop*, (Springer, Cham, 2018, September), pp. 311–320
26. S. Pereira, A. Pinto, V. Alves, C.A. Silva, Brain tumor segmentation using convolutional neural networks in MRI images. IEEE Trans. Med. Imaging **35**(5), 1240–1251 (2016)
27. S. Pereira, R. Meier, V. Alves, M. Reyes, C.A. Silva, Automatic brain tumor grading from MRI data using convolutional neural networks and quality assessment, in *Understanding and Interpreting Machine Learning in Medical Image Computing Applications*, (Springer, Cham, 2018), pp. 106–114
28. S. Roy, S.K. Bandyopadhyay, Detection and quantification of brain tumor from MRI of brain and it's symmetric analysis. Int. J. Inform. Commun. Technol. Res. **2**(6) (2012)
29. N.V. Shree, T.N.R. Kumar, Identification and classification of brain tumor MRI images with feature extraction using DWT and probabilistic neural network. Brain Inform **5**(1), 23–30 (2018)
30. K. Sivanantham, Deep Learning-Based Convolutional Neural Network with Cuckoo Search Optimization for MRI Brain Tumour Segmentation, in *Computational Intelligence Techniques for Green Smart Cities*, (Springer, Cham, 2022), pp. 149–168
31. K. Sivanantham, I. Kalaiarasi, B. Leena, Brain tumor classification using hybrid artificial neural network with chicken swarm optimization algorithm in digital image processing application, in *Advance concepts of image processing and pattern recognition*, (Springer, Singapore, 2022), pp. 91–108
32. S.R. Telrandhe, A. Pimpalkar, A. Kendhe, Detection of brain tumor from MRI images by using segmentation & SVM, in *2016 world conference on futuristic trends in research and innovation for social welfare (startup conclave)*, (IEEE, 2016, February), pp. 1–6
33. G. Wang, W. Li, M.A. Zuluaga, R. Pratt, P.A. Patel, M. Aertsen, et al., Interactive medical image segmentation using deep learning with image-specific fine tuning. IEEE Trans. Med. Imaging **37**(7), 1562–1573 (2018)

Expert Systems for Improving the Effectiveness of Remote Health Monitoring in COVID-19 Pandemic: A Critical Review

S. Umamaheswari, S. Arun Kumar, and S. Sasikala

Introduction

Viruses that cause diseases like influenza, pneumonic plagues, and COVID-19 transfer the infection from person to person who are in close contact. Both public and health professionals are affected majorly due to this contagious disease. For the past 2 years, COVID-19 (SARS-CoV-2) infectious lung disease has been a major problem all over the world. The economic and social disruption caused by this pandemic puts nearly half of the world's 3.3 billion workforce at risk of losing their jobs. Many of us are still suffering from this deadly disease. The above factors necessitate to investigate the various methods and technologies available to combat this disease.

Practicing some steps such as vaccination, wearing face mask, washing hands frequently, avoiding close contact with infected people, avoiding unwanted travel, following guidelines given by government, and increasing immune system by eating healthy food are certain protection methods to get away from COVID-19.

Another best method in public health scenario is making use of the technological applications and initiatives listed in Fig. 1.

The lockdown makes it more difficult for infected patients to reach the hospital faster, and the day-to-day problems faced by healthcare professionals while attending COVID patients become more severe. Further, during this pandemic, medical personnel experienced emotional stress, depression, insomnia, and respiratory illness.

To address all the above issues, remote treatment added value to the existing medical infrastructure by reducing the infection rate, cost, and treatment time.

S. Umamaheswari (✉) · S. Arun Kumar · S. Sasikala
Department of ECE, Kumaraguru College of Technology, Coimbatore, India
e-mail: umamaheswari.s.ece@kct.ac.in; arunkumar.s.ece@kct.ac.in; sasikala.s.ece@kct.ac.in

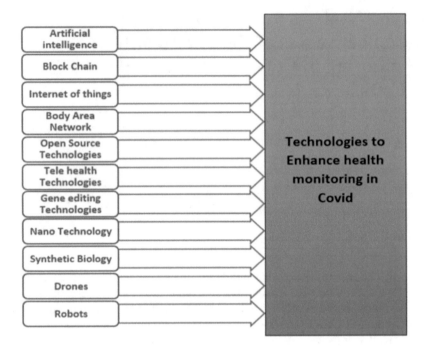

Fig. 1 Different technologies in public health emergencies

Technological evolution from wired to wireless devices, reduction in size, and development of wearable devices and sensors has led to the rapid use of remote health monitoring systems.

Remote health monitoring market of pandemic disease can be analyzed by splitting the examining area into disease, location of the patient, and instrument based. Triggering forces of the market are pandemic diseases and changes in the living style, and due to comfort treatment at homes, most instruments in remote monitoring are handy with only cost as a controlling factor. A lot of studies and research shows that patient monitoring request is in increasing mode from 2017 to 2025 and further hike in the market is possible due to the present consequence of COVID-19 variant, black fungus, Zika, etc. According to the WHO report, many people are infected by the current COVID-19 variant, and thus there is a large market for respiratory disease in the global market from 2020 to 2025.

Since India is the second largest overpopulated country, mortality rate is also higher. It is observed from various studies that remote monitoring management in India will be elevated more in the near future as compared to other countries.

The above influencing factors motivated us to focus toward reviewing the effectiveness of remote health monitoring in the pandemic under telehealth technologies.

Rapid growth in technologies such as IoMT Internet of Medical Things), Artificial Intelligence (AI) techniques, Wireless Body Area Networks (WBAN), sensor technologies, and medical robotics have paved way for the effective use of remote health monitoring for COVID-19 in the pandemic.

Internet of Things

Information from a patient can be transmitted using communication devices such as Zigbee, Bluetooth, ultrawideband, and short-range wireless communication. Various modules could be used to analyze blood pressure, heartbeat, body temperature, etc. IoT-based systems for remote monitoring improve the accuracy. Communication overhead and energy consumption are majorly less due to the Internet of medical things. Throughput, packet loss rate, and end-to-end delay are comparatively better than existing technology in remote health monitoring.

Artificial Intelligence (AI) and Robotics

Deep learning and image/signal processing techniques have been used along with smartphones to analyze vital parameters such as heart rate, cough, etc. When traditional measurement methods are compared to AI-based measurement methods, it is observed that most of the results in AI techniques are better with the least cost setup.

Medical robotics have been widely used in electronic health record creation and maintenance, mass production of vaccines and drugs, surgery, and telemonitoring.

Wireless Body Area Networks

Even if COVID patients have recovered from the disease, people with mild COVID symptoms and some individuals must be monitored on a regular basis. By integrating some features with their mobile phones, doctors can easily monitor patients from a distance, allowing infected people to receive treatment in complete comfort. To process the patient data, sensors, controllers, gateways, mobile application platforms, and web application platforms will be used on both sides.

The use of a coronavirus body area network, wearable biosensors, and machine learning techniques resulted in a high degree of accuracy in diagnosing COVID in earlier conditions.

The significant contributions of this chapter include:

- Analysis of need of remote health monitoring in COVID-19 pandemic.
- Analysis of the impact of use of remote health monitoring in improving the treatment of COVID-affected people.

- A review on the use expert systems such as Wireless BAN (Body Area Network), IoT (Internet of Things), Artificial Intelligence (AI), and robotics to improve the effectiveness of remote health monitoring in a pandemic like COVID.

COVID-19 Pandemic

The severe acute respiratory Syndrome coronavirus 2 (SARS-CoV-2) virus had a significant social impact. The virus-caused disease (COVID-19) has spread throughout the world, disrupting people's daily lives. Several studies indicate that COVID-19 is formed during experimentation in a research laboratory, and it is not a variation of an existing virus [1].

Being feverish, coughing, and difficulty in breathing are the most known reported symptoms. Coronavirus infection mostly affects the lungs, but the extensive distribution of enzyme receptors in organs can impact the cardiovascular, gastrointestinal, renal, liver, central nervous system, and eyes, all of which must be closely watched.

Appropriate treatment at early stage is required to save the lives of people infected with COVID-19 virus. This chapter proposed expert system-based solutions to improve the effectiveness of COVID-19 in remote health monitoring.

Remote Health Monitoring System

Remote health monitoring will be the best option for the elderly, the disabled, those with early symptoms of COVID, people in quarantine, and patients whose homes are away from hospitals, to avoid the unnecessary spread of viruses and provide continuous support. We all know that many physicians lost their lives during different COVID waves. This technology will be safe for health professionals also.

Advantages of Remote Health Monitoring System for COVID-19

- Minimizing frequent visits to hospitals.
- Reducing travel time to the hospital.
- Allowing educational videos to be distributed and updated instantaneously.
- Patient-reported outcomes are derived from survey questions that have been carefully constructed.
- Data input by the user, such as blood pressure or temperature, is incorporated into the workflow through cloud technology.

- The monitoring platform is controlled from a central location and is updated in real time to reflect new disease information or updated symptom questionnaires.
- Feasibility of obtaining exact details via live video.
- Features such as secure bidirectional conversation are included.
- A patient can ask for a follow-up call or, in other words, call back for assistance.

While treating patients infected with COVID-19 viral disease, the sensor technology provides one of the most efficient and secure remote treatment options without exposing healthcare workers or infected patients to becoming easy targets or infected with any type of virus. This sensor records the environment's physical condition as well as the COVID-19 patient's health parameters such as are temperature, respiratory problem, and oxygen saturation and heartbeat through wearable sensors.

Vital parameters [2] are very important for health officials in remote to monitor COVID patients. Integration of hardware and software modules in remote health monitoring task will provide better results. Modules used in hardware section are depicted in Fig. 2.

The Pan-Tompkins algorithm (PTA) for detecting QRS peak detection in ECG signal and support vector machine for abnormality classification in the software module play an important role in remote monitoring technology. PTA will be used to process the electrocardiographic signals. Noise elimination and smoothing will be done by PTA algorithm. Support vector machines are used to differentiate between non-QRS waves and QRS waves from ECG signals.

Table 1 summarizes the more effective hardware and software modules for remote monitoring technology.

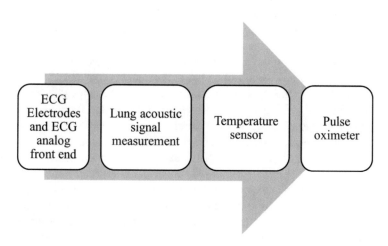

Fig. 2 Important modules in hardware section

Table 1 Summary of hardware and software in remote health

Hardware and software used in remote health	More effective	Less effective
Air-coupled sensors	✓	
Contact sensors		✓
Condenser microphone	✓	
Piezo-microphone		✓
Dynamic microphone		✓
Infrared-based temperature sensor – Contact		✓
Infrared-based temperature sensor – Noncontact	✓	
PTA	✓	
SVM classifier	✓	

Wireless Body Area Network for Remote Monitoring of SARS-CoV-2

Wireless body area networks consist of sensors that are placed either near or in the human body. It consists of three sections, viz., sensor section, data collection section, and user section. It can be used for both medical and nonmedical applications. For infectious diseases like COVID-19, WBAN will be very supportive. This WBAN will be helpful to alert soldiers in nonmedical applications.

In [3], a WBAN architecture is proposed to combat COVID-19 virus. First, the user must register, which can be done in the same way as regular registration in a web portal/mobile application. After successfully enrolling, the user must fill out all the health-related conditions, stored in the cloud. The data collected from sensors is subjected to machine learning algorithm, to determine if the person is suffering from a common cold or the infectious disease COVID-19. Once a person's COVID-positive status is confirmed, sensors are placed on their bodies to monitor their health. The body state will be measured using Arduino microcontroller and My Signal Hardware chip portion, and the obtained data will be sent to a remote server of a physician for therapy using LoRa. The architecture is shown in Fig. 3.

Algorithms such as the logistic regression algorithm, the naive Bayes algorithm, the random forest algorithm, the support vector machine algorithm, and the multilayer perceptron algorithm are all used for classification. For these five classifiers, precision, recall, error rate, accuracy, and Brier score are evaluated. Random forest (RF) and multilayer perceptron (MLP) algorithms outperformed over other algorithms.

In [4], quarantine management and remote monitoring of infected patient is experimented. Sensors such as the electrocardiogram (ECG), oxygen measuring medical device (SpO2), body temperature, respiration sensor, accelerometer, and gyroscope are used to extract the patient's physiological data. Wi-Fi is used for data transmission from the body of the patient to Raspberry Pi microcontroller. Based on the disease severity, boundary limits can also be fixed for the patient. Location of the patient is also checked here to manage quarantine. If the patient exceeds the

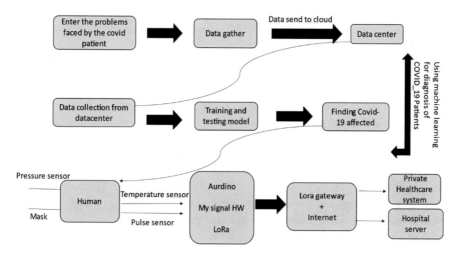

Fig. 3 Intelligent wireless network with sensors integrated with artificial intelligence technique and LoRa gateway

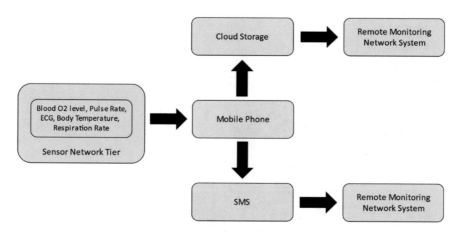

Fig. 4 A Distributed wireless body area network

coverage area, an alarm will be sent to both patient and health professional. The real-time data obtained from body sensors is fed as input to machine learning algorithm for disease identification and further treatment. The system architecture of [4] is depicted in Fig. 4.

Remote monitoring will be the best treatment for COVID-19 in all aspects. Unnecessary spreading will be greatly avoided. For patients who have been sick for a long time, for elderly people, and for emergency situations, this method will be of good choice. Sensor model, prediction model, and remote monitoring model in WBAN are used for remote COVID monitoring [5].

Workflow of WBAN Architecture

The proposed distributed wireless body area network [5] consists of four sections: Wireless medical sensor, wireless sink mode, Android application, and remote monitoring center. All four modules work together to complete the task of remote monitoring and diagnosis. The functions of each module are clearly discussed below. The workflow is illustrated in Fig. 5.

Wireless Medical Sensors

During initialization, the serial timer is fired, and the serial module is opened. The byte is read and will be computed to write a buffer. This buffer will be directed to wireless timer. There, the buffer is read. If the data is present in the buffer, it will be sent to wireless sink mode using wireless transmission.

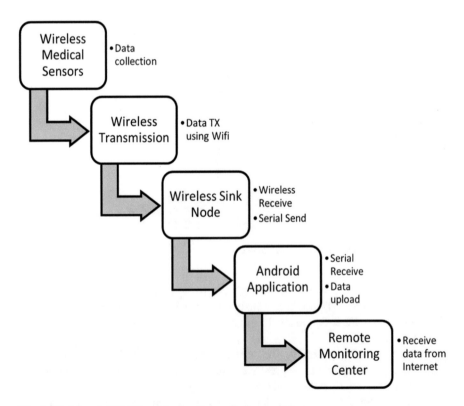

Fig. 5 Workflow in WBAN architecture for medical supervision

Wireless Sink Mode

The data from the buffer will be received and it will be sent to the Android application.

Android Application

The data from the previous module will be received serially. The data received is displayed in a Liquid Crystal Display (LCD) screen. Then, the data is checked based on the byte it encloses. If the data is found dangerous, a warning is displayed in the LCD screen. If the data is safe, it is stored and uploaded to remote monitoring center.

Remote Monitoring Center

Upon initializing the module, a new thread is created and a socket is produced. Using the socket produced, the data from the Android application is received. The socket is then closed to avoid overlapping or contamination of any other data. Once the socket is closed, the data will be displayed on the screen, and the data is successfully stored in a cloud-based storage platform.

Security Constraints in Wireless Body Area Network

Security of medical data is a concern in WBAN. In a remote monitoring setup, security is to be maintained to avoid intruders altering the data collected from sensors. Mainly attackers will affect the WBAN at three levels [6].

- Data collection level – Data is collected from various sensors which are placed on different parts of the body.
- Transmission level – Data is transmitted from patient to healthcare professional.
- Storage level – Data is stored for further treatment.

Using intrusion detection systems in conjunction with machine learning algorithms, attacks can be avoided [7]. Prediction of attack will also be made instantly by identifying the attacks based on the attribute information collected from the body area network [8]. Stronger routing algorithms and shortest path discovery methods provide correct results, which make diagnosis and treatment perfect for a patient in remote [9, 10]. Implementation of cluster and key generation architectures also provides better results [11, 12]. Even though there are many intrusion detection and security algorithms for telemedicine technology, there are also many threatening factors. In designing a remote technology, high security is needed to avoid failure of the system and to give better treatment for remote patient.

IoT in COVID-19 Remote Health Monitoring

Internet of Things (IoT) is an interconnection of devices, objects, and people provided with unique identifiers. IoT systems possess inherent ability to transfer data over a network without human intervention. The thing in IoT refers to a person with an implant, animal with a transponder, automobile with a sensor, or a thing (natural/man-made) which can transfer data over a network when assigned to an Internet Protocol (IP) address.

IoT in conjunction with Artificial Intelligence (AI) makes more easier, dynamic, and meaningful decisions.

Internet of Medical Things (IoMT) refers to interconnection of medical devices, hardware infrastructure, and software in a healthcare scenario. IoMT helps in remote devices to communicate over the Internet for transferring medical data. Thus, IoMT or IoT in healthcare enables building of efficient remote health monitoring systems in COVID-19 pandemic. The IoMT architecture is shown in Fig. 6.

Many works in literature [13–23] focused on using remote health monitoring systems using IoT for contactless treatment and telemonitoring.

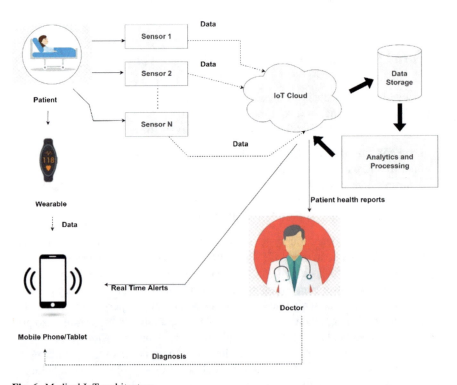

Fig. 6 Medical IoT architecture

IoMT is used in [13] to remote monitor the vitals and for rapid diagnosis, contact tracking, screening, reducing the workload of healthcare professionals, and disease containment and control. The use cases are depicted in Fig. 7.

Remote Monitoring of Vitals

Blood pressure, glucose, heart rate, pulse rate, and oxygen saturation are the vital parameters collected from wearable IoT sensors placed in the patients. The data collected from the sensors can be connected to the Internet, enabling the clinicians, healthcare workers, and caregivers to remote monitor the COVID-19 patients. This could prevent infection and save time.

Rapid Diagnosis

IoT enables sharing of rapid diagnosis results of COVID-19 obtained from patients with travel history to the officials to take possible actions. Persons with travel history can be connected through network applications to afford services for fast diagnosis.

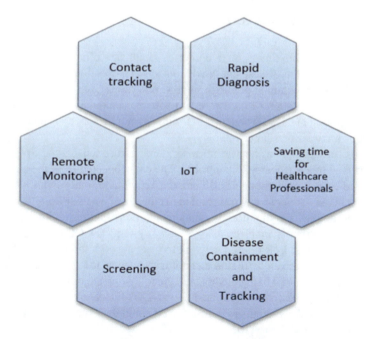

Fig. 7 Use cases of IoT-enabled healthcare in COVID-19 pandemic

Contact Tracking

Health authorities can track positive cases by accessing the location history of patients stored in a database. Location- and zone-wise case details can be obtained if the healthcare units are connected via IoT.

Screening

Facial recognition data collected through thermal imaging sensors at various entry points in a city can be used to effectively screen the patients if data is shared via a common network. Screening can reduce the movement of confirmed positive cases.

Reducing the Workload of Healthcare Professionals

Remote health monitoring using fusion of AI and IoT and telemedicine can reduce the workload of healthcare professionals.

Disease Containment and Tracking

Use of IoT can enable timely intervention by healthcare officials and corporation officials to contain the disease and track contacts. The positive cases in proximity can be notified to a common public through various apps (Aarogya Setu in India).

In [14], a combination of hardware and software modules is used to automate health monitoring in COVID patients. IoT module, mobile app, and cloud server are the various modules used in the study.

Various sensors such as heartbeat sensor, temperature sensor, and SpO2 sensor are connected to a Raspberry Pi controller. The data collected from the sensors are transmitted to a mobile phone via Bluetooth. Activities of daily living (ADL) are monitored in mobile phone and transmitted to cloud over a network connection. The mobile app notifies the monitoring status to the user. Further, the collected data from the cloud server is analyzed using a fuzzy system. The COVID safe platform is supplemented with LoRa-based network to meet network failure in rural areas.

Telemedicine is driven by digital technologies such as IoT, AI, block chain, and big data. IoT can be used in telemedicine in the following areas to contain the infection in COVID times: rural healthcare, post-COVID care, remote monitoring, chronic disease management, system-initiated reminders for follow-ups, elderly care, and mobile healthcare [15].

A robust IoT platform with layered architecture is proposed in [16] for effectively combating the spread and containment of COVID-19 pandemic. Layered architecture includes four different layers such as perception layer, network layer, fog layer, and cloud layer as shown in Fig. 8.

Perception layer collects data from the sensors placed in the patient, hospital/clinic, and environment.

In network layer, the sensed data is transmitted to the fog node using Wi-Fi, or a network connection (4G/5G).

Fog layer uses higher-end computing resources to reduce the latency in real-time analysis. In fog layer, computations related to non-pharmaceutical interventions (NPIs) for effective COVID tracking, monitoring, and isolation can be implemented.

Cloud layer is used to compute complex prediction use cases such as COVID forecasting and identifying virus mutation changes with powerful resources.

Social distancing is one of the effective means to control COVID. An end-to-end IoT architecture depicted in [17] is presented in Fig. 9. Data acquisition setup includes body sensors and environmental sensors. Wi-Fi and GPS are used for patient localization in indoor and outdoor environment, respectively. Communication module is used to transmit data from the acquisition unit to controller in the handheld mobile unit. Mobile unit can be used for contact tracking through a Bluetooth module and alert creation based on the sensor data. IoT gateway is used to forward the data to the cloud server. Cloud platform performs essential services based on the desired use case.

In developing countries, shortage of healthcare professionals and limited medical infrastructure to cater large population necessitate the need of expert systems in COVID-19 pandemic [18]. Three different approaches are proposed for COVID screening.

The first approach focuses on building COVID-19 screening device using low-cost wearable sensors to measure heart rate, SpO2, and temperature. The acquired data is processed by an Arduino microcontroller and transmitted to Ubidots cloud using Wi-Fi. Data visualization can be done from cloud data for further actions and follow-ups by the clinician/caretaker.

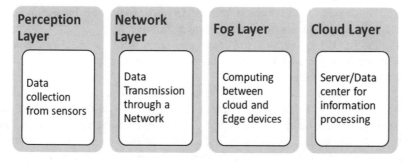

Fig. 8 Layered architecture in IoT-enabled healthcare in COVID-19 pandemic

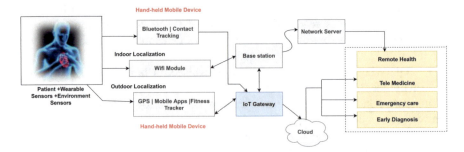

Fig. 9 IoT architecture for building expert systems. Expert systems in COVID-19 pandemic

Table 2 Digital technology for IoT-enabled health care in COVID

S. no	Digital technology	Usage
1.	Big data	Used to store COVID data in digital form. Data stored can be used to make quick decisions. Electronic health records can be maintained.
2.	Cloud	Data description using internet. On-demand data storage for remote diagnosis.
3.	Sensor technology	Data acquisition. Health monitoring.
4.	Actuators	Parameter control. Maintains accuracy.
5.	Artificial intelligence	Detection and classification. Prediction. Data visualization.
6.	Software	Improves patient care. Disease diagnosis. Medical history.
7.	Virtual/augmented reality	Digital imagery/audio information. Improves patient safety and service quality.

In the second approach, rule-based methodology based on the collected data is proposed. A rule base is created based on the expert's opinion and clinical guidelines. Symptoms are matched with the data in rule base to grade the severity of COVID-19 patients. Data collected from sensors is transmitted using a cloud infrastructure for data visualization and real-time tracking.

Authors in [19] review the application use cases of IoT-enabled healthcare in COVID pandemic. Further the use of various digital technologies for IoMT during COVID is listed in Table 2.

In [20], a Health 4.0 framework is formulated to improve the treatment and prevention of COVID-19 disease. To enhance the diagnosis, a four-stage IoT pipeline is proposed. Data collection from wearable, data transmission over a network, data processing using feature engineering, and assisted decision-making using AI are the steps involved in the pipeline. The framework is illustrated in Fig. 10. In using medical robotics in assisted surgery, emergency ambulatory care is also analyzed.

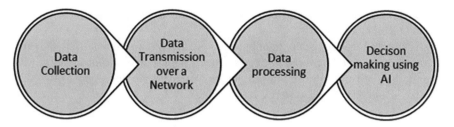

Fig. 10 Health 4.0 framework for building expert systems in COVID-19 pandemic

Table 3 Technologies used in Health 4.0 framework

S. no	Actors	Technology	Usage
1.	Caretaker	Smartphones	Remote monitoring
2.	Hospital	Software	Data entry and tracking
3.	Patient	Sensors and smart implants	Data collection
4.	Robot	AI and computer vision	Surgery
5.	Cloud	Higher-end computing resources	Data storage

The technologies used in IoT architecture at various actors, in a Health 4.0 framework, are listed in Table 3.

In [21], IoT and early warning system are used to strengthen the remote health monitoring of COVID-19 patients. In addition, the challenges associated with remote monitoring are analyzed and listed as follows:

- Precise identification of health deterioration and risk conditions.
- Patient-specific analysis based on the health condition and previous medical history.
- Customizing assessment methods and devices in a wireless infrastructure.
- Scalability – To support concurrent monitoring of COVID patients, as disease spreading is quick.
- Component failure in IoT framework.
- Reliability of network infrastructure in rural areas.
- Accuracy of prediction and issuing early warning signs.
- Data confidentiality while sharing data from sensors to cloud.
- Integrating the sensor data to legacy systems available in hospitals.
- Usage of low-cost IoT framework that suffers from speed, memory, and processing issues.
- Power and energy requirement of sensors and controllers used.

A mobile-based framework COVIDApp in [22] is used for early detection and rapid tracking of cases in COVID-19 pandemic. Further, remote monitoring using mobile application is also proposed for remote deployment of protocols. The details of the patients are collected through a questionnaire. Based on the options given in the questionnaire, a rule-based approach is used to grade the presence or absence of

COVID based on collected symptoms. Further follow-ups and treatment are suggested based on the severity.

A mobile-based m-health monitoring system used for monitoring the vital parameters in elderly people is experimented in [23]. Video consultations, vital monitoring, self-tracking, and informing the caregivers are the services offered by mobile health monitoring systems.

Robotics and AI Technologies in COVID-19 Pandemic

Robotics and AI were vastly used for the betterment of the situations during COVID-19 pandemic in various use cases as shown in Fig. 11. A detailed literature in [24] analyzes the impact and use of robotics and AI in COVID-19 pandemic in a remote monitoring scenario. An overview of Robotics and AI technologies presented in [24] is discussed in the following section.

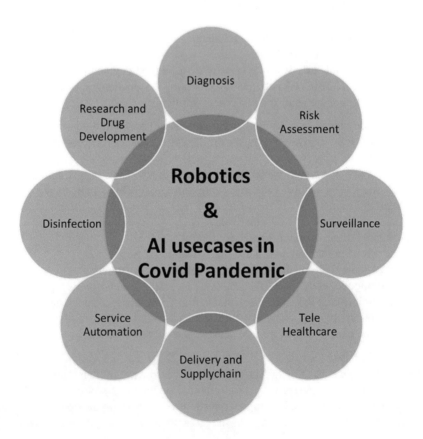

Fig. 11 Robotics and AI use cases in COVID pandemic

In diagnosis, rapid testing was extremely useful in diagnosing the infection. Though it is very much essential to identify the infected people, it was the most challenging task during the pandemic as the direct contact with the affected people increases the chance of getting viral infection and also lack of medical resources. To overcome the difficulties faced in those situations, contactless collection of samples could be done remotely with the help of robotic technology to minimize the chances of getting the infection.

AI algorithms may be used to prioritize and expedite the testing of suspects, allowing for more testing to be done with less labor.

Another way of combining medical imaging modalities such as X-ray, CT, and processing techniques along with AI algorithms can be used to assess the persons with suspected symptoms [25].

Many literatures suggested various learning-based classification models incorporating linear/nonlinear classification models using CT and/or X-ray images for early detection of COVID-19 infection and reported good results. In the same way, many deep learning-based models for COVID detection have been proposed and revealed promising results. Also, some of the researchers have introduced some hybrid techniques combining normal machine learning models and customized deep CNN architectures to improve the performance of the detection. Few of the transfer learning methods also proved to be better for detection. Another set of researchers have focused on combining the features of both lung CT and chest X-ray images to improve the detection performance.

Apart from the features from those images, for COVID-19 screening, AI algorithms have been used to combine some of the acoustic signal properties such as cough, speech, breathing, voice, and so on. The COVID Symptom Study is used to predict COVID symptoms by comparing user's symptom with COVID-positive patient symptoms. More than three million users used the app to report their health issues, indicating that it was well received.

Lab-on-a-chip device integrated with laboratory functions can be used for analyzing the sample and making quick decision for COVID screening in a single chip.

COVID-19 Risk Assessment

Coronavirus has different effects on different people. Some people, for example, may not require extensive medical care, treatment, or consultation. Other individuals, particularly the elderly and the frail, require extra attention and a timely reaction from the service provider to survive. However, determining the severity of COVID-19 is a difficult task. AI-based approaches (ML or DL) have also been expanded to detect high-risk patients based on their preexisting health issues, respiratory difficulties, and chest X-ray and/or CT image results, and a vulnerability index or score has been created.

Many of the AI methods created can reliably identify whether newly infected COVID-19 patients will develop severe respiratory illness or whether they will have problems.

Surveillance During COVID-19

Following the discovery of the first incidence of coronavirus, many countries had major healthcare crises as a result of this unexpected risk, since it was impossible to estimate the virus's transmission, identify infection hot spots, and predict death due to the virus's mutation over time. The government's lack of preparation had exacerbated the problem.

It would be beneficial for policymakers to act proactively and take the appropriate procedures if it were feasible to foresee the spread. In this regard, AI approaches can be quite beneficial in evaluating the geographical distribution of viral infection and identifying groups and hot spots. These data may be used to identify susceptible zones in various zones.

Individuals have been monitored using AI-powered contact tracking applications to identify risk and anticipate the disease's future course of action. In comparison to the traditional medical data reporting system, which can establish effective strategies for preventing the spread, epidemiological data may be analyzed swiftly by an AI tool to detect the COVID-19 transmission networks.

To monitor social distancing, a variety of AI-enabled smartphone applications, vision-based robotic solutions, and wearable devices were developed.

Customized, fully autonomous patrol robots have been developed to replace human patrols, particularly in risky areas to run inspections. They can monitor body temperature and social distancing and also check whether people are wearing facial mask and alert the concerned authorities to take real-time initiatives.

Guangzhou Gosunch Robot Company developed an IoT-based 5G patrol robot equipped with infrared thermometers and five high-resolution cameras deployed in China to monitor the prevention measures of COVID-19, which can scan high temperatures of about ten people within a 5-meter radius. Steps involved in social distance monitoring are presented in Fig. 12.

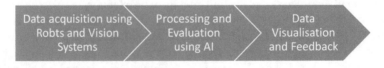

Fig. 12 Steps involved in social distance monitoring in real time

Telehealth Care Services During COVID-19

During the COVID-19 crisis, telemedicine was regarded one of the most crucial necessities. Tele-robotics has aided frontline employees in a variety of activities, reducing the transmission of disease by reducing intimate contact with patients.

Telehealth services including telesurgery, teleconsultation, teleultrasound, self-checker services, telepresence robots, and AI chatbots have been widely employed in hospitals to relieve demand in healthcare departments.

CRUZR, an interactive robot created by the Belgian firm Zo-raBots, can approach guests, detect temperature, and converse with them in one of 53 languages. It can also do and learn the repeated tasks that medical personnel must perform.

Drug and fluid delivery into the blood vessels can be achieved using robotic tabletop designed by Rutgers.

Medical robotic devices in conjunction with AI and image acquisition systems can perform the above tasks in less time.

Delivery and Supply Chain During COVID-19

Autonomous delivery robots are used in hospitals for various tasks to enhance the transfer of drugs, collection of samples, and dissemination of medical reports. Integrating self-driving robots into the supply and delivery chain can help to protect patients and medical workers while also easing the burden on healthcare professionals.

Phollower 100, an autonomous mobile delivery robot developed by Photoneo, a Slovakian company, is used to distribute medicines, laundry, etc. in hospitals and healthcare centers. Delivery robots are also used for enhancing delivery and supply chain. Steps involved in RPA in supply chain management are shown in Fig. 13.

RPA, often known as software robotics, is a method of automating business processes while eliminating the need for human participation. RPA replaces frontline staff's repetitive, monotonous, and time-consuming duties such as testing and diagnosis, ensuring more efficient use of human resources. To deliver advanced governance services, it also ensures enhanced efficiency and scalability while lowering

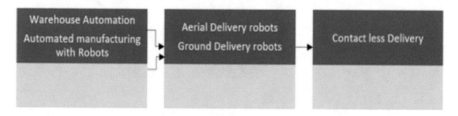

Fig. 13 Use of robots in supply chain management in COVID-19 service automation

operational expenses and reducing the frequency of mistakes. Use of RPA in COVID-19 scenario is depicted in Fig. 14.

RPA is used for medical record collection from patients and transferring records to concerned department for reducing manual errors.

The advantages of RPA are enlisted below:

- Automating appointment.
- Electronic health record maintenance through patient registration.
- Remote health monitoring.
- Fasten vaccine development.
- Enhance stock and supply chain management.
- Automating paperwork and reducing workload.
- Ease payment-related tasks.

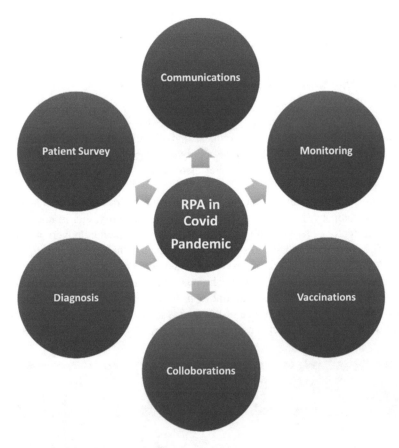

Fig. 14 Use of RPA in COVID pandemic

Disinfection

Robots can be deployed for spraying disinfectant to control infection in the possible disease-contaminated areas. Many disinfectant robots manufactured by UVD Robots, Nimbus robot, Xenex, and Youibot are currently used as disinfectant robot in market.

Research and Drug Development

Robotics can be used in mass manufacturing of drugs and vaccines to contain COVID-19 infection at a faster rate. Data collected from patients can be processed using AI algorithms such as machine learning and deep learning to aid decision-making from structured and unstructured data. Vaccine research, protein structure analysis, and analysis of drug target interaction can also be empowered using AI techniques.

Conclusion

COVID-19 is a deadly disease which created a huge impact in the lives and the medical infrastructure of developed and developing nations. The use of WBAN, IoT, AI, and robotics technology to enhance remote monitoring is detailed in this chapter.

It is observed that sensors in wireless body area networks play a very important role in closely monitoring the patient's body condition during COVID-19 remotely.

Most wireless body area network and IoT applications integrate with microcontroller and Android applications for processing and real-time display work. Different machine learning algorithms are used to identify whether the patient is affected or not affected. Cellular networks and LoRa technology are implemented in some systems to transmit the sensed information to the office of the health professional. Fast history access of the patient by the physician is also possible. Due to the equivalent development of wearable technology, infected patients can go and do their regular routines. A lot of research is going on to combine WBAN with virtual reality, cognitive radio, and 5G technology. By incorporating stronger security algorithms into WBAN, it makes the work of health professionals easier and tries to make patients also work during the quarantine, thus increasing the country's economic growth.

The use of IoT for improving the health infrastructure in remote health monitoring through data collection, data analysis and processing, and data transmission to cloud is the basic step in IoT framework irrespective of the architecture.

AI and robotics technology are used for various use cases in COVID-19 pandemic. Disease diagnosis and prediction is enhanced using machine learning and deep learning algorithm. Robotics technology is used for disease containment, accelerating medical research and mass production of vaccine.

Future work is to develop an expert system by integrating WBAN, IoT, AI, and robotics for betterment of people suffering from pandemic and epidemic diseases.

References

1. M. Ciotti, M. Ciccozzi, A. Terrinoni, W.-C. Jiang, C.-B. Wang, S. Bernardini, The COVID-19 pandemic. Crit. Rev. Clin. Lab. Sci (2020)
2. D.S. Rajeswari, J. Hitha Shree, A.L.N. Simha, M.N. Subhani, B.G. Shivaleelavathi, V. Yatnalli, A review on remote health monitoring sensors and their filtering techniques. Glob. Trans. Proceed. **2**(2), 392–401 (2021)
3. N. Bilandi, H.K. Verma, R. Dhir, An intelligent and energy-efficient wireless body area network to control coronavirus outbreak. Arab. J. Sci. Eng (2021)
4. F. Ullah, H.U. Haq, J. Khan, Arslan Ali Safeer, Usman Asif and Sungchang lee, wearable IoTs and geo-fencing based framework for COVID-19. Remote Patient Health Monitoring and Quarantine Management to Control the Pandemic **10** (2021)
5. C. Wang, Q. Wang, S.Z. Shi, A distributed wireless body area network for medical supervision, in *2012 IEEE International Instrumentation and Measurement Technology Conference Proceedings*, (2022)
6. R. Nidhya, S. Karthik, Security and privacy issues in remote healthcare systems using wireless body area networks. Body Area Netw. Challen. Sol., 37–53 (2018)
7. S. Umamaheswari, S. Arun Kumar, S. Sasikala, Towards building robust intrusion detection system in wireless sensor networks using machine learning and feature selection, in *2021 International Conference on Advancements in Electrical, Electronics, Communication, Computing and Automation (ICAECA)*, (2022)
8. S. Umamaheswari, K.H. Priya, S.A. Kumar, Technologies used in smart city applications–An overview, in *2021 International Conference on Advancements in Electrical, Electronics, Communication, Computing and Automation (ICAECA)*, (2021), pp. 1–6
9. Umamaheswari, S. Hybrid optimization model for energy efficient cloud assisted wireless sensor network. Wirel. Pers. Commun. **118**(1), 873–885 (2021)
10. S. Umamaheswari, C. Kavitha, S.M. Chandru, Machine learning for connecting humans for different applications. Int. J. Pure Appl. Math. **117**(8), 167–170 (2017)
11. M. Mathankumar, S. Karthikeyani, S.G. Kumar, N. Mahesh, N.J. Savitha, R. Rajaguru, An efficient dynamic key generation architecture for distributed wireless networks, in *2021 third international conference on intelligent communication technologies and virtual Mobile networks (ICICV)*, (2021), pp. 157–160
12. M. Mathankumar, U. Rajkanna, C. Mohanraj, Implementation of optimised wireless sensor network using cluster architecture, in *2019 innovations in power and advanced computing technologies (i-PACT)*, (2019), pp. 1–4
13. S. Swayamsiddha, C. Mohanty, Application of cognitive internet of medical things for COVID-19 pandemic. Diabetes Metab. Syndr. Clin. Res. Rev. **14**(5), 911–915 (2020)
14. S.S. Vedaei, A. Fotovvat, M.R. Mohebbian, G.M. Rahman, K.A. Wahid, P. Babyn, et al., COVID-SAFE: An IoT-based system for automated health monitoring and surveillance in post-pandemic life. IEEE Access **8**, 188538 (2020)
15. S. Bahl, R.P. Singh, M. Javaid, I.H. Khan, R. Vaishya, R. Suman, Telemedicine technologies for confronting COVID-19 pandemic: A review. J. Indus. Integra. Manag. **5**(04), 547–561 (2020)
16. Y. Dong, Y.D. Yao, IoT platform for COVID-19 prevention and control: A survey. IEEE Access **9**, 49929–49941 (2021)

17. S. Siddiqui, M.Z. Shakir, A.A. Khan, I. Dey, Internet of things (IoT) enabled architecture for social distancing during pandemic. Front. Commun. Netw. **2**, 6 (2021)
18. H. Mukhtar, S. Rubaiee, M. Krichen, R. Alroobaea, An IoT framework for screening of COVID-19 using real-time data from wearable sensors. Int. J. Environ. Res. Public Health **18**(8), 4022 (2021)
19. M. Javaid, I.H. Khan, Internet of things (IoT) enabled healthcare helps to take the challenges of COVID-19 pandemic. J. Oral Biol. Craniofac. Res. **11**(2), 209–214 (2021)
20. C.I. Loeza-Mejía, E. Sánchez-DelaCruz, P. Pozos-Parra, L.A. Landero-Hernández, The potential and challenges of health 4.0 to face COVID-19 pandemic: A rapid review. Heal. Technol. **11**(6), 1321–1330 (2021)
21. A.I. Paganelli, P.E. Velmovitsky, P. Miranda, A. Branco, P. Alencar, D. Cowan, et al., A conceptual IoT-based early-warning architecture for remote monitoring of COVID-19 patients in wards and at home. Internet of Things **100399** (2021)
22. P. Echeverría, J. Puig, J.M. Ruiz, J. Herms, M. Sarquella, B. Clotet, E. Negredo, Remote health monitoring in the workplace for early detection of COVID-19 cases during the COVID-19 pandemic using a Mobile health application: COVIDApp. Int. J. Environ. Res. Public Health **19**(1), 167 (2022)
23. S. Abbaspur-Behbahani, E. Monaghesh, A. Hajizadeh, S. Fehresti, Application of mobile health to support the elderly during the COVID-19 outbreak: A systematic review. Health Pol. Technol. **100595** (2022)
24. S. Sarker, L. Jamal, S.F. Ahmed, N. Irtisam, Robotics and artificial intelligence in healthcare during COVID-19 pandemic: A systematic review. Robot. Autonom. Syst. **146**, 103902 (2021)
25. M. Bharathi, S.A. Kumar, S. Sasikala, Deep learning architectures for improving effectiveness of Covid detection–a pilot study, in *2021 International Conference on Advancements in Electrical, Electronics, Communication, Computing and Automation (ICAECA)*, (IEEE, 2021), pp. 1–5

Artificial Intelligence-Based Predictive Tools for Life-Threatening Diseases

Vijay Jeyakumar, Prema Sundaram, and Nithiya Ramapathiran

Abbreviations

5G	Fifth generation
AI	Artificial intelligence
AIDS	Acquired immune deficiency syndrome
ANAM-NET	Anamorphic depth embedding-based lightweight CNN
ANN	Artificial neural network
AUC	Area under the curve
BERT	Bidirectional Encoder Representations from Transformers
CI	Confidence interval
CNN	Convolutional neural network
CNN-AE	Convolutional neural network-autoencoder
COPD	Chronic obstructive pulmonary disease
COVID-19	Coronavirus disease 2019
COVNet	COVID-19 detection neural network
CRP	C-reactive protein
CT	Computerized tomography
DHIS2	District Health Information Software into a single-window

V. Jeyakumar (✉)
Sri Sivasubramaniya Nadar College of Engineering, Chennai, India
e-mail: vijayj@ssn.edu.in

P. Sundaram
PSNA College of Engineering and Technology, Dindigul, India
e-mail: premas@psnacet.edu.in

N. Ramapathiran
Agni College of Technology, Chennai, India
e-mail: nithiya.bme@act.edu.in

© The Author(s), under exclusive license to Springer Nature Switzerland AG 2023
G. R. Kanagachidambaresan et al. (eds.), *System Design for Epidemics Using Machine Learning and Deep Learning*, Signals and Communication Technology, https://doi.org/10.1007/978-3-031-19752-9_8

DICOM	Digital Imaging and Communications in Medicine
DL	Deep learning
DNA	Deoxyribonucleic acid
DNN	Deep neural network
DST	Department of Science and Technology
EHR	Electronic health records
EN	Elastic net model
FDA	Flexible discriminant analysis
GLDM	Gray level dependence matrix
GLSZM	Gray level size zone matrix
GRU	Gated recurrent unit
GUIDE	Graphical User Interface Development Environment
HIV	Human immunodeficiency virus
HMC	Hamiltonian Monte Carlo
ICU	Intensive care unit
INR	International normalized ratio
IoT	Internet of Things
K-NN	K-nearest neighborhood
LASSO	Least absolute shrinkage and selection operator
LDH	Lactate dehydrogenase
LR	Linear regression
LSTM	Long short-term memory
MATLAB	Matrix Laboratory
MCHC	Mean corpuscular hemoglobin concentration
MERS-CoV	Middle East respiratory syndrome coronavirus
ML	Machine learning
MOGA	Multi-objective genetic algorithm
MRMR	Maximum relevance minimum redundancy
NA	Not applicable
NBML	National Brain Mapping Laboratory
OWL	Web Ontology Language
pH	Potential of hydrogen
PLS	Partial least square regression
RF	Random forest
RNA	Ribonucleic acid
RNN	Recurrent neural network
RT-PCR	Reverse transcriptase-polymerase chain reaction
SARS	Severe acute respiratory syndrome
SARS-CoV	Severe acute respiratory syndrome coronavirus
SARS-CoV-2	Severe acute respiratory syndrome coronavirus 2
SIR	Susceptible-infected-removed
SMOTE	Synthetic Minority Oversampling Technique
SOP	Standard operating procedures
SORMAS	Surveillance Outbreak Response Management and Analysis System
SpO_2	Partial saturation of oxygen
SVM	Support vector machine

SVM-RFE	Support vector machine-recursive feature elimination
SWRL	Semantic Web Rule Language
TELINET	Telefax Library Network
VGG	Visual Geometry Group
WASH	Water, sanitation, and hygiene
WHO	World Health Organization
XGBoost	Extreme Gradient Boosting

Origin and Background of Diseases

A medical condition that generally affects the normal structure or function of an organism and is related to specific signs and symptoms is termed a disease. This may be due to any external factor or internal body disorder resulting in pain, dysfunction, injury, or syndrome. It represents the impairment of the body's normal homeostatic balance.

The different stages of a disease are its:

- Etiology
- Pathogenesis
- Morphological changes
- Corresponding functional alterations associated with the changes

Classification

Diseases are classified into majorly four types:

1. Infectious diseases are illnesses caused by pathogens and their toxic products such as bacteria, viruses, fungi, or parasites, e.g., COVID-19.
2. Deficiency disease or malnutrition disease is caused due to deficiency, excess, or imbalance of nutrients affecting body tissues, e.g., anemia.
3. Hereditary disease or metabolic disease gives rise to alterations in the gene or abnormality in chromosomes. The two subtypes under this category are genetic and nongenetic diseases, e.g., hemophilia.
4. Diseases caused by abiotic factors (cold, high temperature, low pH) as well as nutritional imbalances are termed physiological diseases. The organs and organ systems of the body do not function properly leading to illness, e.g., diabetes.

There are other ways of disease classification.

1. Based on spread, diseases are classified as follows:
   - *Communicable disease* involves the transmission of the pathogen from an infected host through various modes of transmission, e.g., HIV infection.
   - *Noncommunicable diseases* do not spread from individual to individual, e.g., cancer.

2. Based on the time frame, diseases can be classified as follows:
   - The *acute disease* appears suddenly and persists only for a short term from a few days to weeks, e.g., common cold.
   - The *chronic disease* develops gradually and persists for long periods usually from months to years, e.g., arthritis.
3. Based on the cause of the disease, the disease can be classified as follows:
   - A *primary disease* that occurs due to some initiating cause of illness, e.g., common cold.
   - *Secondary disease* arises due to the complication caused by the primary disease or its underlying cause, e.g., rhinitis can be due to a common cold or bacterial infection.
4. Based on the body system, diseases are classified as follows:
   - *Insanity* on *mental illness* comprises a broad range of diseases which includes emotional imbalance, behavior disturbance, logical dysfunction, or cognitive impairment and can be biological or psychological, e.g., depression.
   - *Organic diseases* can be brought about by the structural or functional changes to the organ systems of the body, e.g., stroke.
5. Based on the extent, diseases can be classified as follows:
   - A *localized disease* is confined to one part of the body, e.g., eye infection.
   - *Disseminated* disease indicates the spread of disease from the site of its origin to a distant site, e.g., cancer.
   - The *systemic disease* affects the entire body leading to illness, e.g., blood pressure

The course of a disease in an individual is the time taken from the inception of the disease until its complete recovery or eventual death. The progression of a disease is a set of biological events right from its etiology (cause) to the outcome (recovery or death). The important perspectives to characterize the history of a disease are that of the family doctor who can analyze the presence of health issues in an individual and that of an epidemiologist who can discover the occurrence of new diseases and their solutions by using health records and biostatistical information [1].

Phases of Disease

There are three phases in the progression of the disease.

1. *Pre-pathogenic period* – In this period, the disease arises but the person will not present any symptoms related to the disease in their body. So, the body conditions, causative agent, and the environment play a major role.

2. *Pathogenic period* – In this period, alteration in the person's body tissue originates but the person doesn't yet find out any clinical signs of the disease. It includes two sub-phases.

    - The incubation period is a fast-evolving phase from hours to days and is the time taken for the disease-causing agent to propagate and produce symptoms after exposure to the pathogen in the host.
    - The latency period or pre-infectious period is a very-slow-evolving phase lasting from months to years and is the time taken to become infectious and capable of transmitting the disease.

3. *Clinical period* – In this period, the patient shows clinical signs and changes, and the pathology of the disease keeps continuing without treatment and can result in recovery, disability, or fatality. It includes three sub-phases.

    - Prodromal – Denotes the clinical beginning of the disease where the first symptoms appear
    - Clinical – Indicates the appearance of specific symptoms which could be identified by the physicist to choose the right treatment protocol either to treat the patient or to avoid any long-term damage
    - Resolution – Represents the terminal phase where the disease can completely resolve or progress to an advanced stage or can result in death

Transmission of Infection

This process follows the three factors mentioned below:

- An infected individual.
- A vulnerable individual.
- An effective contact between the infected and the vulnerable individual is such that the infected individual affects the vulnerable individual.

The number of effective contacts made in unit time in a given population is termed effective contact rate (β). It is nothing but the multiplication of total contact rate (γ) (whether effective or not) and the risk of infection transmission (p) and is given by the expression

$$B = \gamma^* p \tag{1}$$

Infectivity is the ability of an infectious agent to get access and amplify in the host causing an infection. Transmissibility is the chance of transmitting an infection from the infected one to the susceptible individual and can spread either by the community or local transmission. In community transmission, the epidemiological link among a group of people causing the spread of infection is not known, whereas in local transmission, the origin of infection within a specified location can be identified.

Routes of Transmission

The routes of disease transmission between different populations are essential to know about the patterns of contact and the spread of the disease based on social-economic and cultural conditions. The disease-causing agent can be transmitted in either of the following ways:

- *Horizontal disease transmission* – Infection can be acquired from the environment or unrelated people in the same generation either through direct or indirect contact.
- *Vertical disease transmission* – It is the passage of the infectious agent from the mother to the offspring which can be intracellular or extracellular.
- *Mixed-mode disease transmission* – Disease transmission can be vertical as well as horizontal depending upon the host density which can be low or high, respectively.

Mode of disease transmission can be in the following ways:

1. *Airborne infection* – Refers to the transmission of very small dry and wet aerosols of size less than 5 μm that spread through evaporated droplets which can remain living in the environment for long periods and can affect the upper and lower respiratory tract, e.g., tuberculosis.
2. *Droplet infection* – Transmission of a respiratory droplet is the most common route for respiratory infections produced by coughing, sneezing, or talking by infected hosts, wherein small and wet particles of size larger than 5 μm remain in the environment for a limited period over minimum distances. It can be transmitted either directly to the susceptible mucosal surface or indirectly through contact with the contaminated area, e.g., coronavirus.
3. *Direct physical contact* – Direct contact happens through skin-to-skin touch, kissing, and sexual contact and can lead to a variety of infectious and contagious diseases, e.g., syphilis.
4. *Indirect physical contact* – Also referred to as vehicle-borne transmission characterizes the spread of infection through the contamination of insensate objects, which can act as vehicles transmitting the infection either through a vector or an intermediate host, e.g., malaria.
5. *Transmission by other organisms* – Transmission is usually through a vector that may be of mechanical or biological origin and is not responsible to cause disease on its own but can spread infection by transmitting pathogens from one person to another, e.g., rabies.
6. *Fecal-oral transmission* – This mode of transmission poses a serious health risk for people where the fecal particles pollute food and water so that the pathogen transmits from one person to the mouth of another due to poor sanitation and personal hygiene, e.g., cholera.

Morbidity and Mortality Rates

The two important and commonly used terms in epidemiology are morbidity and mortality which are denoted as a proportion or rate and represent the frequency and severity of a specific disease condition [2].

- Morbidity is defined as a state of having a particular illness or complication which is an unnatural consequence of a disease or treatment. It can be acute or chronic and can be presented either as the incidence or prevalence of a disease, e.g., heart disease, stroke, diabetes, obesity, and infection.
- The morbidity rate represents the rate of disease occurrence in a population and evaluates the overall health of a population and their health care requirements:

$$\text{Morbidity rate} = \frac{(\text{Number of cases of disease or injury or disability})}{(\text{Total population})} \quad (2)$$

- Mortality indicates the number of deaths caused due to a specific illness or disease condition, e.g., in 2020, COVID-19 will be a remarkable cause of mortality.
- Mortality or death rate measures the count of deaths in a specific population scaled to the total population per unit of time.

Increased human and animal interaction due to expanded global trade events has resulted in the transmission of zoonotic pathogens and facilitated the continuous transmission of infections among mankind. The progressive population escalated the exposure and spread of novel illnesses to the increased risk for outbreaks, epidemics, and pandemics [3].

Let us review the significant terms for disease occurrence and transmission in various geographical regions [4].

- An endemic refers to the predictable rate of a disease condition that is present consistently among the population, e.g., malaria.
- An outbreak is a sudden rise in the count of people presenting a disease. It may occur in one place or extend widely and can last for days to years. It may be new to the community or has been absent for a long period, e.g., influenza.
- An epidemic spreads quickly to a large population over an extended geographic area and is considered an outbreak, e.g., polio.
- A pandemic spread across countries and continents affecting mankind globally and is an epidemic, e.g., COVID-19.

The mechanism of cross-species pathogen transfer relies on different phases.

– Phase 1 – The infectious agent infects animals particularly.
– Phase 2 – The pathogen progresses and enters the human system, but without human-to-human transference.
– Phase 3 – A few cycles of secondary infection occur between humans.

- Phase 4 – Infection persists in animals although long periods of secondary infection exist among humans but without the presence of animal hosts.
- Phase 5 – Infection persists in humans exclusively.

Pathogens of Bacteria and Virus

The risk of pathogen transmission, in turn, depends upon the animal host carrying the infectious agent, the type of cross-species interaction, and its probability. The most notable past pandemics that have distressed mankind in world history include plague, cholera, influenza, smallpox, HIV and AIDS, and coronavirus disease [5] which are shown in Table 1.

Plague or Black Death

Gram-negative rod-shaped facultative anaerobic bacteria *Yersinia pestis* causes plague which infects rodents and mammals through fleas. Fleas feed on infected rodents, receiving the bacteria which then multiplies in the flea's gut. It regurgitates the blood to new rodent hosts and spreads the infection in three different routes.

1. Bubonic – The most common form which is fatal due to an infected flea with flu-related symptoms (50–90%).
2. Septicemic – The rare form affecting 10–25% of the host resulting in progressive infection of the bloodstream.
3. Pneumonic – It occurs when the bacteria lodges in the lungs and is a rapidly fatal condition when untreated.

The three pandemic plague episodes are:

1. The initial pandemic which occurred between 541 and 543 is the plague of Justinian which originated in Egypt and passed across Rome causing a high mortality rate of 100 million people.
2. In the early nineteenth century, the second plague pandemic wave called Black Death started in Europe and eventually caused the death of 200 million people.
3. During the nineteenth century, the third plague pandemic existed in China and was endemic throughout the world in later years [6]. It is considered as a re-emerging infection by WHO affecting different parts of the world in a variety of periods and is proved to be highly fatal without immediate treatment and can be a major potential public threat.

Table 1 Life-threatening diseases and their origin

Years	Epidemics/pandemics	Pathogens	Vectors	Death toll	Location
541–543	Plague of Justinian	*Yersinia pestis*	Fleas associated with wild rodents	15–100 million	Europe and West Asia
1347–1351	Black Death	*Yersinia pestis*	Fleas associated with wild rodents	75–200 million	Europe, Asia, and North Africa
1817–1824	First cholera pandemic	*Vibrio cholerae*	Contaminated water	1–2 million	Asia, Africa
1827–1835	Second cholera pandemic	*Vibrio cholerae*	Contaminated water	Less than a million	Europe, Asia, America
1839–1856	Third cholera pandemic	*Vibrio cholerae*	Contaminated water	1–2 million	Asia, Europe, Africa, and North America
1863–1875	Fourth cholera pandemic	*Vibrio cholerae*	Contaminated water	600,000	Russia, Europe, Africa, and North America
1881–1886	Fifth cholera pandemic	*Vibrio cholerae*	Contaminated water	Less than a million	Worldwide
1885–ongoing	Third plague	*Yersinia pestis*	Fleas associated with wild rodents	12–15 million	Worldwide
1889–1893	Russian flu	Influenza A/H3N8	Avian	1 million	Worldwide
1899–1923	Sixth cholera pandemic	*Vibrio cholerae*	Contaminated water	Less than a million	Europe, Asia, and North Africa
1918–1919	Spanish flu	Influenza A/H1N1	Avian	17–100 million	Worldwide
1957–1959	Asian flu	Influenza A/H2N2	Avian	1–4 million	Worldwide
1961–ongoing	Seventh cholera pandemic	*Vibrio cholerae*	Contaminated water	3–5 million	Worldwide
1968–1970	Hong Kong flu	Influenza A/H3N2	Avian	1–4 million	Worldwide
2002–2003	Severe acute respiratory syndrome	SARS-CoV	Bats, palm civets	Less than a million	China, Hong Kong, Canada
2009–2010	Swine flu	Influenza A/H1N1	Pigs	Less than 3 lakhs	Worldwide
2015–ongoing	Middle East respiratory syndrome	MERS-CoV	Bats, dromedary camels	Less than a lakh	Worldwide
2019–ongoing	Coronavirus disease	SARS-CoV-2	Bats, pangolins	5.7–23.8 million (as of February 2022)	Worldwide

Cholera

A Gram-negative comma-shaped facultative anaerobic bacteria *Vibrio cholerae* acutely infects the gastrointestinal tract and causes the most fatal disease called cholera. The bacteria reside in the small intestine producing cholera toxin leading to rapid dehydration resulting in hypovolemic shock and fatality. It involves the waterborne transmission of the infection which can be mild or asymptomatic [7].

Cholera remained endemic in Asia up to 1817 and then became a pandemic spreading and infecting different parts of the world leading to seven cholera pandemics due to increased globalization and foreign trade resulting in a fatal condition. Cholera cannot be completely eradicated, and its persistence is due to poor living conditions and proper sanitation and inefficient sewage systems. Also, changes in the ecosystem and climate favored genetic exchange protocols in *Vibrio cholerae* making them more virulent causing mild to life-threatening infections leading to a potential threat for mankind.

Influenza or Spanish Flu

Influenza viruses are enveloped RNA viruses (single, negative sense) belonging to the *Orthomyxoviridae* family coding for ten structural and nonstructural proteins causing severe illness and death worldwide. Influenza virus consists of four strains: A, B, C and D. Strains A and B types cause outbreaks in tropical areas and seasonal epidemics in temperate areas. They show asymptomatic or mild or classical illness and cause approximately 5 lakh deaths. They may also show severe illness and pneumonia along with secondary bacterial infection with *Streptococcus* and *Staphylococcus* species and *Haemophilus influenzae*. Strain A is endemic in humans, birds, and pigs [8].

Reassortments and genetic rearrangements lead to the antigenic shift resulting in the origination of new subtypes of virus influencing spontaneous human transmission and may result in a pandemic. The hit of a pandemic was majorly due to transmission and pathogenicity of the different types of strains and the vulnerability of the people which varied among different age groups and their earlier exposure to the virus. The constant modification and interchange of genes between different species of the influenza virus along with cross-species transmission is a critical challenge for the origin of new strains of avian virus causing low pathogenic and highly pathogenic avian influenza virus strains.

Smallpox

It was an acute, contagious, and deadly infectious disease caused by two strains of variola virus, namely, *Variola major* and *Variola minor*, belonging to the *Orthopoxvirus* family. Initial symptoms of infection were common to all viral diseases and the smallpox virus attacks skin cells leading to the formation of characteristic pimples which then spreads throughout the body ranging from ordinary, modified, malignant, or hemorrhagic forms. Pieces of evidence showed that the disease occurred in outbreaks and there were 500 million deaths in the last hundred years of its existence and it was completely eradicated globally in 1980.

HIV or AIDS

Human immunodeficiency virus falling under retrovirus family causing acquired immune deficiency syndrome (AIDS) is considered a global epidemic infecting 37.9 million people including adults and children less than 15 years of age as of 2018. The most affected region is Sub-Saharan Africa. The pandemic is heterogeneous within regions, with some regions more affected than others. After the initial infection, the person may experience a short period of influenza-like symptoms followed by a long incubation period with the progression of infection, and the immune system gets weakened, thereby elevating the risk of other common infections, inviting opportunistic infections and tumors associated with severe weight loss. This disease has a large impact on society as well as the economy.

Coronavirus

The novel coronavirus termed severe acute respiratory syndrome coronavirus 2 (SARS-CoV-2) belongs to the *Coronaviridae* family infecting animals and humans. They have enveloped RNA virus (+ sense, single-stranded) and include four genera – Alpha, Beta, Gamma, and Delta variants. The virus was identified from an outbreak in China in Wuhan city causing the coronavirus or COVID-19 pandemic. The virus is of zoonotic origin from bats and related mammals. Human coronavirus can lodge in the upper and lower respiratory tract causing severe respiratory system diseases and sometimes to a lower extent can also cause gastroenteritis, although it is rarely fatal. It spread globally to more than 390 million people causing 5.72 million fatalities making COVID-19 one of the deadliest diseases in world history. The symptoms range from mild to deadly conditions including fever, dry cough, and tiredness and are transmitted by small airborne particles enclosing the virus. Virus-infected people can transmit the disease for 10 days even if symptoms do not develop. So, vaccination, social distancing, wearing of face mask, and quarantining are the recommended preventive measures to combat the coronavirus [9].

The common cold is caused by the Alpha-coronavirus genus, whereas the Beta-coronavirus genus causes severe respiratory tract infection. In addition, Beta-coronavirus includes three pathogenic strains of virus, namely:

1. Severe acute respiratory syndrome coronavirus (SARS-CoV)
2. Middle East respiratory syndrome coronavirus (MERS-CoV)
3. Severe acute respiratory syndrome coronavirus 2 (SARS-CoV-2), the causative factor of COVID-19 inducing dreadful pneumonia

SARS-CoV originated in China and the natural reservoirs were bats and intermediary hosts were palm civets before human infection. The transmission was nosocomial and caused influenza-related symptoms. The major cause of fatality was respiratory failure and patients infected also showed pneumonia and watery diarrhea-causing serious threats. MERS-CoV showed its first emergence in Saudi Arabia. Bats were the prospective animal reservoirs and Arabian camels were the intermediary hosts infecting humans showing clinical illness from moderate to drastic pulmonary disease.

SARS-CoV-2 pandemic causing COVID-19 involving bats as an animal reservoir and pangolins as animal host before virus transmission to humans. COVID infection is asymptomatic and can show a range of mild symptoms to common complications affecting the major organs like the heart, lungs, and liver and can result in life-threatening conditions.

Disease Management System

The spillover of zoonotic organisms and the transmission dynamics of infection to mankind are remarkably escalating due to various factors such as globalization, trade of animals, animal-based food products, land use and urbanization, modifications in the living habits of the pathogen, and increased animal-human interaction [10].

This may pose new threats and challenges to public health, and there will be recurrence of epidemic and pandemic diseases. To control the spread of various diseases and to have a check over the increase, numerous protocols have been devised for disease management.

- Water, sanitation, and hygiene (WASH) programs to ensure safe drinking water access, effective sanitation methods, and hygiene practices.
- Vector control program targeting immature or adult stages of vector to control the spread of infection.
- Global surveillance program for quick detection of pathogen spillover to avoid cross-species transmission.

- Global virome project began to encounter viral transmission and to develop pathogenicity markers for life-threatening viruses.
- Next-generation sequencing of viral genome analysis to enhance novel virus detection and characterization of the virome in the respiratory system.
- Vaccine development and their clinical trials.

In the pandemics, healthcare companies have initiated the use of big data analytics and prediction tools to better understand the pathogen and cross-species infection transmission. Thus, healthcare settings expanded the use of predictive algorithms and models to gain insight into the risks and outcomes of disease and the potential impact of the pathogen on humans.

Role of Expert Systems

The expert system is one of the major applications in predicting the pandemic and epidemic illness. An expert system predicts the thoughts and behaviors of an individual or organization having experience in a specific sector. It contains the prior knowledge and also a set of procedural guidelines as a base for each unique case. The major qualities of an expert system are a representation of the user data, inference, and detailed explanations which are all terms that come to mind when thinking about the user interface, etc. The advantages of an expert system are higher dependency, fewer errors, lower costs, a smart database, and lower risk. Even though there are many benefits, certain limitations lack common sense without artificial intelligence (AI) [11].

The ultimate focus of an expert system-based medical decision tool is to protect, cure, and identify diseases. The evidence obtained through such a system can be taken as a second opinion which could support the doctors and medical specialists in clinical decision-making. Among the existing algorithms and predictive techniques, AI is the most promising one, where the infectious disease dataset will be collected in various forms and given as input. Based on the inputs, AI can predict disease like how mankind thinks and acts. However, in a few scenarios, unpredicted parameters are evolved during the transmission of infectious diseases such as influenza, severe acute respiratory syndrome (SARS), etc. Hence, it is difficult for AI to predict results in the early stage, especially in cancer and lymphoma diagnosis. In such conditions, AI encompasses machine learning as a subdomain in the medical expert system for the early prediction of infectious disease using Bayesian distribution, artificial neural network (ANN), and so on. From Fig. 1, the expert system containing mathematics modeling, machine learning, and AI can be used to forecast numerous types of diseases. To reduce the spread of contagious diseases, standard operating procedures (SOP), self-testing, and quarantine are not sufficient. Rather, mass screening through a noncontact ecosystem would be the best alternative by adopting AI.

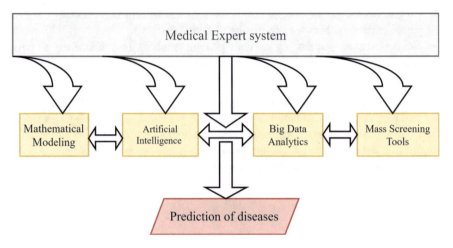

Fig. 1 Medical expert system

Mathematical Model for Predictive Modeling

Epidemic and pandemic diseases spread easily. Their outburst in the environment is due to the emergence of mass level interaction of pathogens and host bacteria in the atmosphere. To predict the pandemic disease, different types of modeling are available. Some of the specific components of spread can be predicted by mathematical models like compartment-based susceptible, infectious, and/or recovered (SIR) model, contact network model, disease control model, and many more. Mathematical modeling will follow particular rules depending on the behavior of diseases; it will also help us for the prediction of disease easily.

Compartment Model

Since 1921, the compartment model has been used to detect infectious diseases like influenza, Ebola, and end-level kidney disease. In this model, different compartments are combined and the comparative study on the different compartments from the predicted results can be easily done. SIR is the most important model used to predict measles and Nipah viruses accurately compared to other mathematical models.

SIR Model

The most widely used compartment model for infectious disease is the susceptible-infected-removed model [12]. Since individuals fall into any one of these categories, the SIR model is a basic predictive tool, primarily functioning on individual

Table 2 SIR model-based prediction tools

Predictive tools in a compartment model	Diseases predicted	Prediction accuracy (%)
SIR model (pandemic disease)	Measles, Nipah virus infection, Asian influenza, and so on	93
SIS model (disease not having permanent immunity like a seasonal disease)	Viral fever, cold, cough	96
Vertical transmission (where children got infected from parents)	AIDS and hepatitis	93.2
Vector transmission (not spread by human to a human directly)	Malaria, swine flu	94

concern reports. This model represents the probability of the disease spreading using the data of affected $S(x)$, prone to get infected $I(x)$, and recovered $R(x)$ individuals. The SIR model has been tested with the COVID-19 dataset to predict the test results [13]. The SIR model starts to work when there is a combination of the number of people who got infected and people having the possibility of infection and runs until there is a change in this combination. The result is obtained from the count of the patient cured and the death rate of patients affected by this pandemic disease and is statistically represented. If the epidemic disease is spread worldwide in one shot or even if the mortality rate is very high, the SIR model can be recommended as a predictive tool. Thus, the model can estimate the rate of recovered individuals, thereby determining the rate of infectious disease. Table 2 shows the predictive disease accuracy done on various predictive tools in the SIR model.

Limitations:

- The pathogen's characteristics change due to age, environmental conditions, and genetic and environmental factors.
- It does not consider the latent period followed by exposure.
- It severely assumes the population with no migration and the number of deaths and birth apart from epidemics.
- Quantification of uncertainty cannot be expected in this model.

Other Mathematical Models

As shown in Table 3, mathematical modeling can be used as a predictive tool in a variety of ways [14].

The Implication of Machine Learning Algorithms

In recent years, machine learning algorithms have been utilized as a predictor of infectious disease during pandemics and epidemics. Machine learning is the best use of AI in which all the input is given to the computer, which then learns and

Table 3 Mathematical modeling used for predictions

S. no	Types	Methodology/algorithm	Applications	Accuracy (%)
1	Mathematical tools for biochemical biomarkers	Receiver operator curve analysis, logical regression analysis	Ebola, AIDS, influenza	88
2	Dynamic modeling	Discrete-time epidemic modeling	Measles	95
3	Epidemic chain models	Chain model	Chicken pox, measles, mumps	93.2
4	Reversible jump Markov chain Monte Carlo methods	Bayesian network	*Staphylococcus*	94.3

begins to react based on the data and is also capable of predicting future disease progression. Unsupervised and supervised algorithms are two types of machine learning algorithms [15].

Supervised Algorithm

A supervised algorithm predicts an undefined disease based on the input information that the expert trains over the output. Examples of supervised algorithms include Bayesian, ANN, support vector machine (SVM), K-nearest neighbor, convolutional neural network (CNN), multimodal logistic regression, and linear regression (LR).

The Bayesian Networks

The Bayesian network model is a fundamental and one of the most effective machine learning algorithms with 97% accuracy for predicting and interpreting diseases [16]. It represents the numerous connections between nodes, where each node has its own set of variables. Both statistical data and simply accessible algorithm frameworks, such as STAN, Web Ontology Language (OWL), Semantic Web Rule Language (SWRL), naive Bayes, and the random forest method are used in Bayesian analysis. For convenience, graphical data can be depicted to deliver the right prediction for various forms of terrible diseases as shown in Fig. 2 [17].

The Bayesian network is mostly used to analyze unpredictably large amounts of data as well as to develop forecasting algorithms for specific diseases. The STAN Bayesian network has been built using the available medical dataset and the knowledge of experts. HMC sampling is the primary tool used in STAN to diagnose epidemic and pandemic diseases quickly and accurately. When compared to other Bayesian networks, the result obtained with this probabilistic programming approach is accurate [18]. The expert must anticipate the disease using two web

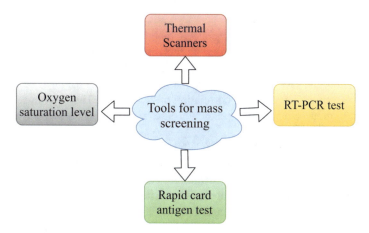

Fig. 2 Diagnostic tools for mass screening

languages, OWL and SWRL, based on medical facts [19]. Both web languages are knowledge-based prediction tools, and they can be combined with a Bayesian network to provide an outcome.

Other Machine Learning Methods

There are various other machine learning methods for disease prediction. They are as follows:

(i) Artificial Neural Network (ANN)

An ANN based on the Internet of Things (IoT) was created to forecast diseases like typhoid and severe acute respiratory syndrome (SARS). The development of an ANN network was based on the user's perception to improve the quality of life for those suffering from life-threatening diseases [19]. It is the algorithm that will revoke the working of the human brain as a network to find a solution from it. It was built using ten types of networks and different hidden layers for the early diagnosis of Middle East respiratory syndrome (MERS).

(ii) Support Vector Machine (SVM)

SVM works on the available input data and can classify the disease conditions into two categories of infected and not infected groups. There are two optimizations in SVM, namely, linear and quadratic, based on the division of data into groups. If the data are separated equally, it will be classified under linear optimization otherwise quadratic optimization [20]. In quadratic optimization, kernel values are used to obtain different results. SVM classifier can be used as a predictive tool so that it can identify the pandemic disease-related microRNA [21] and DNA variation of the specified disease. Therefore, these are the two important vital parameters needed to identify or classify at the molecular level for the prediction of the spread of disease.

(iii) K-Nearest Neighbor (KNN)

The KNN classification model can be used even when the dataset is unknown. It is completely based on the K values of the nearest neighbor data values, which are determined using the Euclidean distance. Once the dataset is available, the "K" similar neighbor in the unknown dataset can be identified and classified based on the correlation of "K" values. The K-nearest neighbor algorithm has been used to predict diseases such as Parkinson's and acute leukemia [22].

(iv) Convolutional Neural Network (CNN)

Convolutional neural networks (CNN) are automatically made up of numerous levels such as pooling, convolution, and fully connected layers, and with these features, disease prediction can be extracted from a back-projection algorithm. The input data for the network includes a dataset of symptoms. In comparison, the results showed that CNN is 85% more accurate than KNN because other factors, such as time and memory, were required in the K-nearest neighbor method.

(v) Multimodal Logistic Regression

Once trained, this network is the best method in biological sciences as the multimodal LR mostly uses the dependent variables, namely, regression and classification variables [23]. From each modal, common features can be chosen for multiple variables. Multimodal or multi-task logistic regression finds application in the study of Alzheimer's disease and cardiac arrest [24].

(vi) Linear Regression

Usually, independent variables can work on linear regression. If there are two variables present in the same application, then linear regression can be used so that a comparative study could be made between them [25]. Depending on the type of application employed, the algorithm can differentiate between linear and logistic regression. In Table 4, the various machine learning tools used for the prediction of the pandemic disease with their accuracy level are depicted [26].

Unsupervised Algorithm

The unsupervised algorithm is used to analyze and aggregate unlabeled symptom datasets of diseases. Using this algorithm, the identification of hidden patterns and data grouping can be accomplished without the assistance of a human being. The two techniques involved in unsupervised algorithm are as follows:

Clustering

It is the process of combining similar datasets into one cluster and dissimilar datasets into another cluster. Depending on the common characteristics, clustering can be done easily for the prediction of the disease, e.g., chronic diseases like diabetes.

Table 4 Machine learning tools used for the prediction of disease

S. no	Machine learning tools	Techniques	Predicted disease	Percentage of prediction
1	ANN	Three-layered network with 1000 hidden layers, under the curve (AUC) specificity, and predictivity are determined	Breast cancer, Naples plague, SAARC, H1N1 Flu	P curve value almost accurate to expert result AUC = 0.939 ($P < 0.001$)
2	SVM	Select the set of variables and classify the individual into two categories. C-I (infected) vs C-II (not infected/maybe infected). The classification was done on common variables for pandemic diseases	Respiratory syndrome, MERS, Ebola, flu	93.34%
3	K-nearest neighbors	Alignment-free method for the prediction of new virus by a comparative study of the sequence of molecules	SARS, H1N1, MERS, West Nile fever	94.30%
4	CNN	Classification using 16 layers, visual group network, mobile net, U-Net on imaging	Malaria, smallpox, SAARC, influenza H1N2	93%
5	Multimodal LR	The classifier network will classify the dataset into four different layers of classes so that prediction can occur	SARS, ARDS, malaria, influenza	96.2%
7	Linear regression	Tenfold cross-validation techniques using Synthetic Minority Oversampling Technique (SMOTE) data	Malaria, influenza, heart disease	Accuracy = 95.2% AUC = 99%

Association

It is one of the unsupervised algorithms which can predict disease from the specified symptoms by the technique of association, e.g., genetic disease.

Deep Learning Model for Big Medical Data Analytics

According to the World Health Organization, 12.8 million people died worldwide because of past pandemic diseases. This pandemic has generated a large amount of data, which is either structured or unstructured; the main job of Big Medical Data Analytics is to work on this large dataset and improve the efficiency of data processing to provide useful information to the public to prevent epidemic diseases such as influenza, flu, and malaria [27].

Big data processing includes data consolidation and fine-tuning and removing unwanted data to generate the required data in various forms. Multi-objective genetic algorithm (MOGA) is the algorithm used to generate big data in various efficient forms. This allows technicians to speed up data processing for early prediction of pandemic disease but is the most time-consuming step [28].

The Internet of Things (IoT) and big data analytics are playing an important role in the prediction against pandemic disease to collect enormous amounts of data, to view disease information, dissipate pandemic disease risk, and take precautions against disease prevention. For processing all this data, a neural network model can be employed which provides 98% accuracy when compared to other machine learning models [29].

Another type of big data analytics is the gene prediction algorithm, where most of the predictive analysis for the epidemic disease is dependent on the type of gene prediction. Particularly, the genes that are coded like protein-coding genes will be collected from the infected person and studied for the identification of a specific gene responsible for a disease using an National Brain Mapping Laboratory (NBML) algorithm. According to the findings, big data analytics can predict disease with an accuracy of 96.05% [30].

Big data is simply a massive database gathered from the public in various scenarios. The main challenge in big data analytics is maintaining the privacy of public data. Digital Imaging and Communications in Medicine (DICOM), electronic health records (EHR), or IoT-based tools were deployed to store the data in the appropriate location for future analysis and diagnostic purposes. STATA and MATLAB R2021 are the tools used to maintain the privacy of the big data that are used in big data analytics [29].

Tools Used for Mass Screening

According to the modeling study shown in Fig. 2, mass screening techniques utilized can reduce the spread of pandemic disease by 60% and the mortality rate can be reduced from 0.66% to 0.19%. As a result, most experts believe that mass screening could reduce the spread of infectious diseases [31].

Predictive Tool for Mass screening

(a) Lyfas COVID Score is a DST-funded Android application developed by Bangalore-based Acculi Labs. It is a mobile phone application in which the individual places his/her index finger on the camera, and it analyzes 95 biomarkers, namely, capillary pulse, blood volume variations, etc., using different processors and sensors to track the small changes in the physiological and path-

Table 5 Mass screening software for prediction

S. no	Name of the software	Developer	Year	Technology
1	DHIS2 (District Health Information Software)	University of Oslo	2020	National information system platform for data integration around 70 countries. Case-based surveillance to track the situation easily
2	SORMAS	Helmholtz Centre for Infection Research	2020	Mobile e-health systems are mainly for disease control systems
3	Go. Data	WHO and GOAN	2020	It is the data collection tool for Ebola, MERS, and COVID-19. From the pathological data collected by this app, contact list tracking can be done

ological conditions of the body. It can be used as a predictive app for mass screening.

(b) Graphical User Interface Development Environment (GUIDE) is a platform that combines many predictive software tools, such as District Health Information Software into a single-window (DHIS2), Surveillance Outbreak Response Management and Analysis System (SORMAS), and GO. The various tools introduced by the vendors are shown in Table 5.

Thus, these expert systems for predicting pandemic and epidemic diseases help in the management and prevention of COVID-19 as follows.

COVID-19 Prediction Tools

In 2019 SARS-CoV-2 is impacting global health and becoming a life-threatening disease. Many countries impose curfews and lockdown based on the impact of the COVID-19 virus and its variants. These restrictions by central and state public administrations affect the daily routines of individuals, professionals, and both private and public organizations. It creates a major impact on the global economy, thereby affecting all the sectors like education, tourism, manufacturing, automobile, etc. Many COVID-19 medication solutions like vaccines, drugs, self-testing home kits, diagnosis, and treatment procedures are being proposed by healthcare researchers and professionals in various instances. As the SARS-CoV-2 virus is mutating into different characteristics and spreading as an airborne disease, the rate of morbidity and mortality across the countries has become more critical to estimate [32]. The statistical data about the variants of coronavirus is very rare and almost not available for prediction and estimation. The evolving field of radiomics provides knowledge extraction from the clinical images that are acquired from different sources along with biological results.

AI plays a major role in the prediction and diagnosis of COVID-19 infections using various sources of datasets like CT X-ray images, reverse transcriptase-polymerase chain reaction (RT-PCR) examination results, the blood sample features, and the symptoms identified from the individuals. Many machine learning (ML) algorithms and CNN-based frameworks have been developed and published by researchers since January 2020. Apart from COVID-19-related predictions, recent technologies like the Internet of Things (IoT), fifth generation (5G) communication, and blockchain technologies are also adopted for the effective diagnosis and treatment of coronavirus-affected patients. AI-based noncontact measurement techniques of physiological parameters of an individual or group have become another research avenue during this pandemic situation [33]. Both ML and deep learning-based algorithms are applied to predict the spread of the disease, disease classification (pneumonia, non-pneumonia, COVID-19, and healthy), diagnosis, mortality risk, ICU admission, survival rate, and discharge period as illustrated in Fig. 3.

Machine Learning Algorithm-Based Predictive Tools

COVID-19 disease management is being carried out by many professionals to find out the mortality rate, ICU admission, prediction of disease, disease classification, and survival rate of the severely affected persons. To accomplish these tasks, LR, Extreme Gradient Boosting (XGBoost), SVM, neural networks (NN), random forest (RF), recurrent neural network (RNN), long short-term memory (LSTM), and least absolute shrinkage and selection operator (LASSO) have been considered either individually or as a combined model with others to arrive at the best results [34]. The performance measures like sensitivity, specificity, F1-score, accuracy, and AUC are incorporated in the proposed system to justify their outcomes.

Li et al. [35] collected a total of 413 patient data such as age, CT scan results, cough and fever signs, and blood sample results. These significant features were considered to distinguish influenza and COVID symptoms using the XGBoost model. They achieved a sensitivity and specificity of 92.5% and 97.9%, respectively. A similar dataset was collected [36] from the University Medical Centre Ljubljana to predict COVID-19 diagnosis using random forest (RF), deep neural network (DNN), and XGBoost. These data were collected from 5333 patients. They concluded that the MCHC, eosinophil ratio, prothrombin, INR, prothrombin percentage, and creatinine are the important factors that differentiate COVID infections from other bacterial infections.

Many articles related to COVID-19 are published based on machine learning and deep learning frameworks. Some of them are listed in Table 6.

Few researchers utilized LR to differentiate COVID infections from other respiratory disorders. Most of the datasets, considered as inputs to the expert systems, are patient-related information such as age; medical history; smoking habits; self-estimated results like cough, fever, sore throat, smell, and taste sensations; and complete blood count components [45, 48, 49]. Apart from this, LR has been adopted by

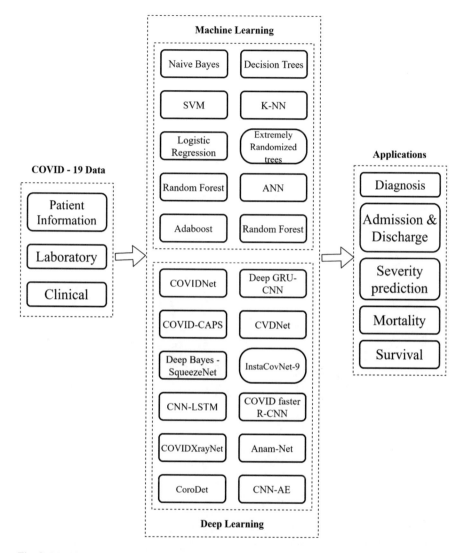

Fig. 3 Machine learning and deep learning approaches used for COVID-19 applications

many for the early prediction of COVID patients' mortality rate. Hu et al. [44] considered more than ten algorithms to find the mortality rate based on the data derived from 183 patients. Finally, they concluded that LR, partial least square (PLS) regression, elastic net, RF, and FDA yielded the best results by comparing the percentages of AUC. An interesting fact is that most of the non-survivors belong to the male gender and are older. From the results obtained by [50, 51], the proposed predictive tools suggest a few important factors that cause severe illness to coronavirus-infected patients. They are elevated heart rate, chronic obstructive pulmonary disease (COPD), comorbidities, respiration rate, CRP, partial saturation of oxygen (SpO_2), and LDH.

Table 6 ML and DL in COVID-19 diagnosis

Source	Sample size	Features	Algorithms/methodology	Performance
Chest CT image [37]	Training/validation: 106	Shape features, gray level size zone matrix (GLSZM), gray level dependence matrix (GLDM)	Feature selection: Maximum relevance minimum redundancy (MRMR)	AUC: 0.95 ± 0.029
				Accuracy = 88% ± 4.6 (95% CI: 0.88–0.89)
	Testing: 46		Classification: XGBoost	Sensitivity = 88% ± 6.6 (95% CI = 0.87–0.9)
				Specificity = 89% ± 7 (95% CI = 0.87–0.9)
Chest CT images [38]	Testing: 322	Visual features	COVID-19 detection neural network (COVNet)	AUC: 0.96
	Training: 3000			Sensitivity: 90% [95% CI: 83%, 94%]
				Specificity = 96% [95% CI: 93%, 98%]
Routine blood tests [39]	600 samples	Leukocytes, platelets, monocytes, eosinophils, and patient age quantile	DNN, CNN, RNN, LSTM	Accuracy: 92.5%
				Precision: 86.96%
				Sensitivity: 100%
				Specificity: 85%
				F1-score: 92.20%
Clinical and demographic data [40]	628 samples	Noninvasive features: S_pO_2, age, and cardiovascular disorders	Support vector machine-recursive feature elimination (SVM-RFE)	AUC: 0.92 ± 0.03
				Sensitivity: 0.81 ± 0.08
				Specificity: 0.91 ± 0.05
Chest X-ray images [41]	Pneumonia infected: 1628	NA	Ensemble deep convolutional neural network model	Precision: 98.33%
	COVID-19-positive patients: 1628			Recall: 98.33%
	Healthy patients: 2345			Accuracy: 99.71%
Chest X-ray images [42]	Normal: 1583	NA	Deep Bayes-SqueezeNet	Correctness: 98.26%
	Pneumonia: 4290 COVID-19: 76			Recall: 98.25%
				Accuracy: 98.26%
				F1-score: 98.25%

Source	Sample size	Features	Algorithms/methodology	Performance
Routine blood tests [43]	235 samples	Lymphocytes, leukocytes, and eosinophils	SVM	AUC: 85% Sensitivity: 68% Specificity: 85%
Patient data [44]	183 samples	Demographic, clinical, and laboratory data	Linear regression (LR), partial least square (PLS) regression, elastic net model (EN), flexible discriminant analysis (FDA)	AUC: 89.5% Sensitivity: 89.2% Specificity: 68.7%
Patient information [45]	43,752 samples	Age, gender, prior medical conditions, smoking habits, fever, sore throat, cough, shortness of breath, loss of taste or smell	Linear regression (LR)	AUC: 73.7%
CT and patient data [46]	413 samples	Age, CT scan result, temperature, lymphocyte, fever, coughing	XGBoost	Sensitivity: 92.5% Specificity: 97.9%
Patient information [47]	3524 samples	Sex, age	LR	AUC: 83%

Multiple algorithms are also considered for COVID data analytics by the researchers for the early prediction of disease diagnosis and the survival rate of the patients [38, 52]. Many methods have been deployed with a set of COVID data to predict the results. Each of their results ends up with certain predictions, cannot be taken as a universal solution for the same cause.

Deep Learning-Based Predictive Tools

Generally, the predictions can be performed through statistical approach and medical data analytics. As the number of COVID morbidity, diseased, recovered, and death rates is increasing day by day across the countries, the traditional methods such as mathematical modeling and statistical-based approaches are not encouraging to deal in a huge volume. Hence, the recent approach like deep neural network-based models is being imposed by many researchers. Many deeper neural network models with optimizers are adopted for COVID applications.

Karthik, R et al. [34] proposed a pixel-based upsampling module that encompasses an encoder to segment the chest CT images. This model provides a dice score of 85.43% and a recall of 88.10% for a dataset containing 50 samples of 3D CT scans chosen selectively from 1110 studies. A fuzzy rank-based algorithm along with the CNN model has been used to classify COVID and non-COVID cases from the CT scan images [53]. To rank the decision scores, three neural network models, namely, Visual Geometry Group (VGG), Wide ResNet, and Inception, were utilized. Optimized data augmentation and hyperparameter tuning techniques associated with CovidXrayNet yield 95.82% accuracy with only 30 epochs of training in finding the COVID disease classification [54].

A dynamic CNN model constructed from the modification of MobileNet and ResNet finds COVID-19 features from both chest CT and X-ray images. It has provided 99.6% test accuracy [55]. Anamorphic depth embedding-based lightweight CNN (Anam-Net) is a lightweight CNN [56] to find the anomalies from COVID-19 chest CT images. It extracts very few parameters to attain its task. This model has been implemented in Raspberry Pi, and other mobile-based Android applications to make it a point of care solution. Many COVID research articles explore the implications of deeper neural networks (DNN) on 3D chest images. To name a few, 3D DNNs are COVID-Nets, CNNBERT, LuMIRa, Telefax Library Network (TELINET), etc.

Summary

In this chapter, a complete overview of pandemic and epidemic diseases, disease transmission ways, and various pathogens evolved across the globe at different instances was discussed. The pandemic data can be analyzed through some statistical tools or mathematical models to predict the spread of disease and mortality and morbidity rates. During the mid-nineteenth century, mathematical models were imposed to know the severity of infectious diseases. During the interpretation by mathematical modeling, data inconsistency, nonavailability of global data, and lack of clinical and nonclinical data dropped the efficiency of the predicted results. Due to its simplicity, understanding of the data had been done through various assumptions. Constructing the mathematical model and execution time to arrive at the prediction results were not cost-effective. Data preprocessing and the removal of outliers are time-consuming processes. To overcome these limitations, machine learning-based algorithms have been adopted for various findings like severely infected person recovery rate, ICU admission, discharge rate, demographic widespread rate, etc. Such results helped both private and public sectors to take necessary steps before announcing night curfews and lockdowns across the country or part of it. Nowadays, the predictive peaks in data visualization alert the government to plan for healthcare establishments, procurement of drugs, and recurring and non-recurring medical facilities.

The analytics on COVID data supports the governments to know the number of citizens who have taken up first, second, and booster shots (if required). It also helped the pharmaceutical companies to know their vaccine efficacy during drug trials. The major factor to be considered while imparting machine learning-based predictive tools is data inconsistency due to variants of pathogens. During this COVID pandemic, almost 42 crore people were infected and around 58 lakhs were deceased. This is the highest pandemic infection rate after the French flu. This data is publicly available and announced by various governments daily. Apart from that, many have not been revealed to the outside world. Still, data collection is a crucial part of medical data analytics and predictions. To handle billions and billions of CT chest data, patient information, and blood-related features, in which machine learning algorithms were not capable of handling in a large volume, many researchers are proposing deeper neural networks to handle high-dimensional data. Still, a benchmark network to handle heterogeneous medical data is a golden opportunity for data analysts to explore. However, during this pandemic situation, the public is being advised to follow all safety procedures and protocols like social distancing, sanitizing the hands often, wearing masks, and vaccinating to help everyone to "stay safe."

Acknowledgments The authors would like to sincerely thank reviewers for their thoughtful comments and efforts toward improving this chapter. Also, they would like to extend their gratitude to the editors for considering this chapter and including it in the book.

References

1. M. Porta (ed.), *Natural history of disease. A Dictionary of Epidemiology*, 5th edn. (Oxford University Press, 2014), pp. 193–194
2. L. Shaw-Taylor, An introduction to the history of infectious diseases, epidemics and the early phases of the long-run decline in mortality. Econ. Hist. Rev. **73**(3), E1–E19 (2020)

3. J.F. Lindahl, D. Grace, The consequences of human actions on risks for infectious diseases: A review. Infect. Ecol. Epidemiol. **5**, 30048 (2015). https://doi.org/10.3402/iee.v5.30048
4. D. Grennan, What is a pandemic? JAMA **321**(9), 910 (2019). https://doi.org/10.1001/jama.2019.0700
5. J. Piret, G. Boivin, Pandemics throughout history. Front. Microbiol. **11**(631736), 1–16 (2021). https://doi.org/10.3389/fmicb.2020.631736
6. I. Ansari, G. Grier, M. Byers, Deliberate release: plague – A review. J. Biosaf. Biosecur. **2**, 10–22 (2020). https://doi.org/10.1016/j.jobb.2020.02.001
7. F.R. Chowdhury, Z. Nur, N. Hassan, L. von Seidlein, S. Dunachie, Pandemics, pathogenicity and changing molecular epidemiology of cholera in the era of global warming. Ann. Clin. Microbiol. Antimicrob. **16**, 10 (2017). https://doi.org/10.1186/s12941-017-0185-1
8. J.H. Beigel, F.G. Hayden, Influenza therapeutics in clinical practice-challenges and recent advances. Cold Spring Harb. Perspect. Med. **a038463** (2020). https://doi.org/10.1101/cshperspect.a038463
9. M.A. AlBalwi, A. Khan, M. AlDrees, U. Gk, B. Manie, Y. Arabi, et al., Evolving sequence mutations in the middle east respiratory syndrome coronavirus (MERS-CoV). J. Infect. Public Health **13**, 1544–1550 (2020). https://doi.org/10.1016/j.jiph.2020.06.030
10. A. El-Sayed, M. Kamel, Climatic changes and their role in emergence and re-emergence of diseases. Environ. Sci. Pollut. Res. **27**, 22336–22352 (2002). https://doi.org/10.1007/s11356-020-08896-w
11. M.A. Kadhim, M.A. Alam, H. Kaur, Design and implementation of fuzzy expert system of back pain diagnosis, international journal of innovative technology & creative. Engineering **1**(9), 16–22 (2011)
12. T. Di Noia, V.C. Ostuni, F. Pesce, G. Binetti, D. Naso, F.P. Schena, E. Di Sciascio, An end stage kidney disease predictor based on an artificial neural networks ensemble. Expert Syst. Appl. **40**(11), 4438–4445 (2013)
13. J.C. Boyd, Mathematical tools for demonstrating the clinical usefulness of biochemical markers. Scand. J. Clin. Lab. Invest. **57**(sup227), 46–63 (1997)
14. B.F. Finkenstädt, B.T. Grenfell, Time series modeling of childhood diseases: A dynamical systems approach. J. R. Stat. Soc.: Ser. C: Appl. Stat. **49**(2), 187–205 (2000)
15. M.I. Jordan, T.M. Mitchell, Machine learning: Trends, perspectives, and prospects. Science **349**(6245), 255–260 (2015)
16. H.A. Karaboga, A. Gunel, S.V. Korkut, I. Demir, R. Celik, Bayesian network as a decision tool for predicting ALS disease. Brain Sci. **11**(2), 150 (2021)
17. D. Akila, D. Balaganesh, Semantic web-based critical healthcare system using Bayesian networks. Mater. Today Proc. (2021). https://doi.org/10.1016/j.matpr.2021.01.870
18. V. Jackins, S. Vimal, M. Kaliappan, M.Y. Lee, AI-based smart prediction of clinical disease using random forest classifier and Naive Bayes. J. Supercomput. **77**(5), 5198–5219 (2021)
19. K. Ganji, S. Parimi, ANN model for users' perception on IOT based smart healthcare monitoring devices and its impact with the effect of COVID 19. J. Sci. Technol. Policy Manag. **13**(1), 6–21 (2021)
20. W. Yu, T. Liu, R. Valdez, M. Gwinn, M.J. Khoury, Application of support vector machine modeling for prediction of common diseases: The case of diabetes and pre-diabetes. BMC Med. Inform. Decis. Mak. **10**(1), 1–7 (2010)
21. Q. Jiang, G. Wang, S. Jin, Y. Li, Y. Wang, Predicting human microRNA-disease associations based on support vector machines. Int. J. Data Min. Bioinform. **8**(3), 282–293 (2013)
22. N.Z. Supardi, M.Y. Mashor, N.H. Harun, F.A. Bakri, R. Hassan, Classification of blasts in acute leukemia blood samples using k-nearest neighbor, in *2012 IEEE 8th International Colloquium on Signal Processing and Its Applications* (2012), pp. 461–465.
23. L. Prompers, N. Schaper, J. Apelqvist, M. Edmonds, E. Jude, D. Mauricio, L. Uccioli, V. Urbancic, K. Bakker, P. Holstein, A. Jirkovska, Prediction of outcome in individuals with diabetic foot ulcers: Focus on the differences between individuals with and without peripheral arterial disease. The EURODIALE study. Diabetologia **51**(5), 747–755 (2008)

24. D. Zhang, D. Shen, Alzheimer's disease neuroimaging initiative. Multi-modal multi-task learning for joint prediction of multiple regression and classification variables in Alzheimer's disease. NeuroImage **59**(2), 895–907 (2012)
25. X.D. Zhang, Machine learning, in *A matrix algebra approach to artificial intelligence*, (Springer, Singapore, 2020), pp. 223–440
26. P.S. Kohli, S. Arora, Application of machine learning in disease prediction, in *2018 4th International conference on computing communication and automation (ICCCA)* (IEEE, 2018), pp. 1–4.
27. K. Indhumathi, K.S. Kumar, A review on prediction of seasonal diseases based on climate change using big data. Mater. Today Proc. **37**, 2648–2652 (2021)
28. A. Kumar, T.V. Kumar, Multi-objective big data view materialization using MOGA. Int. J. Appl. Metaheuristic Comput. **13**(1), 1–28 (2022)
29. R. Chauhan, H. Kaur, V. Chang, An optimized integrated framework of big data analytics managing security and privacy in healthcare data. Wirel. Pers. Commun. **117**(1), 87–108 (2021)
30. O.A. Sarumi, C.K. Leung, Adaptive machine learning algorithm and analytics of big genomic data for gene prediction, in *Tracking and Preventing Diseases with Artificial Intelligence*, (Springer, Cham, 2022), pp. 103–123
31. N. Johanna, H. Citrawijaya, G. Wangge, Mass screening vs lockdown vs combination of both to control COVID-19: A systematic review. J. Public Health Res. **9**(4), 523–531 (2020)
32. P. Schwab, A.D. Schütte, B. Dietz, S. Bauer, Predcovid-19: A systematic study of clinical predictive models for coronavirus disease 2019. arXiv preprint arXiv:2005.08302 (2020)
33. J. Vijay, K. Nirmala, S.G. Sarate, Chapter 5: Non-contact measurement system for COVID-19 vital signs to aid mass screening – An alternate approach, in *Cyber-Physical Systems*, ed. by R. C. Poonia, B. Agarwal, S. Kumar, M. S. Khan, G. Marques, J. Nayak, (Academic Press, 2022), pp. 75–92
34. R.M. Karthik, M. Hariharan, D. Won, Contour-enhanced attention CNN for CT-based COVID-19 segmentation. Pattern Recogn. **125**, 108538 (2022)
35. L. Li, L. Qin, Z. Xu, Y. Yin, X. Wang, B. Kong, J. Bai, Y. Lu, Z. Fang, Q. Song, K. Cao, D. Liu, G. Wang, Q. Xu, X. Fang, S. Zhang, J. Xia, J. Xia, Using artificial intelligence to detect COVID-19 and community-acquired pneumonia based on pulmonary CT: Evaluation of the diagnostic accuracy. Radiology **296**(2), E65–E71 (2020). https://doi.org/10.1148/radiol.2020200905
36. M. Kukar, G. Guncar, T. Vovko, S. Podnar, P. Cernelc, M. Brvar, M. Zalaznik, M. Notar, S. Moskon, M. Notar, COVID-19 diagnosis by routine blood tests using machine learning. Sci. Rep. **11**, 10738 (2020)
37. I. Shiri, M. Sorouri, P. Geramifar, M. Nazari, M. Abdollahi, Y. Salimi, B. Khosravi, D. Askari, L. Aghaghazvini, G. Hajianfar, A. Kasaeian, H. Abdollahi, H. Arabi, A. Rahmim, A.R. Radmard, H. Zaidi, Machine learning-based prognostic modeling using clinical data and quantitative radiomic features from chest CT images in COVID-19 patients. Comput. Biol. Med. **132**, 104304 (2021)
38. S. Li, Y. Lin, T. Zhu, M. Fan, S. Xu, W. Qiu, C. Chen, L. Li, Y. Wang, J. Yan, et al., Development and external evaluation of prediction models for mortality of covid-19 patients using the machine learning method. Neural Comput. Applic., 1–10 (2020)
39. S.B. Rikan, A.S. Azar, A. Ghafari, J.B. Mohasefi, H. Pirnejad, COVID-19 diagnosis from routine blood tests using artificial intelligence techniques. Biomed. Signal Process. Control **72**, 103263 (2021). https://doi.org/10.1016/j.bspc.2021.103263
40. M. Mahdavi, H. Choubdar, E. Zabeh, M. Rieder, S. Safavi-Naeini, Z. Jobbagy, A. Ghorbani, A. Abedini, A. Kiani, V. Khanlarzadeh, R. Lashgari, E. Kamrani, A machine learning-based exploration of COVID-19 mortality risk. PLoS One **16**(7), e0252384 (2021). https://doi.org/10.1371/journal.pone.0252384
41. P. Kedia, R.K. Anjum, CoVNet-19: A deep learning model for the detection and analysis of COVID-19 patients. Appl. Soft Comput. **104**, 107184 (2021)

42. F. Ucar, D. Korkmaz, COVIDiagnosis-net: Deep bayes-squeezenet based diagnosis of the coronavirus disease (COVID-19) from X-ray images. Med. Hypotheses **140**(2020), 109761 (2019)
43. A. F. De Moraes Batista, J.L. Miraglia, T.H.R. Donato, A.D.P. Chiavegatto Filho, COVID-19 diagnosis prediction in emergency care patients: A machine learning approach.medRx (2020). https://doi.org/10.1101/2020.04.04.2005209
44. C. Hu, Z. Liu, Y. Jiang, O. Shi, X. Zhang, K. Xu, et al., Early prediction of mortality risk among patients with severe COVID-19, using machine learning. Int. J. Epidemiol. **49**(6), 1918–1929 (2020)
45. S. Shoer, T. Karady, A. Keshet, S. Shilo, H. Rossman, A. Gavrieli, et al., A prediction model to prioritize individuals for sars-cov-2 test built from national symptom surveys. Med **2**(2), 196–208 (2020). https://doi.org/10.1016/j.medj.2020.10.002
46. W.T. Li, J. Ma, N. Shende, G. Castaneda, J. Chakladar, J.C. Tsai, L. Apostol, C.O. Honda, J. Xu, L.M. Wong, T. Zhang, A. Lee, A. Gnanasekar, T.K. Honda, S.Z. Kuo, M.A. Yu, E.Y. Chang, M.R. Rajasekaran, W.M. Ongkeko, Using machine learning of clinical data to diagnose covid-19: A systematic review and meta-analysis. BMC Med. Inform. Decis. Mak. **20**, 247 (2020). https://doi.org/10.1186/s12911-020-01266-z
47. A.K. Das, S. Mishra, S.S. Gopalan, Predicting covid-19 community mortality risk using machine learning and development of an online prognostic tool. PeerJ **8**, e10083 (2020)
48. R.P. Joshi, V. Pejaver, N.E. Hammarlund, H. Sung, S.K. Lee, A. Furmanchuk, H.-Y. Lee, G. Scott, S. Gombar, N. Shah, S. Shen, A. Nassiri, D. Schneider, F.S. Ahmad, D. Liebovitz, A. Kho, S. Mooney, B.A. Pinsky, N. Banaei, A predictive tool for identification of sars-cov-2 PCR-negative emergency department patients using routine test results. J. Clin. Virol. **129**, 104502 (2020). https://doi.org/10.1016/j.jcv.2020.104502
49. M. Tordjman, A. Mekki, R.D. Mali, I. Saab, G. Chassagnon, E. Guillo, R. Burns, D. Eshagh, S. Beaune, G. Madelin, et al., Pre-test probability for sars-cov-2-related infection score: The Paris score. PLoS One **15**(12), e0243342 (2020). https://doi.org/10.1371/journal.pone.0243342
50. Z. Zhao, A. Chen, W. Hou, J.M. Graham, H. Li, P.S. Richman, H.C. Thode, A.J. Singer, T.Q. Duong, Prediction model and risk scores of ICU admission and mortality in covid-19. PLoS One **15**, e0236618 (2020)
51. H. Huang, S. Cai, Y. Li, Y. Li, Y. Fan, L. Li, C. Lei, X. Tang, F. Hu, F. Li, X. Deng, Prognostic factors for covid-19 pneumonia progression to severe symptoms based on earlier clinical features: A retrospective analysis. Front. Med. **7**, 643 (2020). https://doi.org/10.3389/fmed.2020.557453
52. M. Nemati, J. Ansary, N. Nemati, Machine-learning approaches in COVID-19 survival analysis and discharge-time likelihood prediction using clinical data. Patterns **1**, 100074 (2020)
53. R. Kundu, H. Basak, P.K. Singh, et al., Fuzzy rank-based fusion of CNN models using Gompertz function for screening COVID-19 CT-scans. Sci. Rep. **11**, 14133 (2021). https://doi.org/10.1038/s41598-021-93658-y
54. M.A. Maram, J.P. Monshi, V. Chung, F.M. Monshi, CovidXrayNet: Optimizing data augmentation and CNN hyperparameters for improved COVID-19 detection from CXR. Comput. Biol. Med. **133**, 104375 (2021)
55. G. Jia, H.-K. Lam, X. Yujia, Classification of COVID-19 chest X-Ray and CT images using a type of dynamic CNN modification method. Comput. Biol. Med. **134**, 104425 (2021)
56. N. Paluru, A. Dayal, H.B. Jenssen, T. Sakinis, L.R. Cenkeramaddi, J. Prakash, P.K. Yalavarthy, Anam-net: Anamorphic depth embedding-based lightweight CNN for segmentation of anomalies in COVID-19 chest CT images. IEEE Trans. Neural Netw. Learn. Syst. **32**(3), 932–946 (2021). https://doi.org/10.1109/TNNLS.2021.3054746

Deep Convolutional Generative Adversarial Network for Metastatic Tissue Diagnosis in Lymph Node Section

J. Arun Pandian, K. Kanchanadevi, Dhilip Kumar, and Oana Geman

Deep Convolutional Generative Adversarial Network

A generative adversarial network (GAN) is an unsupervised learning-based neural network [1]. The GANs are commonly used as a data augmentation technique in computer vision applications [2]. Also, the GANs are used to create unique animation characters on animation and gaming applications. Getting a larger dataset is one of the most reliable ways to improve the performance of classification techniques [3]. The GANs create new data without the collection of new real data for enhancing the training data. The GAN is a pair of deep neural networks, such as generator and discriminator [4]. The generator network in GAN generates new images based on the training data provided and a discriminator that attempts to distinguish between original and generator-produced data [5]. In every epoch, the generator and discriminator networks try to improve their performance. The new images are created by the generator to become more and more realistic than the previous epochs [6].

The objective of the GAN training process is to create a new image with more realistic image that cannot be identified as a fake image by the discriminator. If the

---

J. Arun Pandian (✉)
School of Information Technology and Engineering, Vellore Institute of Technology, Vellore, India

K. Kanchanadevi · D. Kumar
Computer Science and Engineering, Vel Tech Rangarajan Dr. Sagunthala R&D Institute of Science and Technology, Chennai, TN, India
e-mail: vdhilipkumar@veltech.edu.in

O. Geman
Stefan Cel Mare, University of Suceava, Suceava, Romania
e-mail: Oana.geman@usm.ro

© The Author(s), under exclusive license to Springer Nature Switzerland AG 2023
G. R. Kanagachidambaresan et al. (eds.), *System Design for Epidemics Using Machine Learning and Deep Learning*, Signals and Communication Technology, https://doi.org/10.1007/978-3-031-19752-9_9

generator creates a realistic image, then it means the discriminator will fail to differentiate between the real and fake image [7]. The training loss of the generator should be reduced in each epoch against the discriminator. Until achieving the minimum training loss for the generator, the training process of the GAN will be continued [8]. The simple GAN architecture was shown in Fig. 1.

The discriminator is generally known as a binary classifier, and it is trained to classify the real and fake input data [9]. It also uses the convolutional layers for extracting the features for the classification process. There are several GANs that are proposed for various applications [10]. The deep convolutional generative adversarial network (DCGAN) is one of the commonly used GANs for the data augmentation process [11]. The DCGAN is a type of GANs that uses the sequence of convolutional layers to generate and classify the images [12]. Simple DCGAN architecture is illustrated in Fig. 2. The left part of the figure shows the architecture of the generator network and the right part shows the architecture of the discriminator.

Transposed convolutional layers and dense layers are used to construct the generator in the GANs. The transposed convolutional layers are used for up-sampling the input features to the sample data in GANs [13]. Furthermore, the convolutional

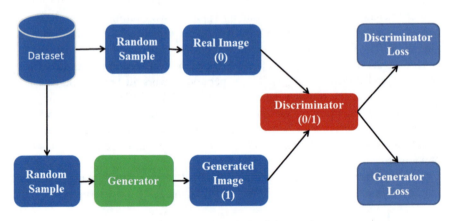

Fig. 1 The simple architecture of the generative adversarial network

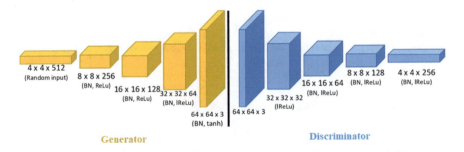

Fig. 2 The simple architecture of the deep convolutional generative adversarial network

and max-pooling layers are used to classify the real and fake data in the discriminator network of the GANs [14]. To balance the number of images and increase the number of samples in both classes, the DCGAN model was proposed in this research. The subsequent section discussed the implementation of the DCGAN for data augmentation on the PCam dataset.

Data Augmentation on PatchCamelyon Dataset Using DCGAN

A custom DCGAN model was proposed to generate augmented images on the PatchCamelyon (PCam) dataset in this section. The number of layers and filter or kernel size of each layer in the custom DCGAN model was optimized concerning the PCam dataset. Development of data augmentation process using DCGAN on PCam dataset was implemented on GPU environment. The PCam dataset preparation and DCGAN model development and training were discussed in the subsequent subsections.

PCam Dataset Preparation

The PatchCamelyon (PCam) dataset consists of 327,680 scanned lymph node section images [15]. Each image in the dataset is annotated with a binary label indicating the presence of metastatic tissue. The PCam dataset will be used to train the machine learning or deep learning model for the detection of metastatic tissues on lymph node section images. Figure 3 shows the random sample images on the PCam dataset.

Images on PCam dataset were resized to 64×64 pixels for training the DCGAN model. Also, the data are split with a batch size of 64 for efficient training. The data preparation part of the proposed work was developed using ImageDataGenerator in the TensorFlow keras package.

DCGAN Model Design and Parameter Optimization

Design and development of proposed DCGAN were developed using Python programming tool with TensorFlow keras library. Initially, one convolutional transpose layer was used to develop the model. The proposed DCGAN model receives 64×64 pixel sized images and generates the same resolution images. The binary cross-entropy loss technique was used in the proposed DCGAN model. The convolutional layers in the model have used the stride size of 2×2 pixels. The zero-padding technique was used after the completion of each convolutional transpose function. The LeakyReLU activation function was used in the convolutional layers of the

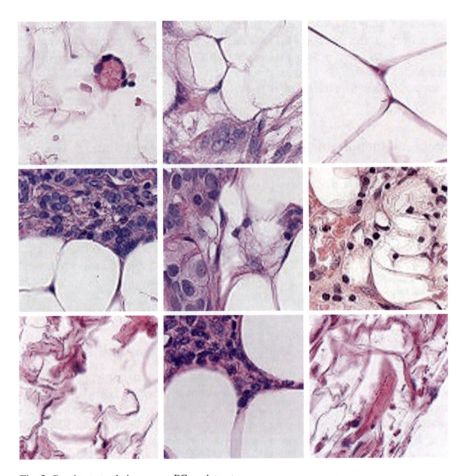

Fig. 3 Random sample images on PCam dataset

discriminator of the DCGAN network. One fully connected or dense layer was used in the discriminator of the DCGAN to classify the real and generated fake image.

The developed initial model was trained on the preprocessed PCam dataset. The initial DCGAN model was trained up to 100 epochs on GPU environment. The model achieved a training loss of 1.376 on the 100th training epoch. The initial model was extended using additional pair of convolutional transpose layer and batch normalization layer. The two convolutional transpose layer networks achieved a training loss of 1.079 on the 100th epoch, which is better than the initial model. After that, the model got updated using three pairs of convolutional transpose layers and a batch normalization layer. The updated model received the training loss of 0.792, after the completion of 100 epochs.

Furthermore, the number of convolutional transpose layers in the model was updated to four layers in the DCGAN model for PCam data augmentation. The four convolutional transpose layer DCGAN networks achieved 0.627 as a training loss

Table 1 Optimized hyperparameters for proposed DCGAN

Hyperparameters	Optimized value
Batch sizes	16
Optimizer	Adam
Learning rate	0.001

after the 100 epochs. But the training loss of the five convolutional transpose layer DCGAN networks was lesser than the four convolutional transpose layer DCGAN networks. The five convolutional transpose layer DCGAN networks received only 0.861 as a training loss after the completion of 100 training epochs.

The convolutional transpose layer extension process was ended with the four convolutional transpose layer DCGAN networks, since it achieved very less training loss than other variations of the DCGAN model on the PCam dataset. Also, the learning rate, batch size, and optimizer were tuned using random search hyperparameter optimization technique. Randomly selected hyperparameters were used to train the DCGAN model up to 100 epochs. Comparing several random selections, the optimization technique identified the most suitable combination of hyperparameter for training DCGAN on PCam dataset. The optimized hyperparameter values are illustrated in Table 1.

Figure 4 illustrates the complete layered architecture of the proposed four convolutional transpose layer DCGAN networks. The proposed DCGAN model for PCam data augmentation was trained up to 300 epochs on GPU environment. The training process of the proposed DCGAN model was discussed in the subsequent section.

Training the DCGAN on PCam Dataset

The proposed DCGAN model was trained up to 300 training epochs using optimized hyperparameter on PCam dataset for generating augmented images. The model used 90 percent of data for training and 10 percent of data for the validation process. Sample augmented images were visualized after completion of every 60 epochs while training. Also, the model weights were stored after the completion of every 60 training epochs. Nine random images were generated for the visualization after the completion of each 60 epochs.

The DCGAN model achieved the training loss of 0.453 after the completion of the first 60 epochs. The Matplotlib package was used to visualize the sample images after every 60 epochs and training plot of the proposed DCGAN model in this research. Figure 5 shows the sample augmented images that are generated by the DCGAN model after the training of 60 epochs.

The visual quality of the generated image after the first 60 epochs is very low. The discriminator effortlessly detected the generated fake images at this stage. The training loss of the discriminator is 0.168 at the stage of 60 training epochs. The visual quality of the sample images after the 120 training epochs was improved

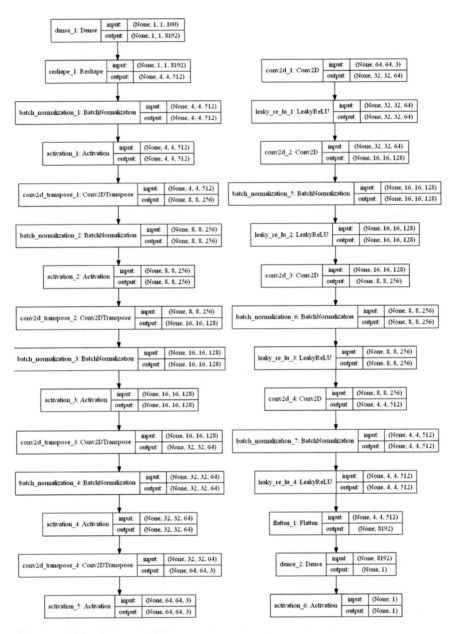

Fig. 4 The layered structure of proposed DCGAN

from the previous sample. Also, the training loss of the DCGAN model was 0.327 on the 120th training epoch, which is better than the previous checkpoint epoch.

The discriminator of the DCGAN model produced the training loss of 0.273 at the 120th training epoch. The positive changes in generator loss, discriminator loss,

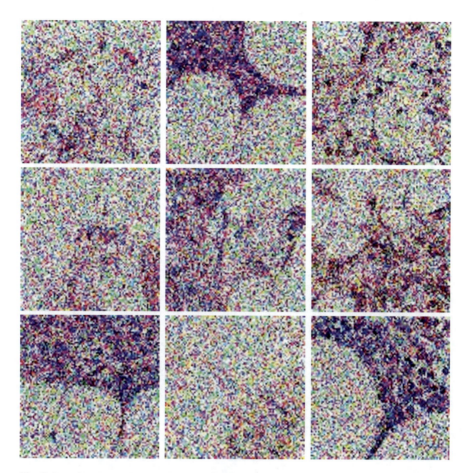

Fig. 5 Sample generated image after 60 training epochs

and the generated image quality gave the confidence to continue the training process of the DCGAN network on the PCam dataset for image augmentation. The trained weights of the proposed model were saved after the completion of 120 training epochs. The generated sample images after the completion of 120 training epochs were shown in Fig. 6.

The sample generated images after the completion of 180 epochs were illustrated in Fig. 7. Also, the image quality became improved compared with the previous epochs. The training loss of the generator at the stage of 180 epochs was 0.263.

The training loss of the model was reduced compared with the previous epochs. Figure 8 shows the sample generated images after completion of 240 training epochs with a training loss of 0.218.

Figure 9 illustrates the sample generated images after the completion of 300 training epochs on the GPU environment.

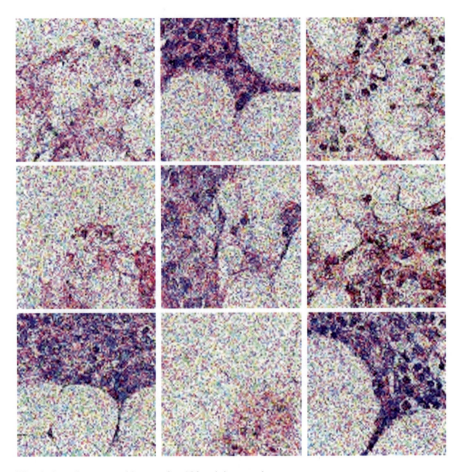

Fig. 6 Sample generated image after 120 training epochs

The model trained till 300 training epochs achieves the generator training loss of 0.137. The training loss of discrimination was increased because of the improvements in the generated image qualities. The sample generated image shows the improvement in image visibility compared with previous stages. Training loss changes in the entire training process were illustrated in Fig. 10.

The weights and architecture of the trained model were stored for future developments and testing processes. The trained model generated 37,856 unique augmented images. The image quality and performance of the proposed DCGAN model were discussed in the subsequent section.

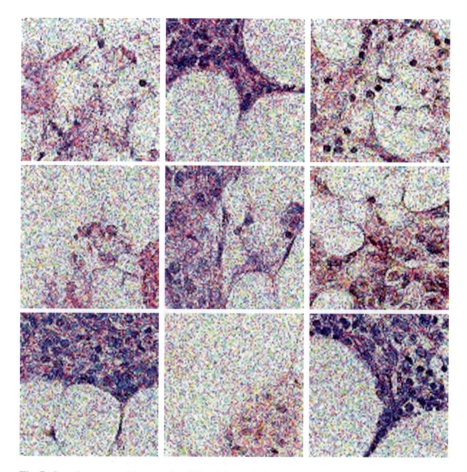

Fig. 7 Sample generated image after 180 training epochs

DCGAN Performance Testing Using Frechet Inception Distance

Frechet Inception Distance (FID) is a widely used performance measurement technique for GANs. The FID value of the proposed DCGAN was compared with existing state-of-the-art GAN techniques. The following figure compares the FID value of the proposed DCGAN model with existing techniques (Fig. 11).

The comparison result shows that the proposed DCGAN model performs superior to the existing GAN models. The subsequent section discussed the significance of the augmented dataset using the proposed DCGAN model.

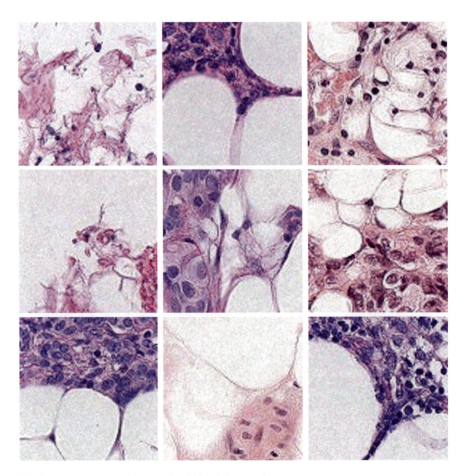

Fig. 8 Sample generated image after 240 training epochs

Development of Classification Models for Metastatic Tissue Detection

The augmented dataset was used to train the standard pre-trained models such as VGG19 Net and InceptionV3 Net. The classification models were used to examine the significance of the augmented dataset using the DCGAN model. Training and testing of both pre-trained models were performed in a GPU environment. The training and validation performance of the VGG19 Net was shown in Fig. 12.

After the completion of 300 training epochs, the model weights and architecture are stored for the testing process. Also, Fig. 13 illustrated the training and validation progress of the InceptionV3 Net.

In addition, the pre-trained models were trained on the original dataset. Around ten percentages of data was used to test the performance of the pre-trained models. The classification accuracy of the pre-trained models using original and augmented datasets was compared in the subsequent section.

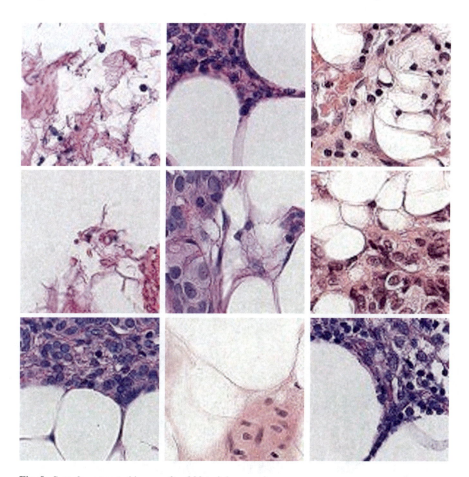

Fig. 9 Sample generated image after 300 training epochs

Results and Discussions

Classification accuracy of the pre-trained models using original and augmented datasets was compared in this section. And the classification accuracy of the models was measured using test data on the GPU environment. 1500 images are used to test the trained classification models. Figure 14 compares the classification accuracy of the VGG19 Net and InceptionV3 Net using original and augmented data.

The VGG19 Net model with an augmented dataset produced 96.48 percentages, and the InceptionV3 Net model achieves 99.26 percent of classification accuracy on test data. The comparison result shows that the augmented dataset used classification models produced superior classification accuracy to the non-augmented dataset used models.

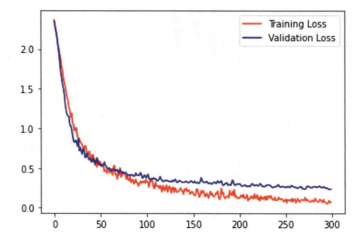

Fig. 10 Training loss of proposed DCGAN model

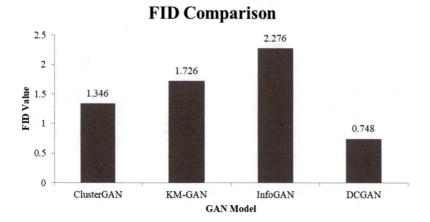

Fig. 11 Comparison of FID values

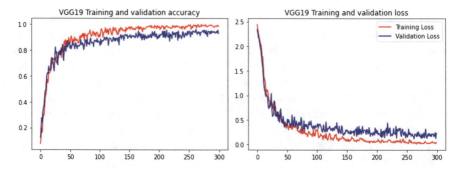

Fig. 12 Training progress of VGG19 Net

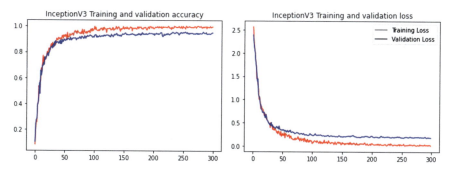

Fig. 13 Training progress of InceptionV3 Net

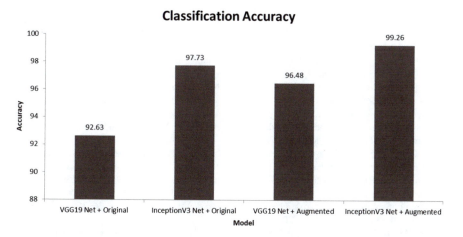

Fig. 14 Comparison of classification accuracy

Conclusion

Data augmentation is one of the commonly used approaches to increase the data samples without collecting new data. Data augmentation techniques can overcome the insufficient data issues in deep learning applications. The DCGANs are convolutional neural network-based GAN; it creates new data from the set of existing samples. A novel DCGAN was proposed in this chapter to generate additional samples on the PCam dataset for enhancing the performance of the classification models for detecting metastatic tissue on the lymph node section. There are four convolutional transpose layers that were used in the DCGAN model. The DCGAN model achieved an FID value of 0.748. The FID value of DCGAN was better than other standard GANs. Also, the importance of the augmented dataset was proved using state-of-the-art transfer learning-based classification techniques. The augmented dataset-based classification models performed superior to the original dataset-based model. The VGG19 Net and IncepptionV3 Net produced classification accuracy using augmented data were 97.73 and 99.26 percentages, respectively. In the future, the research will consider other recent data augmentation techniques also to enhance the performance of the metastatic tissue diagnosis model.

References

1. Z. Zheng, L. Zheng, Y. Yang, Unlabeled samples generated by GAN improve the person re-identification baseline in vitro, in *Proceedings of the IEEE International Conference on Computer Vision* (2017), pp. 3774–3782. https://doi.org/10.1109/ICCV.2017.405
2. J. Yang, A. Kannan, D. Batra, D. Parikh, LR-GAN: Layered recursive generative adversarial networks for image generation, in *5th International Conference on Learning Representations, ICLR 2017 – Conference Track Proceedings* (2017)
3. W. Fang, F. Zhang, V.S. Sheng, Y. Ding, A method for improving CNN-based image recognition using DCGAN. Comput. Mater. Contin. **57**, 167–178 (2018). https://doi.org/10.32604/cmc.2018.02356
4. P.L. Suarez, A.D. Sappa, B.X. Vintimilla, Infrared image colorization based on a triplet DCGAN architecture, in *IEEE Computer Society Conference on Computer Vision and Pattern Recognition Workshops* (2017), pp. 212–217. https://doi.org/10.1109/CVPRW.2017.32
5. X. Liang, L. Chen, D. Nguyen, Z. Zhou, X. Gu, M. Yang, J. Wang, S. Jiang, Generating synthesized computed tomography (CT) from cone-beam computed tomography (CBCT) using CycleGAN for adaptive radiation therapy. Phys. Med. Biol. **64** (2019). https://doi.org/10.1088/1361-6560/ab22f9
6. J. Chang, S. Scherer, Learning representations of emotional speech with deep convolutional generative adversarial networks, in *ICASSP, IEEE International Conference on Acoustics, Speech and Signal Processing* (2017), pp. 2746–2750. https://doi.org/10.1109/ICASSP.2017.7952656
7. X.-L. Tang, Y.-M. Du, Y.-W. Liu, J.-X. Li, Y.-W. Ma, Image recognition with conditional deep convolutional generative adversarial networks. Acta Automat. Sin. **44**, 855–864 (2018). https://doi.org/10.16383/j.aas.2018.c170470
8. K. Nazeri, E. Ng, M. Ebrahimi, Image colorization using generative adversarial networks, in *International Conference on Articulated Motion and Deformable Objects* (Springer, Cham, 2018). https://doi.org/10.1007/978-3-319-94544-6_9
9. F. Gao, Y. Yang, J. Wang, J. Sun, E. Yang, H. Zhou, A deep convolutional generative adversarial networks (DCGANs)-based semi-supervised method for object recognition in synthetic aperture radar (SAR) images. Remote Sens. **10** (2018). https://doi.org/10.3390/rs10060846
10. G. Hu, H. Wu, Y. Zhang, M. Wan, A low shot learning method for tea leaf's disease identification. Comput. Electron. Agric. **163**, 104852 (2019). https://doi.org/10.1016/j.compag.2019.104852
11. S. Lu, T. Sirojan, B.T. Phung, D. Zhang, E. Ambikairajah, DA-DCGAN: An effective methodology for DC series arc fault diagnosis in photovoltaic systems. IEEE Access **7**, 45831–45840 (2019). https://doi.org/10.1109/ACCESS.2019.2909267
12. G. Hu, J. Huang, Q. Wang, J. Li, Z. Xu, X. Huang, Unsupervised fabric defect detection based on a deep convolutional generative adversarial network. Text. Res. J. **90**, 247–270 (2020). https://doi.org/10.1177/0040517519862880
13. Y. Gao, B. Kong, K.M. Mosalam, Deep leaf-bootstrapping generative adversarial network for structural image data augmentation. Comput. Civ. Infrastruct. Eng. **34**, 755–773 (2019). https://doi.org/10.1111/mice.12458
14. H. Salehinejad, E. Colak, T. Dowdell, J. Barfett, S. Valaee, Synthesizing chest X-ray pathology for training deep convolutional neural networks. IEEE Trans. Med. Imaging **38**, 1197–1206 (2019). https://doi.org/10.1109/TMI.2018.2881415
15. B.S. Veeling, J. Linmans, J. Winkens, T. Cohen, M. Welling, Rotation equivariant CNNs for digital pathology, in *International Conference on Medical Image Computing and Computer-Assisted Intervention* (Springer, Cham, 2018). https://doi.org/10.1007/978-3-030-00934-2_24

Transformation in Health Sector During Pandemic by Photonics Devices

Jyoti Ahlawat, Archana Chaudhary, and Dinesh Bhatia

Introduction

Optical technologies pervade practically every facet of society, from microscopy to optical communications. As a result, it's not surprising that concepts presented have been identified in optical technologies and created by optical professionals to address the concerns of a global pandemic. Despite the fact that work from home conditions have hampered endeavors in research and development and manufacturing has been hampered by supply chain shortages, by modifying current systems and inventing new technologies, researchers and companies operating in photonics have significantly improved diagnostics and personal safety gear (PPE).

Many governments accelerated the approval of certain technologies or provided emergency use authorization in the context of the pandemic. As a response, the medical world had access to these precautionary measures within months.

Furthermore, to better meet COVID-19 standards, technologies were reconfigured or changed.

A development of systems for tracking and accelerating pharmaceutical remedies was highlighted in the mid- and long-term solutions. In order to decrease and manage COVID-19 transmission, a mix of software and technology is required to

J. Ahlawat
ECE Department, Faculty of Engineering & Technology, SGT University, Gurugram, Haryana, India

A. Chaudhary (✉)
Department of Environmental Science, Faculty of Science, SGT University, Gurugram, Haryana, India

D. Bhatia
Department of Biomedical Engineering, North Eastern Hill University, Shillong, Meghalaya, India

reliably track infected persons (diagnostics). While software solutions were immediately developed, effective diagnoses have been more difficult to adopt, owing to the various unanswered questions surrounding COVID-19's pathophysiology. As a consequence, numerous diagnoses, notably diagnosis using light (optical diagnostic), are being used to determine the disease's type right away.

In the meantime, scientists are working on developing therapeutics and vaccines. Several prospective solutions are being researched, but they are outside the scope of this perspective, in the hopes that one may be shown effective fast.

This viewpoint will address the function of optics in healthcare, including disinfection and diagnostic technology. A brief background is provided for both themes, followed by a more in-depth review of contemporary inventions and their societal influence. Finally, we explore the field's future potential and unresolved questions.

It's also worth mentioning that the basic strategy to vaccination and treatment studies has been rethought, potentially reducing time to market.

Existing Technologies for Healthcare Monitoring

Disease diagnosis has been important in medicine and healthcare since Hippocrates' time. Palpation and analysis of physical signs, such as temperature, were used in the early stages. Medical professionals and researchers developed more sophisticated diagnostic techniques as technology developed, such as analyzing the color and form of red blood cells. From the cellular to the molecular level, medical diagnosis has progressed in the current era, and device development is often facilitated by an integrated transducer platform. With the emergence of equipment like ex vivo and in vitro, there are now additional imaging methods besides MRI, NMR, and CT.

Integrated diagnostic platforms has shown the possibility to identify both molecular and protein signs of disease via mechanical, electrical, and photonic transmission methods. In scientific research, all three types of sensors have seen a lot of action. Individual cancer cells have been weighed. To test the efficacy of various therapies, cantilever-based mechanical sensor arrays were employed. Optical sensors built on photonics were used to explore specific antibody binding interactions, while DNA analysis and sequencing have both been done using electrical sensors built on nanopore arrays. Technology based on optics, on the other hand, is used in the majority of marketed diagnostic systems used in medical settings for illness diagnosis due to their simplicity and their ability to work with several different types of samples. As photonic biosensors have made the sickness diagnosis precision and accuracy, optical detectors have allowed illness monitoring, while laser-based medications and therapies have enhanced treatment effectiveness and lowered recovery period.

Many contemporary technologies have been quickly reconfigured for COVID-19 and are now being used for both self-development and self-illness progression tracking and diagnostics in a clinical environment.

As a result, before a diagnostic can be produced, the RNA or DNA must be obtained and sequenced, or the antibody responsible for the response must be identified. The former is more straightforward from a diagnostic standpoint because it identifies the illness directly. Furthermore, is it RNA or DNA? Tools that exist to identify sufferers' (who are not yet sick) active circulation infections.

An antibody-based diagnostic, contrasted with, depending on how the body's immunological system responds, implies the existence of the virus.

As a result, false positives are much more likely because it's an indirect indicator of illness. That also necessitates an understanding of the pathogen's particular antibody. Importantly, antibody-based approaches are used because they would only indicate a proper diagnosis. Despite the immune system's response, illnesses that have not yet manifested symptoms cannot be detected (Fig. 1).

As a result, it's not unexpected that an RNA-based test was developed and widely adopted far before an antibody-based assay in the case of COVID-19.

The nasal swab's viral RNA specimen was converted to DNA using conventional DNA techniques including reverse transcriptase chain of events. Following standard sample processing and handling techniques (RT-PCR), the DNA concentration was amplified to trace levels that use RT-PCR (Fig. 2).

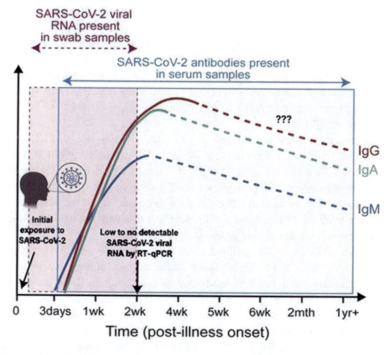

Fig. 1 Over time, the RNA and antibody levels that indicate a SARS-CoV-2 infection can change. Front. Immunol. 11, 879, Lee et al., used with permission (2020). (The writers, Copyright 2020, have agreed to abide under the conditions of an Open Source licenses Attribution 4.0 License)

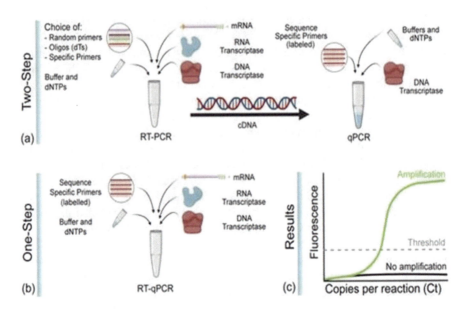

Fig. 2 It's crucial to remember in this method that RT-PCR and qPCR are two separate processes. Real-time concentration measurements can be made possible by combining qPCR with RT-PCR though. Real-time RT-PCR is the abbreviation for this technique (or RT-qPCR)

While RT-PCR improves sample concentration, a fluorescence-based sensing technology, called quantification PCR (qPCR), is commonly used for detection.

It's crucial to remember that qPCR and RT-PCR combine two independent processes. RT-PCR and qPCR can both be run simultaneously in this technique, allowing for real-time concentration. In brief, this method is known as RT-PCR in real-time (or RT-qPCR).

A comparison of PCR techniques for COVID-19 diagnosis. (a) PCR with two steps. RNA is first transformed using RT-PCR to DNA. So, using qPCR, the DNA is measured. This method enables the improvement of both reactions, although it takes longer than a single-step process. (b) PCR done in one step. Simultaneously, qPCR and RT-PCR are carried out exactly on the same vial at the same time. The two reactions are not optimal, despite the fact that this way is faster. (c) A graphic illustrates the many sorts of data generated and analyzed.

qPCR (and RT-qPCR) has profited enormously from several improvements on optical technology, including light sources, detectors, and novel fluorophores, that focuses particularly on fluorescent-based detection techniques. LEDs have a smaller footprint and a longer lifespan than traditional bulbs, which has resulted in smaller systems and lower maintenance and operating expenses. Signal multiplexing in high-performance systems has been facilitated by the accessibility of wide spectral range, sources with small linewidths, and detectors with great sensitivity. When paired with robotic sampling for autonomous handling, a single equipment can analyze hundreds of sample per hour with low false-positive/false-negative interest

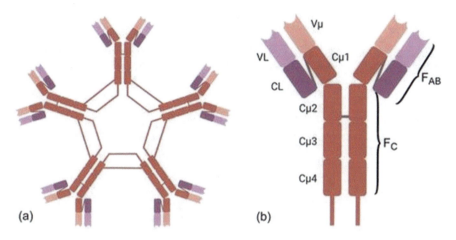

Fig. 3 Structure of immunoglobulin. (**a**) The IgM molecule is made up ten binding sites and five monomers are present. (**b**) There are two binding sites on a single monomer of IgG. At the conclusion of the FAB region, in the variable region of the monomer, are the binding sites

rates. Even though the technology needed for PCR has advanced greatly, PCR can only detect active infections since the RNA and DNA of the virus are instantly recognized and not infections that have occurred before the patient has recovered.

The largest antibody is IgM (Fig. 3), with ten binding sites made up of five monomers organized in a ring. A wide range of applications can use short linewidth sources and highly sensitive detectors. It's polyreactive and low-avid, so it can respond swiftly to unknown insults. IgM's activity depends on its low avidity; this enables it to be the immune system's antibody with the quickest response time. In the context of diagnostics, there's a chance that this feature will produce a lot of random positives.

While doing so, because of their short lifetime, the quick creation of these IgMs allows them to be used as a signal of active or recent infection. IgMs take about a week to develop in the immune system, and they only last about a week in the circulatory system.

IgG, on the other hand, is a dimer that has two flexible binding locations (Fig. 3). It takes that insult with a moderate to high avidity as it was created as a reaction to a particular offense. While IgG antibody concentrations take a few weeks to rise and stabilize, for months or even years, IgGs might circulate at a steady concentration. As a result, they are an excellent indicator of previous exposure.

It's worth noting, however, that the concentration and avidity of IgGs produced are linked to the severity of the original offense and the immunological response of the host. Because neither of these variables is known, the concentration observed for COVID-19 is not a reliable measure of how long after contact. Additionally, IgGs are crucial for the long-lasting immunity-boosting effects of customized vaccines. At this moment, it is unknown if the existence of COVID-19 IgGs denotes lifetime immunity.

Table 1 Description of typical COVID-19 diagnostic procedures

Test	Mechanism	Time for the test	Antibody presence	Concentration of antibodies	Effectiveness of antibodies
Rapid diagnostic test	Substrate changes color to indicate the presence of antibody	10–30 min	Yes	No	No
Neutralization assay test	Patient sample and virus are mixed with cells to determine the presence and efficacy of protecting cells	3–5 days	Yes	No	Yes
ELISA Chemiluminescent immunoassay	Substrate changes or emits color a series to indicate the presence of antibody of dilutions are run to obtain concentration	2–5 h	Yes	Yes	No

Most optical sensors used to detect COVID-19 antibodies have focused on recycling already-used signal readout technology, including such microplate scanners or fluorescent image sensors, and constructing simple colorimetric indications for point-of-care devices. IgG and IgM identifying approaches, data processing and chemical complexity, duration to results, and data that can be provided are all different between these procedures (Table 1). The precision and accuracy of the finding are demonstrated by all of these factors that have an impact on the false detection rates (or dependability). Because there are so many different diagnostic procedures, it's crucial to understand that "antibody test" relates to a broad category of testing that depends on finding antibodies.

A most common type of rapid diagnostic test (RDT) widely recognized antibody diagnostic procedure among the several antibody diagnostic tests.

Figure 4 depicts an RDT in a typical arrangement. With a little sample of blood, the user can make a diagnosis in 10–30 min by only keeping an eye on the two detecting strips' colors (as well as the control strip). These tests have swiftly grown in popularity given their low price and ease of use, and quick response time.

RDTs are one source of information that can be used, but until more reliable and better affinity antibodies are developed, healthcare decisions should not be made only on the basis of test results.

A basic set of physical signs has been established for identifying and keeping track of COVID-19 development, comprising, among many other things, oxygen saturation levels and temperature.

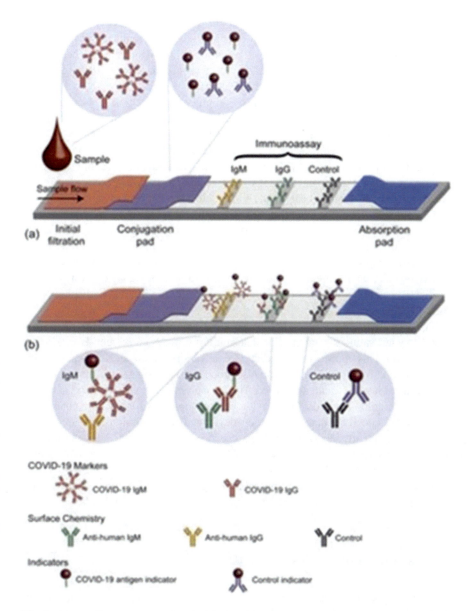

Fig. 4 shows a diagram representing the RDT. (**a**) The RDT has one control lane, two diagnostic lanes, and one diagnostic lane. On the conjugation pad, a metal nanoparticle is attached to both COVID-19 antigens and a control antibody. Following the three lanes, the material is dispersed throughout the conjugation pad. (**b**) The presence of the antibody is shown if a coloring of a strip changes

Despite the fact that both readings can suggest a variety of other conditions, they can give information quickly and cost-effectively without requiring costly equipment, blood tests, or nasal swabs. Furthermore, after a condition has been diagnosed, the measures can be used to track illness progression by performing it from home, thereby lessening the load on the healthcare system.

Since quite some time, the scientific community has widely used thermal imaging with standoff cams with infra (8–14 m) detectors, especially in the meteorological and aviation fields, but they are also used in environmental research to track climate change on a worldwide scale. On the other hand, these detectors were incredibly expensive and large. In reaction to SARS, standoff scanning methods rely on thermal imaging cameras that were created at airports and other high-traffic places several years ago to easily and swiftly detect the temperatures of passengers.

On the other hand, the switch to handheld devices required both a major reduction in size and cost and the inclusion of self-referencing capabilities. It was only lately that this precise combination was accomplished. Currently, standoff temperature measurements play a significant role in numerous businesses and governments observing COVID-19 initiatives. Internal temperature, though, is not always a good predictor because symptomatic carriers can transmit the virus while displaying no signs of illness.

Pulse oximetry, sometimes known as pulse-ox, is a technique for measuring blood oxygen saturation method of determining how much oxygen is carried by hemoglobin. This metric is a predictor of a variety of physical characteristics, including lung function. The most precise procedure is blood gas measurement, it is also the most intrusive and rarely used. The measurement of peripheral oxygen saturation is the gold standard of care. Although technologies for tracking changes in transmission and reflectance have been developed, transmission measurement is used more frequently because of its higher accuracy. Deoxygenated hemoglobin has an optical absorbance that is nearly 620–700 nm, which is a factor of 10 less than the oxygenated hemoglobin found in red blood cells. However, near-IR values (800–940 nm) are practically comparable. As a result, by comparing the two signals, it is possible to calculate the fraction of oxygenated hemoglobin.

Diagnostic Technologies on the Rise

The creation of biological or chemical sensors for the diagnosis of a variety of illnesses is a major area in integrated photonics.

Unlike the approaches previously addressed, the developing technologies utilize direct interactions between light and matter in the detection process and can be used in conjunction with microfluidics to deliver and analyze samples at high throughput. Given the diagnostic test shortages that plagued the COVID-19 pandemic early on, multiplexed or greater capabilities are very crucial.

The measurement of changes in optical transmittance and refractive index and the detection of optical scattering are two extensively used approaches for detecting and identifying specific chemicals in clinical samples.

Additionally, Biacore smart sensing techniques based on silicon-based photonic rings, transmission lines, and plasmonic nanotechnology are continually being developed in an attempt to provide more desirable analytical properties for quick screening and diagnosis. A popular example of these is the plasmon resonance resonance (SPR) biosensor. These platforms are now more mobile, thanks to advancements in optical component integration and nanofabrication technology. These sensors depend on a fundamentally simple idea known as subwavelength field sensing of the index of refraction shift.

They've also served as the cornerstone for portable diagnostic tools for Ebola and malaria virus detection. Due to their proven viability and excellent versatility, photonic biosensor technologies are a desirable option for cutting-edge COVID-19 diagnostics.

After the COVID-19 pandemic, researchers started working on photonic biosensors to discover the genetic material of SARS-CoV-2.

A plasmonic photothermal effect and localized SPR sensing are combined in the gold nanoisland-based sensing Fig. 5a, which improves the selected hybridization of base pairing while minimizing binding of associated targets without distinction. According to Qiu et al., the detection limit for the whole viral RNA strand was around 104 copies/ml, with detection range inside the picomolar (pM) range. Considering the infection rate, the sensitivity of the biosensor should, in theory, be appropriate for directly testing of clinical specimens without PCR as the average copy number of COVID-19 for throat/nasal swab of COVID-19-positive patients is around 105 and 106 copies/ml.

An ultimate goal is to directly identify live virus particles. By equipping the sensing surface with certain sensors (such as antibodies) directed toward the outside protein of the virus membrane, it is possible to collect entire virus entities that move through body fluids without the requirement of RNA extract and/or fragmentation

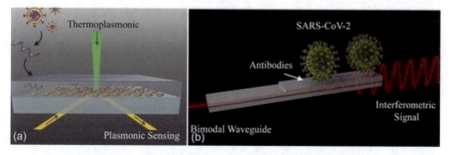

Fig. 5 (a) Schematic of a multifunctional nanostructures biosensing for COVID-19 RNA detection. (Reprinted in Qiu et al., ACS Nano 14, 5268, with permission (2020). The American Chemical Society is the owner of the rights to this composition). (b) A visual depiction of a nanophotonic bimodal waveguide interferometer for use in the detection of intact SARS-CoV-2 viruses

methods. This provides precise information on the live viral load in the patient. It is understandable that no information on SARS-CoV-2 virus detection techniques has been reported with photon biosensors because the analysis shows extremely specialized antibodies, which take longer to create as nucleic acid probes. Many significant projects of research are, nevertheless, currently in the works.

Technologies for Disinfection

While the current crisis serves as a catalyst, there is a global need for new disinfection technologies. Historically, medical settings have been the source of the bulk of antibiotic-resistant bacterial illnesses. In 2019, however, there was a significant change. The frequency of infections that occur in medical settings has decreased as a result of the heroic efforts made by the medical community to enhance disinfection and sterilization.

However, due to community-based transmission, the aggregate numbers have continued to rise. Furthermore, many disinfection techniques presume easy access to chemicals and produce a lot of waste.

Alternative approaches must be developed and assessed to increase the availability of cleaning procedures in areas with limited resources, lessen the impact on the environment, and enhance usage.

An initial stage in developing a disinfection procedure is to assess the biological contaminant's major components. The fundamental components of coronavirus are its envelope proteins, RNA, and spike glycoprotein, in that order, which are responsible for stability, replication, and cell targeting abilities.

A virus will be inactivated if any of these components are eliminated. As a result, most disinfection treatments are tailored to one or more of these components. Thermal, chemical, and radiation approaches are the three broad categories (Fig. 6).

Thermal approaches, predominantly based on the thermal dose, have an impact just on envelope protein via the spike glycoprotein (heat and duration). Thermal disinfection remedies a simple open flame or even boiling hot water, and they may be the first to be developed. On the other hand, more precisely both dry and moist heat can be used in controlled systems, which depend on ovens or even other substantial chambers. They are especially good for linens because they treat a sample equally, but they may be used for a wide range of goods, including surgical equipment.

Targeting a spike's glycoprotein as well as the envelope protein is done chemically using agents like chlorine and hydrogen peroxide.

Both chemical vapor treatments and hand sanitizers have been created. The best disinfection techniques on surfaces or solid objects are wipe-based chemical approaches since they are rapid to remove, are both monolayers, and have greater quantities of pollutants.

Chemical approaches, on the other hand, have the limitation of only destabilizing viruses with which they directly interact. A hybrid system, which combines both

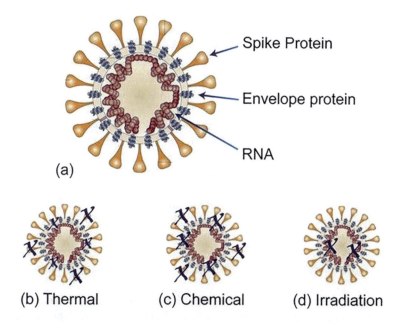

Fig. 6 Shows a virus will be inactivated if any of these components are eliminated. As a result, most disinfection treatments are tailored to one or more of these components. Thermal, chemical, and radiation are the three broad categories

heat and chemical processes, is widely used to increase the effectiveness of material with complex topologies, like linens.

Disinfection with ozone (O_3) is under a different category from chemical disinfection because of its unique mechanism. Ozone, as a potent oxidant, can eliminate all RNA's nucleotide bases, glycoproteins, envelope proteins, and other proteins. The application of ozone on porous or solid surfaces is possible because it is a gas. Furthermore, the method is particularly desirable because it doesn't require high temperatures. Ozone, however, is incredibly reactive and transforms into oxygen gas very quickly (O_2). Consequently, using it is really difficult.

Systems that disinfect using radiation are the most current advancement in disinfection technology. Systems in this category include IR, UV-C, and microwave systems. Infrared and microwave-based devices often work in a circumstantial way. Water is excited by radiofrequency radiation or microwaves, which heats it and thermally breaks down the spike glycoprotein. As a result, it is a form of moist thermal disinfection that uses microwave radiation. Similar reasoning applies to information retrieval systems that can be classified as being either dry or wet steam turbines given that thermal sources include IR sources. Contrarily, systems based on UV-C operate quite differently.

With regard to UV-C, COVID-19 has demonstrated to be effective particularly at sanitizing the PPE, including face masks, face shields, and eyewear, that protects healthcare personnel from airborne pathogens.

This capability has aided in meeting the enormous surge in demand for PPE that has posed a threat to the safety of healthcare workers. Governments tried to loosen import restrictions to lessen the impact on PPE delivery networks during the worst of the initial COVID-19 crisis, but healthcare professionals in numerous countries were nevertheless forced to recycle a significant amount of their PPE. Despite the fact that many nations have passed the peak of COVID-19, outbreaks are predicted to continue until a vaccine is widely accessible. For the time being, as a result, it will be necessary to develop methods that enable safe PPE reuse in emergency situations. This means that hypothetical PPE shortages will actually occur. One technique for cleaning personal protective equipment is UV-C.

However, because UV-C has catastrophic health effects for both people and viruses, including irreversible blindness, DNA and RNA are both destroyed by the universal damage process. Thermal and radiation technologies have a substantial advantage over chemical procedures in that they require very little consumables. This distinction is noteworthy for various reasons. First, when compared to chemical procedures, both the volume of garbage produced and its impact on the environment are reduced. Furthermore, the dependency on supply chains and production is lessened.

Currently, three basic strategies for PPE disinfection are being researched: traditional biosafety cabinets are being reconfigured, covered transportable boxes with only one source of UV-C or a collection sources of UV-C are being made, and broad spaces with powerful sources of UV-C in the middle are being constructed. In contrast to the third approach, the first two methods can only sanitize, however, could disinfect hundreds of N95 masks, whereas the other two methods could only sterilize a few to just a few dozen N95 face masks or face protection at a time simultaneously. A third method, on the other hand, needs much more expensive infrastructure.

Its UV-C dose threshold for degradation processes has been thoroughly studied because of the material's vital role within N95 mask's filtering performance. One study looked at the ratio between the UV-C radiation required to disinfect wounds and the mask's structural stability using biosafety cabinets which serve as the source of UV-C. The effectiveness of the N95 masks' filtering was shown to be unaffected by sterilizer cabinet after 20 cycles (from 95% to 93%). N95 masks were not physically harmed at any dose below 4.5 J/cm^2, although this value varies widely, and in certain cases, levels as high as 120 J/cm^2 could be safe.

This figure develops a "damage threshold" criterion for various PPE types.

During disinfection, the surroundings of the mask could potentially harm it. Because humidity hastens the disinfection process, thermal treatments are typically carried out in a moist or muggy environment. The masks' filtration is reduced to 80% during ten cycles by the humidity, which has the opposite effect.

It is obvious that the environment is an important component to consider and control when compared to an UV sterilization cabinet or the 95% filtering for a dry oven.

The lowest dosage necessary to disinfect a surface sets a lower restriction. In contrast, the damage threshold places a cap on the total dosage. A 17 mW/cm2 for 30 min (30.6 J/cm2) therapies were beneficial in one research.

UV-based disinfection is used exclusively while wearing N95 masks and has a current scientific foundation according to this study.

Future Outlook and Conclusion

Optical technology has directly aided in both the prevention and diagnosis of COVID-19. The pervasiveness of photonics technologies is exemplified by this. Many of the technologies covered here are currently used in society and in medical facilities, although some were in the early stages but have not been realized. High-throughput diagnoses involving photonics, robots, and artificial intelligence and automated disinfection using these technologies will both see significant expansion (AI). Intelligent revolutions are occurring in both robotics and AI as a result of synergistic developments, like the case of automated robots.

Our method of cleaning and diagnosis may be transformed if these sophisticated automated systems are combined using photonic-based diagnostics or disinfection technologies.

Environmental applications, such as air and water purification, were among the early uses of UV-C disinfection, and this sector is still the biggest today. The majority of these units have typically employed filtration which should be used in conjunction with pollutants breakdown and removal to stop the spread of airborne mold or other respiratory problems particles. Because COVID-19 spread through airborne transmission, incorporating the use of UV-C in ventilators is one method to potentially lower transmission in enclosed spaces.

A UV-C would be especially appealing for this use because it has the ability to disinfect without needing direct human participation. The total dose required, operating expenses, and the capacity to resupply the source of UV-C are just a few of the challenges that must be taken into account for long-term, efficient operation. The optimum source would be high-power UV LEDs for this kind of system due to its low operating costs, stable emission intensity throughout time, and lengthy working lifetime. On the other hand, highly powerful UV LEDs initially cost substantially more than mercury lamps. Decision-making in this application will therefore be significantly impacted by developments in photonics production. Finally, direct transmission from one person to another would not be prevented by this method.

The likelihood of pathogen transmission via ventilation systems in this instance is not quite certain.

In a related application, cleaning surfaces with which we have direct contact is labor-intensive. Maintaining cleanliness in crowded settings like public transportation, restrooms, and sporting venues is quite difficult. The danger of transmission at these high-contact locations is therefore very significant. An autonomous robot with the ability to work alone could reduce the risk of transmission through regular disinfecting.

Due to the fact that many seasonal flu viruses are spread via surfaces, this capability will improve future healthcare in addition to reducing infections during the ongoing COVID-19 pandemic. Although there is no doubt that modern technology helps society, it has certain drawbacks.

Recognizing and resolving ethical and safety concerns are equally important.

To prevent them from getting in touch with the UV-C source, for instance, a robotic system that is autonomous and interacts with people and other dogs must have safety features incorporated in and discussions are also being held about the difficult ethical environment that robotics and AI are occupying.

It has become abundantly obvious throughout the COVID-19 pandemic that diagnosis, which depends on biotechnology and sensing techniques, is very challenging. Additionally, many different sample types can be studied. The majority of contemporary antibody testing uses blood, but formerly, nose swabs were the most frequent entry site. Due to this variation, numerous robotic sample handling systems were created, using lower sample quantities and fewer chemicals as per the test. Throughput was greatly boosted by the robotic systems' accelerated sample processing. However, a large portion of these robotic devices depended on microbial pathogens and exclusive polymers. Due to supplier limitations, diagnostic labs have been forced to create their own supply chains by several facilities. The reliance on external vendors, especially for vital reagents, is always something to take into account while designing a new diagnostic.

Antibody testing can produce false positives as well as false negatives, as was previously mentioned. As a result, in order to increase accuracy, it is crucial to look at more than just one test result. Instead, examine the outcome in light of a patient's other symptoms. In addition, time-to-result, or how quickly a diagnostic test delivers a response, is crucial given the high risk of transmission. While optical sensors offer quick responses, extra information is needed to contextualize those results.

By combining these results with an AI powered by machine learning and designed to contextualize the results, doctors will have the resources they need to make faster, more accurate treatment decisions. Such a technology might transform our approach to patient care, in addition to advancing the present COVID-19 treatment plan.

On the other hand, in order for machine learning systems to be effective, they also need extensive learning libraries and a deeper understanding of disease pathophysiology.

Since COVID-19 is so new, it can be challenging to get this important data.

Bibliography

1. J. de Anda, E.Y. Lee, C.K. Lee, R.R. Bennett, X. Ji, S. Soltani, M.C. Harrison, A.E. Baker, Y. Luo, T. Chou, G.A. O'Toole, A.M. Armani, R. Golestanian, G.C.L. Wong, ACS Nano **11**, 9340 (2017). https://doi.org/10.1021/acsnano.7b04738
2. F. Wang, H. Wan, Z. Ma, Y. Zhong, Q. Sun, Y. Tian, L. Qu, H. Du, M. Zhang, L. Li, H. Ma, J. Luo, Y. Liang, W.J. Li, G. Hong, L. Liu, H. Dai, Nat. Methods **16**, 545 (2019). https://doi.org/10.1038/s41592-019-0398-72.3
3. W. Zipfel, R. Williams, W. Webb, Nat. Biotechnol. **21**, 1368 (2003). https://doi.org/10.1038/nbt899
4. D.M. Lukin, C. Dory, M.A. Guidry, K.Y. Yang, S.D. Mishra, R. Trivedi, M. Radulaski, S. Sun, D. Vercruysse, G.H. Ahn, J. Vučković, Nat. Photonics **14**, 330 (2020). https://doi.org/10.1038/s41566-019-0556-6
5. A. Kovach, D. Chen, J. He, H. Choi, A.H. Dogan, M. Ghasemkhani, H. Taheri, A.M. Armani, Adv. Opt. Photonics **12**, 135 (2020). https://doi.org/10.1364/aop.376924
6. A.N. Willner, P. Liao, K. Zou, Y. Cao, A. Kordts, M. Karpov, M.H.P. Pfeiffer, A. Almaiman, A. Fallahpour, F. Alishahi, K. Manukyan, M. Tur, T.J. Kippenberg, A.E. Willner, Opt. Lett. **43**, 5563 (2018). https://doi.org/10.1364/ol.43.005563
7. R. Verity, L.C. Okell, I. Dorigatti, P. Winskill, C. Whittaker, N. Imai, G. Cuomo-Dannenburg, H. Thompson, P.G.T. Walker, H. Fu, A. Dighe, J.T. Griffin, M. Baguelin, S. Bhatia, A. Boonyasiri, A. Cori, Z. Cucunubá, R. FitzJohn, K. Gaythorpe, W. Green, A. Hamlet, W. Hinsley, D. Laydon, G. Nedjati-Gilani, S. Riley, S. van Elsland, E. Volz, H. Wang, Y. Wang, X. Xi, C.A. Donnelly, A.C. Ghani, N.M. Ferguson, Lancet Infect. Dis. **20**, 669 (2020). https://doi.org/10.1016/s1473-3099(20)30243-7
8. M. Satyanarayana, Chem. Eng. News (2020). https://cen.acs.org/analytical-chemistry/diagnostics/Shortage-RNA-extraction-kits-hampers/98/web/2020/03
9. Y.J. Kim, H. Sung, C.-S. Ki, M. Hur, Ann. Lab. Med. **40**, 349 (2020). https://doi.org/10.3343/alm.2020.40.5.349
10. A.S. Fauci, H.C. Lane, R.R. Redfield, N. Engl. J. Med. **382**, 1268 (2020). https://doi.org/10.1056/nejme2002387
11. C. del Rio, P.N. Malani, J. Am. Med. Assoc. **323**, 1339 (2020). https://doi.org/10.1001/jama.2020.3072
12. D. Cereda, M. Tirani, F. Rovida, V. Demicheli, M. Ajelli, P. Poletti, F. Trentini, G. Guzzetta, V. Marziano, A. Barone, M. Magoni, S. Deandrea, G. Diurno, M. Lombardo, M. Faccini, A. Pan, R. Bruno, E. Pariani, G. Grasselli, A. Piatti, M. Gramegna, F. Baldanti, A. Melegaro, and S. Merler, arXiv:2003.09320 [q-Bio] (2020)
13. A.M. Armani, D.E. Hurt, D. Hwang, M.C. McCarthy, A. Scholtz, Nat. Rev. Mater. **5**, 403 (2020). https://doi.org/10.1038/s41578-020-0205-1
14. I. Santiago, ChemBioChem (published online 2020). https://doi.org/10.1002/cbic.202000250
15. L. Liao, W. Xiao, M. Zhao, X. Yu, H. Wang, Q. Wang, S. Chu, Y. Cui, ACS Nano **14**, 6348 (2020). https://doi.org/10.1021/acsnano.0c03597
16. K. J. Card, D. Crozier, A. Dhawan, M. Dinh, E. Dolson, N. Farrokhian, V. Gopalakrishnan, E. Ho, E. S. King, N. Krishnan, G. Kuzmin, J. Maltas, J. Pelesko, J. A. Scarborough, J. G. Scott, G. Sedor, D. T. Weaver, medRxiv:2020.03.25.20043489 (2020)
17. R.C. She, D. Chen, P. Pak, D.K. Armani, A. Schubert, A.M. Armani, Biomed. Opt. Express **11**, 4326 (2020). https://doi.org/10.1364/boe.395659
18. L. Zou, F. Ruan, M. Huang, L. Liang, H. Huang, Z. Hong, J. Yu, M. Kang, Y. Song, J. Xia, Q. Guo, T. Song, J. He, H.-L. Yen, M. Peiris, J. Wu, N. Engl. J. Med. **382**, 1177 (2020). https://doi.org/10.1056/nejmc2001737
19. C.Y.-P. Lee, R.T.P. Lin, L. Renia, L.F.P. Ng, Front. Immunol. **11**, 879 (2020). https://doi.org/10.3389/fimmu.2020.00879

20. C. Wang, W. Li, D. Drabek, N.M.A. Okba, R. van Haperen, A.D.M.E. Osterhaus, F.J.M. van Kuppeveld, B.L. Haagmans, F. Grosveld, B.-J. Bosch, Nat. Commun. **11**, 2251 (2020). https://doi.org/10.1038/s41467-020-16256-y
21. Q.-X. Long, B.-Z. Liu, H.-J. Deng, G.-C. Wu, K. Deng, Y.-K. Chen, P. Liao, J.-F. Qiu, Y. Lin, X.-F. Cai, D.-Q. Wang, Y. Hu, J.-H. Ren, N. Tang, Y.-Y. Xu, L.-H. Yu, Z. Mo, F. Gong, X.-L. Zhang, W.-G. Tian, L. Hu, X.-X. Zhang, J.-L. Xiang, H.-X. Du, H.-W. Liu, C.-H. Lang, X.-H. Luo, S.-B. Wu, X.-P. Cui, Z. Zhou, M.-M. Zhu, J. Wang, C.-J. Xue, X.-F. Li, L. Wang, Z.-J. Li, K. Wang, C.-C. Niu, Q.-J. Yang, X.-J. Tang, Y. Zhang, X.-M. Liu, J.-J. Li, D.-C. Zhang, F. Zhang, P. Liu, J. Yuan, Q. Li, J.-L. Hu, J. Chen, A.-L. Huang, Nat. Med. **26**, 845 (2020). https://doi.org/10.1038/s41591-020-0897-1
22. C. Liu, Q. Zhou, Y. Li, L.V. Garner, S.P. Watkins, L.J. Carter, J. Smoot, A.C. Gregg, A.D. Daniels, S. Jervey, D. Albaiu, ACS Cent. Sci. **6**, 315 (2020). https://doi.org/10.1021/acscentsci.0c00272
23. G. Lippi, M. Plebani, Clin. Chem. Lab. Med. **58**, 1063 (2020). https://doi.org/10.1515/cclm-2020-0240
24. S. Jiang, C. Hillyer, L. Du, Trends Immunol. **41**, 355 (2020). https://doi.org/10.1016/j.it.2020.03.007
25. J. Alijotas-Reig, E. Esteve-Valverde, C. Belizna, A. Selva-O'Callaghan, J. Pardos-Gea, A. Quintana, A. Mekinian, A. Anunciacion-Llunell, F. Miró-Mur, Autoimmun. Rev. **19**, 102569 (2020). https://doi.org/10.1016/j.autrev.2020.102569
26. S.F. Ahmed, A.A. Quadeer, M.R. McKay, Viruses **12**, 254 (2020). https://doi.org/10.3390/v12030254
27. B.E. Young, S.W.X. Ong, S. Kalimuddin, J.G. Low, S.Y. Tan, J. Loh, O.-T. Ng, K. Marimuthu, L.W. Ang, T.M. Mak, S.K. Lau, D.E. Anderson, K.S. Chan, T.Y. Tan, T.Y. Ng, L. Cui, Z. Said, L. Kurupatham, M.I.-C. Chen, M. Chan, S. Vasoo, L.-F. Wang, B.H. Tan, R.T.P. Lin, V.J.M. Lee, Y.-S. Leo, D.C. Lye, Singapore 2019 Novel Coronavirus Outbreak Research Team, J. Am. Med. Assoc. **323**, 1488 (2020). https://doi.org/10.1001/jama.2020.3204
28. X. Tang, C. Wu, X. Li, Y. Song, X. Yao, X. Wu, Y. Duan, H. Zhang, Y. Wang, Z. Qian, J. Cui, J. Lu, Natl. Sci. Rev. **7**, 1012 (2020). https://doi.org/10.1093/nsr/nwaa036
29. S. Sun, X. Cai, H. Wang, G. He, Y. Lin, B. Lu, C. Chen, Y. Pan, X. Hu, Clin. Chim. Acta **507**, 174 (2020). https://doi.org/10.1016/j.cca.2020.04.024
30. J. Shang, Y. Wan, C. Luo, G. Ye, Q. Geng, A. Auerbach, F. Li, Proc. Natl. Acad. Sci. U. S. A. **117**, 11727 (2020). https://doi.org/10.1073/pnas.2003138117
31. G. Li, E. De Clercq, Nat. Rev. Drug Discov. **19**, 149 (2020). https://doi.org/10.1038/d41573-020-00016-0
32. T.T.-Y. Lam, N. Jia, Y.-W. Zhang, M.H.-H. Shum, J.-F. Jiang, H.-C. Zhu, Y.-G. Tong, Y.-X. Shi, X.-B. Ni, Y.-S. Liao, W.-J. Li, B.-G. Jiang, W. Wei, T.-T. Yuan, K. Zheng, X.-M. Cui, J. Li, G.-Q. Pei, X. Qiang, W.Y.-M. Cheung, L.-F. Li, F.-F. Sun, S. Qin, J.-C. Huang, G.M. Leung, E.C. Holmes, Y.-L. Hu, Y. Guan, W.-C. Cao, Nature **583**, 282 (2020). https://doi.org/10.1038/s41586-020-2169-0
33. O. Altay, E. Mohammadi, S. Lam, H. Turkez, J. Boren, J. Nielsen, M. Uhlen, A. Mardinoglu, iScience **23**, 101303 (2020). https://doi.org/10.1016/j.isci.2020.101303
34. S.E. McBirney, D. Chen, A. Scholtz, H. Ameri, A.M. Armani, ACS Sens. **3**, 1264 (2018). https://doi.org/10.1021/acssensors.8b00269
35. S. Frustaci, F. Vollmer, Curr. Opin. Chem. Biol. **51**, 66 (2019). https://doi.org/10.1016/j.cbpa.2019.05.003
36. A. Raj, A.K. Sen, in *Environmental, Chemical and Medical Sensors*, ed. by S. Bhattacharya, A.K. Agarwal, N. Chanda, A. Pandey, A.K. Sen (Springer, 2018), pp. 389–408
37. S. Mehrabani, A. Maker, A. Armani, Sensors **14**, 5890 (2014). https://doi.org/10.3390/s140405890
38. D. Duval, A.B. González-Guerrero, S. Dante, J. Osmond, R. Monge, L.J. Fernández, K.E. Zinoviev, C. Domínguez, L.M. Lechuga, Lab Chip **12**, 1987 (2012). https://doi.org/10.1039/c2lc40054e

39. K.K.-W. To, O.T.-Y. Tsang, W.-S. Leung, A.R. Tam, T.-C. Wu, D.C. Lung, C.C.-Y. Yip, J.-P. Cai, J.M.-C. Chan, T.S.-H. Chik, D.P.-L. Lau, C.Y.-C. Choi, L.-L. Chen, W.-M. Chan, K.-H. Chan, J.D. Ip, A.C.-K. Ng, R.W.-S. Poon, C.-T. Luo, V.C.-C. Cheng, J.F.-W. Chan, I.F.-N. Hung, Z. Chen, H. Chen, K.-Y. Yuen, Lancet Infect. Dis. **20**, 565 (2020). https://doi.org/10.1016/s1473-3099(20)30196-1
40. Y.-F. Chang, W.-H. Wang, Y.-W. Hong, R.-Y. Yuan, K.-H. Chen, Y.-W. Huang, P.-L. Lu, Y.-H. Chen, Y.-M.A. Chen, L.-C. Su, S.-F. Wang, Anal. Chem. **90**, 1861 (2018). https://doi.org/10.1021/acs.analchem.7b03934
41. B. Koo, C.E. Jin, T.Y. Lee, J.H. Lee, M.K. Park, H. Sung, S.Y. Park, H.J. Lee, S.M. Kim, J.Y. Kim, S.-H. Kim, Y. Shin, Biosens. Bioelectron. **90**, 187 (2017). https://doi.org/10.1016/j.bios.2016.11.051
42. H.D. VanGuilder, K.E. Vrana, W.M. Freeman, BioTechniques **44**, 619 (2008). https://doi.org/10.2144/000112776
43. T. Nolan, R.E. Hands, S.A. Bustin, Nat. Protoc. **1**, 1559 (2006). https://doi.org/10.1038/nprot.2006.236
44. Z. Li, Y. Yi, X. Luo, N. Xiong, Y. Liu, S. Li, R. Sun, Y. Wang, B. Hu, W. Chen, Y. Zhang, J. Wang, B. Huang, Y. Lin, J. Yang, W. Cai, X. Wang, J. Cheng, Z. Chen, K. Sun, W. Pan, Z. Zhan, L. Chen, F. Ye, J. Med. Virol. **92**(9), 1518 (2020). https://doi.org/10.1002/jmv.25727
45. H. Zhang, B.L. Miller, Biosens. Bioelectron. **141**, 111476 (2019). https://doi.org/10.1016/j.bios.2019.111476
46. H.K. Hunt, A.M. Armani, IEEE J. Sel. Top. Quantum Electron. **20**, 121 (2014). https://doi.org/10.1109/jstqe.2013.2272916
47. A.L. Washburn, L.C. Gunn, R.C. Bailey, Anal. Chem. **81**, 9499 (2009). https://doi.org/10.1021/ac902006p
48. M. Shen, Y. Zhou, J. Ye, A.A. Abdullah AL-maskri, Y. Kang, S. Zeng, S. Cai, J. Pharm. Anal. **10**, 97 (2020). https://doi.org/10.1016/j.jpha.2020.02.010
49. H.K. Hunt, A.M. Armani, Nanoscale **2**, 1544 (2010). https://doi.org/10.1039/c0nr00201a
50. R. Weissleder, H. Lee, J. Ko, M.J. Pittet, Sci. Transl. Med. **12**, eabc1931 (2020). https://doi.org/10.1126/scitranslmed.abc1931
51. S.K. Vashist, Diagnostics **10**, 202 (2020). https://doi.org/10.3390/diagnostics10040202
52. D. Ferrari, A. Motta, M. Strollo, G. Banfi, M. Locatelli, Clin. Chem. Lab. Med. **58**, 1095 (2020). https://doi.org/10.1515/cclm-2020-0398
53. L.J. Carter, L.V. Garner, J.W. Smoot, Y. Li, Q. Zhou, C.J. Saveson, J.M. Sasso, A.C. Gregg, D.J. Soares, T.R. Beskid, S.R. Jervey, C. Liu, ACS Cent. Sci. **6**, 591 (2020). https://doi.org/10.1021/acscentsci.0c00501
54. S.K. Yong, P.C. Su, Y.S. Yang, Biotechnol. J. **15**, 2000152 (2020). https://doi.org/10.1002/biot.202000152
55. T. Ishige, S. Murata, T. Taniguchi, A. Miyabe, K. Kitamura, K. Kawasaki, M. Nishimura, H. Igari, K. Matsushita, Clin. Chim. Acta **507**, 139 (2020). https://doi.org/10.1016/j.cca.2020.04.023
56. H.W. Schroeder Jr., L. Cavacini, J. Allergy Clin. Immunol. **125**, S41 (2010). https://doi.org/10.1016/j.jaci.2009.09.046

Diagnosis of COVID-19 from CT Images and Respiratory Sound Signals Using Deep Learning Strategies

S. Maheswaran, G. Sivapriya, P. Gowri, N. Indhumathi, and R. D. Gomathi

Introduction

Coronavirus was first originated in Wuhan, China, in 2019. A 55-year-old man from China's Hubei region may have been the first to get COVID-19, a sickness caused by a novel coronavirus that is sweeping the globe. According to the South China Morning Post, the case dates back to November 17, 2019. That's more than a month sooner than physicians in Wuhan, China's Hubei province, reported cases at the end of December 2019. Authorities thought the illness was spread by something sold at a municipal wet market at the time. However, it is now obvious that during the early stages of what is becoming a pandemic, some affected persons had no access to the market. This includes one of the first instances, which occurred on December 1, 2019, in a person who had no connection to the seafood market, according to researchers who published their findings in the journal *The Lancet* on January 20.

Symptoms of COVID

The most frequent symptoms are:

- Fever and cough.
- Tiredness
- Loss of flavor or odor

Symptoms that are less common:

- Throat pain

- Headache
- Pains and aches
- Diarrhea
- A cutaneous rash or discoloration on the fingers or toes
- Eyes that are red colored or inflamed

Severe symptoms:

- Breathing difficulties
- Discomfort in the chest

Economical Impact on the World

The global economy has been impacted in a variety of ways since the COVID-19 epidemic began in March 2020. Poorer nations have suffered the most, while wealthier ones, despite their superior resources, have experienced their own issues. This article examines the influence of COVID-19 in various parts of the world.

First is dividing 171 countries into three groups based on per capita income: low, middle, and high income. Second is looking at health statistics to see how badly these countries were struck by the virus. Then, third is by comparing the International Monetary Fund's (IMF) pre-pandemic economic expectations for 2020 with their actual values and generated estimates for the pandemic's influence on growth and important economic policy variables [1].

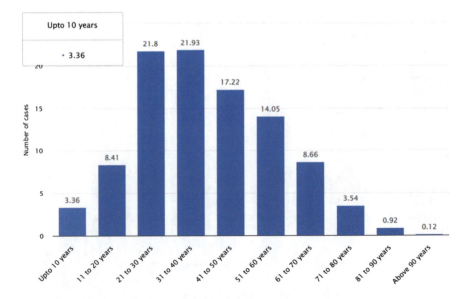

Fig. 1 COVID-19-positive cases in India with age group

The low- and high-income categories each account for 25% of the world's countries, while the middle-income group accounts for 50%. In 2019, the average income per capita in the middle-income category was more than five times that of the low-income group. It was over 20 times higher in high-income countries. Figure 1 shows the COVID-19-positive cases in India with age group.

Economical Impact of India

India has been devastated by the pandemic, particularly during the virus's second wave in the spring of 2021. Despite the fact that the huge drop in GDP is the greatest in the country's history, the economic harm sustained by the poorest households may be understated. From April to June 2020, India's GDP plummeted by a stunning 24.4%. The economy declined by 7.4% in the second quarter of the 2020/2021 fiscal year, according to the most current national income predictions (July to September 2020).

The third and fourth quarters of the recovery (October 2020 to March 2021) were still slow, with GDP increasing by 0.5 and 1.6%, respectively. This indicates that India's total rate of contraction for the fiscal year 2020/2021 was 7.3%. Only four times since independence has India's national GDP declined before 2020 – in 1958, 1966, 1973, and 1980, with the 1980 loss being the most significant. This predicts that the 2020/2021 fiscal year will be the worst in the country's history in terms of economic shrinkage, significantly worse than the worldwide average. The details are presented in Fig. 2. The reduction is principally responsible for reversing the global inequality trend, which had been dropping for three decades but has recently begun to rise again [2–4].

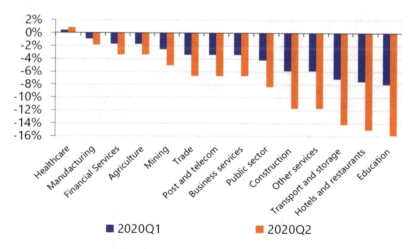

Fig. 2 Economy in different countries

Some Positives of COVID-19

Permits for a proper work and life balance: Many firms, located in large urban areas, and people were historically burdened with long travels, tiresome traffics, or long lines for public transportation. Employees working at home, particularly those with whole families quarantined, get the option to spend time with family members.

Budget-friendly, with improved cost management: Industries can shift their budgets and save money on running expenditures. Expenses are being considered in more realistic and business-oriented manner, notwithstanding the global financial disaster. Workplace supplies, equipment, and leasing costs might be used to aid the existing monetary condition.

Productivity and attention are increasing: Despite the fact that there are distractions at home, the survey concluded that overall attention at work has improved. Stress is minimized when external irritants are eliminated, and projects are finished more resourcefully and correctly. Reduced pressure levels as a result of fewer external irritants permit activities to be completed faster and with fewer mistakes.

Some Drawbacks of Covid

Quarantining: Even while several IT personnel characterize themselves as introverts, the research discovered that they are not truly introverted. There has been no brighter spotlight on this than during quarantine and seclusion. Isolation has had a significant impact on the emotions of employees and executives, and watercooler chatter has proven necessary, even for individuals who self-describe or are thought to be unsociable.

Incompatible with a home office: Not everyone has a great workspace in which to work remotely, and it can be difficult to create an efficient and well-organized workspace. They are unable to create an environment favorable to complete focus, which has a direct impact on staff efficiency. When it comes to production, no man is an island. Autonomy does not work for everybody, and not everybody is capable of professionally self-organizing their job [5].

Electronic communications are prone to being misrepresented: Aside from missing direct physical discussions and meetings, all of those polled were concerned about the essential digital communication methods, such as e-mail, social media, and the possibility for communication gaps. Figure 3 shows the total cases and deaths till 2021.

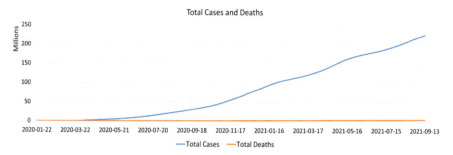

Fig. 3 Total cases and deaths till 2021

Impact on Students

The worldwide lockdowns caused by the global pandemic have had a negative impact on several crucial areas, one of which is education. Because of the epidemic, schools, colleges, and universities were forced to close unexpectedly, exposing pupils to online learning. Changes in classroom to digital learning during the pandemic disrupted the learning of students in low-income regions all across the world. Families that couldn't afford smartphones, Wi-Fi, computers, or laptops had undergone serious depression.

The parents, many of whom lacked the necessary qualifications to become home educators, were forced to take on the task on the spur of the moment. The three primary hurdles to online learning for schoolchildren are poor Internet access, insufficient data, and a lack of resources. The major concern here is whether kids are genuinely learning anything when the process shifts to digital learning and virtual classrooms. Changes in learning techniques have recommended us to shift to approaches that have never been used before, allowing us the opportunity to alter and gain exposure. Initially, the institutions were perplexed, since they had no notion how to continue, but as they established the digital infrastructure, the study pattern began to settle. During the epidemic, most students favored open and distant learning modes, because they foster self-learning and provide opportunity to learn from varied resources as well as personalized learning according to their requirements. Because of the epidemic, most recruiting efforts were limited. Students' placements were also impacted. Many graduating students missed crucial career prospects, and many students and professionals were forced to return home from abroad because to the epidemic, interrupting their work.

This chapter gives detailed description on the chosen datasets, preprocessing techniques adopted, models used to train the network, and different classification method. Finally, different classifiers are compared in terms of various performance measures.

Dataset Description

COVID-CT dataset contains of 349 CT images, which are reported as COVID-19 positive, and these images are collected from 216 patients with different age groups. The non-COVID-CT scan images were considered as negative samples, which are taken from the MedPix database, the LUNA database, and the Radiopaedia website.

SARS-CoV-2 CT scan gives a collection of large datasets with 1252 CT images taken from COVID-19-positive tested people and 1200+ CT images, which are taken from negative tested COVID-19 samples affected with some different pulmonary diseases and shown in Fig. 4. The detailed number of patients with both genders is given in Fig. 2.

Coswara is prepared for the diagnosis of COVID-19 with cough and respiratory sounds and shown in Table 1. There are 1079 healthy subjects and 92 COVID-19-affected subjects available in this dataset. The age group of the subjects included in this dataset is 20–50 years.

Sarcos dataset contains 26 subjects tested negative for COVID-19 and 18 subjects tested positive for COVID-19. This dataset has higher female subjects than the male. The sampling rate for recorded audio sounds is 44.1 kHz.

Proposed Methodology

A new framework was proposed for diagnosing the COVID-19 using CT images and breathing sounds. The entire network is designed to predict the class as normal, COVID-19, bacterial pneumonia, and viral pneumonia using the multiclass classification network MLP. The dataset used for the respiratory sounds are taken from

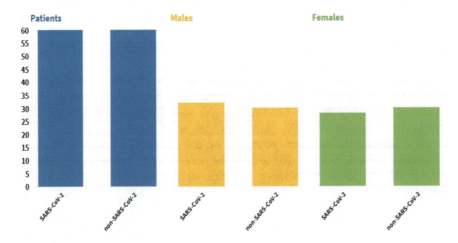

Fig. 4 Number of samples available in SARS-CoV-2 CT-scan

Table 1 Sarcos and Coswara dataset summary

Dataset name	Label type	Size	Audio average per subject	Total recorded audio
Coswara	Positive	92	2.77 s	4.24 min
	Negative	1079	3.26 s	0.98 h
Sarcos	Positive	18	2.91 s	0.87 min
	Negative	26	3.63 s	1.57 min

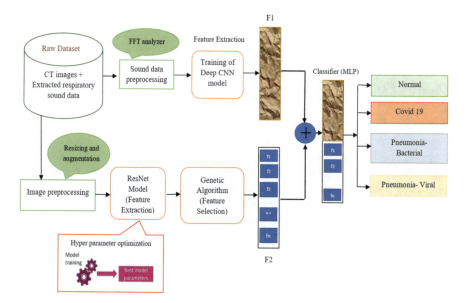

Fig. 5 Block diagram of proposed model for COVID-19 detection

Coswara dataset and Sarcos dataset containing 92 COVID-19-positive samples, 1079 healthy samples and 19 positive, 26 healthy samples respectively. Features like MFCCs, ZCR, log energies, and Kurtosis are needed to be extracted for identifying dry/wet coughs, variability present in the signal, prevalence of higher amplitudes, and for increasing the performance in audio classification. All these features can be extracted with the deep CNN architecture with the series of convolution, pooling, and ReLU layers. Finally, the classification is done with a multilayer perceptron (MLP) classifier. In parallel to this, the diagnosis of the disease is improved by analyzing the CT images. Two publicly available datasets COVID-CT and SARS-CoV-2 CT scan are used for training the proposed network. Various architectures are proposed and used for the classification of images in the literature, but still ResNet-50 helps in providing the promising results. Figure 5 depicts the overview of the proposed framework.

The proposed framework has two modules: (i) respiratory sound analysis framework and (ii) CT image analysis framework. These modules exhibit the workflow for data gathering, data preprocessing, and the development of the deep learning model (deep CNN+MLP). In respiratory sound analysis framework, the gathered audio signals are converted to spectrogram video using FFT analyzer. The resulting video signal are used as dataset for the deep CNN model for feature extraction. In image analysis framework, the acquired CT images are preprocessed and used to train the ResNet model for feature extraction. As the number of layers in ResNet is high, the features extracted will be more, and to select the desirable features, the genetic algorithm is opted. Obtained features from both the frameworks are concatenated and fed to the multiclass classifier. This framework can be implemented in real time, to reduce the number of existing expensive confirmatory tests.

Dataset Preprocessing

Preprocessing is first done to enhance the quality of the image, so that it becomes easier for the network to train faster. Noise and other irrelevant information are discarded in this stage and preserving all the essential information. To reduce the computation cost, the input CT image is first resized to 224 × 224 pixels with the help of OpenCv and converted into NumPy array. Histogram equalization is performed next to adjust the intensity level of each pixel in the image. It is used when the images lack the shadows and highlights.

Data Augmentation

Augmentation is preferred to increase the volume of the input dataset. This makes the network to train with the different versions of the image, and it increases the overall model performance. Random transformations, like image zooming, resizing, shearing, shifting, and rotation at different angles, are done to overcome the insufficiencies of the dataset. Vertical and horizontal flips can also be done where the vertical flip is equal to rotating the image by 180°.

Dataset balancing: Positive COVID-19 samples are not sufficient in the Coswara and Sarcos datasets. To create an equal number of samples in the training process, SMOTE technique of data balancing is adopted here, which helps in overcoming the problem of class imbalance. SMOTE helps in providing the better results compared to the extended versions like borderline-SMOTE. Five different COVID-19-positive samples are chosen randomly for every available sample in the dataset, and Euclidean distance is determined and represented as x_{nn}.

Then, the new positive samples are created with the equation below:

$$X_{SMOTE} = x + u(x_{nn} - x)$$

where u is the multiplication faction distributed in the range (0,1).

Feature Extraction

Figure 6 shows the different features extracted from the preprocessed respiratory and cough dataset.

MFCC

In MFCC, initially the signal is filtered and applied Fourier transform, then the frequencies are warped in mel spectrum. In the next step logarithmic scale is applied to the mel spectrum output followed by Discrete Cosine Transform is applied. The formula to determine the mel frequency is

$$mel(f) = 2595 x \log(1 + f/700)$$

Here, *mel(f)* represents the frequency in mels. The block diagram below represents the overall process carried out in calculating the MFCC. Figure 7 shows the complete process involved in finding MFCC.

The MFCC function is calculated with the formula below:

$$C_n = \sum_{n=1}^{k}(\log S_k)\cos\left[n\left(k-\frac{1}{2}\right)\frac{\pi}{k}\right]$$

The coefficient of mel spectrum is represented by k, output from filter bank is S_k, and C_n represents the output MFCC coefficient.

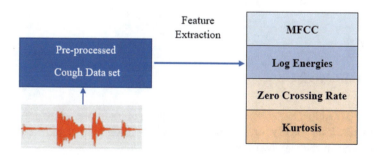

Fig. 6 Feature extraction

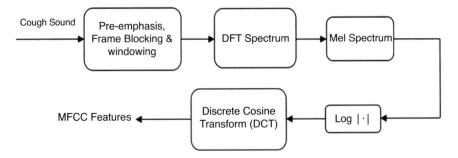

Fig. 7 Complete process involved in finding MFCC

Zero-Crossing Rate

The zero-crossing rate (ZCR) is maximum times the wave moves from positive sign to the negative sign. Voice signals oscillation will be very slow like it takes a 100 cross per second for a frequency of 100 Hz and a non-voice signal takes barely 3000 crossing for the same frequency. The zero-crossing rate is calculated with the formula

$$\text{zcr} = \frac{1}{T-1} \sum_{t=1}^{T-1} 1_{R<0}\left(s_t s_{t-1}\right)$$

T is the length of the signal s and $1_{R<0}$ is an indicator function.

Kurtosis

It is a signal's fourth-order moment which will measure the peak values associated with the given input audio signals.

$$\text{Kurtosis} = \frac{E\left(y_i(t) - \mu\right)^4}{\sigma^4}$$

ResNet-50 Model

ResNet-50 (residual network) is a modified version of traditional convolutional neural network. It has nearly 50 deep layers with 26 million hyperparameters, and the network was introduced by [5–8].

When the network layer goes deeper increases, the performance of the network may reduce because of the vanishing gradient problem. Vanishing gradient is the main reason for the degradation in the accuracy of the models. Residual networks are introduced to solve this problem with the help of skip connection. Skip connection prevents the gradient from vanishing, and it also makes the higher layers to work better than the lower layer by providing identity connections.

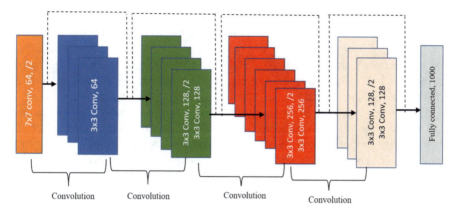

Fig. 8 ResNet-50 model

Fig. 9 Representation of skip connection in residual networks

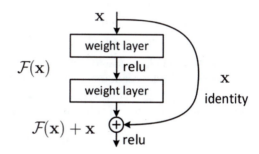

Figures 8 and 9 shows the residual network with identity connection. It is represented mathematically as $y = F(x, W_i) + x$. Here, y is the output of the residual network, x is the input given to the network, and $F(x, W_i)$ is the residual function. The figure shows the architecture of ResNet-50, which has four blocks with different numbers of convolution layers. The input image of size $224 \times 224 \times 3$ is given to the input layer, and ResNet initially performs 7×7 convolution with 3×3 of kernel size. In the first block, the three convolution operation is carried out, where the kernel size is set as 64, 64, and 128, respectively, for the three layers. The dashed line in the architecture represents the identity connection from one block to the next block. As the stride size is fixed as two in the following blocks, the input's height and width gets reduced to half, whereas the channel width will be doubled [9–11].

Feature Selection

Genetic algorithm (GA) is mostly preferred for feature selection; it is a stochastic method for producing the optimal result with the help of biological evaluation. GA makes use of population by evaluating the fitness function. The population with the higher fitness values are carried out for the next genetic process, where the remaining solutions will be removed. These chromosomes carried out for the next stage undergo the process of mutation and crossover to generate new populations. This entire process will be carried forward until till it converges to a solution [12]. Fitness is the most important parameter to be considered in genetic algorithm. The solution of the fitness function determines whether the population continues for the next generation process. Deep learning models, like CNN and ResNet, tend to extract most of the features from the input image. Genetic algorithm is used to select the best features extracted from ResNet-50 architecture. GA is preferred because of its evolutionary process through which it can offer the best solution to classify the CT scanned images as positive or negative [13–16].

- For every input CT images, the features are extracted with the help of proposed method.
- Individuals are represented as zero or one in the population; this indicates the presence of desired attributes in the individual. The size of an individual population depends on the number of features extracted from the image. Figure 10 shows an example for selecting an individual.

Roulette method [8] is used for selecting the parent pair, which involves in the mating process and produces the next new generation. One-point crossover (A. H. Wright) is used for selecting a crossover point for each parent pair. The offspring generated first with the genes present at the right side of the first crossover points and so on.

$$x_{[i]} \leftarrow \begin{cases} P1_{[i]} & if \quad i < \gamma \\ P2_{[i]} & if \quad i \geq \gamma < t \end{cases}$$

Here, x is the child vector, i represents the position index between parent and child, t denotes the parent's size, and γ denotes the randomly chosen crossover points.

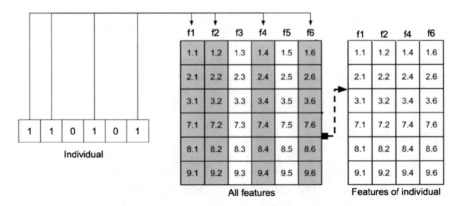

Fig. 10 Creation of individual features

Bitwise Mutation

Bitwise mutation [8] is the mostly preferred operator in case of binary encoding. Each gene is considered individually, and it makes each bit to be inverted within a minimum probability. Elitism is a method used here to generate new population by taking the next individuals from the existing generation. The cycle will continue until it reaches the stopping criteria.

LSTM

Long short-term memory (S. Hochreiter) is introduced for avoiding the problem of vanishing gradient. LSTM contains a cell state to store and covert the input memory cell to an output state. The LSTM architecture shown below has forget, output, input, and update gates. A received information that is sent to the next neuron is decided by the input gate; the information that needs to be forgotten is decided by the forget gate with the help of memory units. These four units interact together and work in a specified manner, where it takes all the long-term inputs and short-term inputs at a given time stamp. The mathematical representation of the input gate is represented as $i_t = \sigma(W_i * [h_{t-1}, x_t] + b_i)$.

The information to be neglected by the forget gate is mathematically given as $f_t = \sigma(W_f * [h_{t-1}, x_t] + b_f)$. The cell states updated with the update gate are represented as $c_t = \tanh(W_c * [h_{t-1}, x_t] + b_c)$, $c_t = f_t * c_{t-1} + i_t * c_t$. The output gate is updated with the equation $o_t = \sigma(W_o * [h_{t-1}, x_t] + b_o)$ and $h_t = o_t * \tanh(c_t)$.

Classification

Classification is a method of grouping given data based on the information found in a dataset, including annotations for which a category has been determined [17]. The CT images were classified as normal, COVID-19, bacterial pneumonia, and viral pneumonia. Cases using several classifiers include a random forest (RF) approach, a multilayer perceptron (MLP), LASSO, elastic net (ENet), a support vector machine (SVM), and an eXtreme Gradient Boosting (XGBoost) algorithm, with the default parameters in each classifier. The classification is verified for the findings using four generally used statistical assessment metrics found in the various literature: Acc (A), recall (R), precision (P), and F-score (F) [18, 19].

Performance Metrics

We can't assert that when a model has a higher level of accuracy, it makes the ideal forecast. The number of true positive (TP), false positive (FP), true negative (TN), and false negative (FN) values defined in the following formula are used to determine the four measures.

$$A = \frac{TP + TN}{TP + TN + FP + FN}$$

$$R = \frac{TP}{TP + FN}$$

$$P = \frac{TP}{TP + FP}$$

$$F = 2 * \frac{R * P}{R + P}$$

Further, the kappa index (K) measures the level of agreement between the proposed methodology's results and the experienced way of ground truth labeling. The area under the receiver operating characteristic (AUROC) curve indicates how successfully the classifier can discriminate between classes based on true positive against false positive numbers. The ratio of number of TP identified to the actual total of TP and FP is measured by the area under the precision-recall curve (AUPRC).

The closer these validation measures' values are to 1, the better the classifier can discriminate between the four distinct class pictures [20]. The suggested model's performance at all categorization thresholds is shown by ROC curve. The area under the ROC curve integrated from (0, 0) to (100, 100) is known as AUC (1, 1). It calculates the total of all potential categorization thresholds. With a range of 0 to 1, AUC is a 100% incorrect categorization. It is appealing for two motives: first, it is scale invariant, which means it evaluates the model's performance irrespective of the magnitude of the absolute values obtained, and second, it is classification threshold invariant, which represents that it evaluates the performance of the model, regardless of the threshold fixed to obtain the various categories used.

Eighty-five characteristics from the lung regions and the cough signal were assessed, and the statistically significant characteristics were those that had a p 0.05 in the univariate analysis. Only ten characteristics were preserved and utilized for COVID-19 detection after this stage. COVID-19 detection was a four-class classification job in the experiment. The classifiers are trained and verified using a tenfold cross-validation procedure based on the attributes obtained from the feature selection techniques [21]. Finally, an external testing dataset is used to put the model to the test. The various classifiers used in the process are analyzed, and the

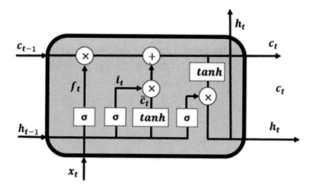

Fig. 11 Architecture of LSTM

tree-based classifier models random forest and XGBoost are found to outperform linear regression-based models in all the metrics. The comparison of the performance of the different model is given in Fig. 11.

Random Forest

RF is a tree-based regression/classification model, in which random samples are chosen from a set of data. The random forest algorithm will then be used to generate a decision tree for each sample. Voting will be done for each expected outcome for each decision tree. Finally, choose the prediction outcome with the highest votes as the final prediction outcome. To classify individuals as positive or negative to COVID-19, a RF classifier comprising of 250 trees was utilized. To split the node, completely grown and unpruned trees are employed, with the Gini index as the criteria. At each split, the features are permuted at random [22].

XGBoost

Gradient boosting is a machine learning-based regression and classification technique that produces a final output based on a group of low prediction decision tree models. The model architecture is framed stage-by-stage similar to other tree-based models such as RF or other boosting approaches; also it broadens the scale of the output by allowing optimization of any differentiable loss function. XGBoost is one of the gradient boosting implementations, but what sets it apart is that it employs a more regularized model formalization to control overfitting, resulting in an improved performance and a reduction in overfitting.

Support Vector Machine

Support vector machine is a frequently applied for classification or regression model that finds lines or boundaries, called hyperplane, using the extreme vectors to correctly identify the training dataset. Then, it chooses the line or boundary with the greatest distance from the nearest data points from those lines or boundaries.

LASSO, Ridge, and Elastic Net Regression

When the model coefficient is very high, the training dataset will be over-fitted. Regularization, which penalizes the bigger coefficient, can be used to solve these difficulties. Ridge regression is a modification of applying a penalty equal to the square of the coefficient values, often known as the L2-norm. Alternatively in the Lasso model, the loss function is changed with the addition of a penalty equal to the magnitude of the coefficient. Elastic net is a combination of both the ridge and LASSO model.

Some respiratory illnesses, like COVID-19, are thought to have a natural defense mechanism in the form of cough. Existing subjective clinical approaches to cough sound analysis were hampered by the human audible hearing range. As illustrated in this work, exploring noninvasive diagnostic options considerably above the audible frequency range (i.e., 48,000 Hz) employed for sample data can overcome this constraint. Signal processing-based techniques face extra hurdles due to the nonstationary properties of cough sound samples. Cough patterns also vary in human beings with the same medical condition. Cough characteristics that are closely related to intensity levels in the temporal domain can differ for the same disease. Figure 12 shows performance score achieved with different classifiers.

When an abnormal occurrence is present, the cough sound is analyzed by the basic frequency and the harmonics component. The instability in the cough sound that makes up the multiples of the fundamental frequencies is caused by airway

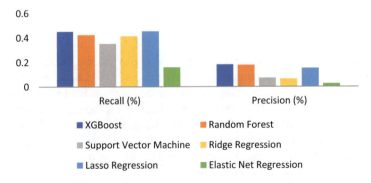

Fig. 12 Performance score achieved with different classifiers

compression. The system that is able to capture various features in the spatial and frequency domain of the cough signal for the complete cycle can accurately predict the variations in the cough due COVID-19 or pneumonia.

Because publicly available databases only include COVID-19-positive and COVID-19-negative examples, this research focuses on distinguishing COVID-19 and other pneumonia-related irregularities in cough sound and lung images from healthy/controls data. The proposed method, on the other hand, may be able to distinguish problematic cough sounds from various pulmonary/respiratory disorders, such as COVID-19, viral pneumonia, and bacterial pneumonia. Cough noises' pathophysiology and acoustic properties can provide valuable information in the frequency domain that can be used to characterize them for multiclass classification tasks. Pneumonia-related diseases make the patient's airways to become irritated and constricted [23, 24]. To demonstrate the distinctiveness of COVID-19, pneumonia, and normal samples, some of their frequency domain features are analyzed. When compared to COVID-19 and samples of asthma cough, the spectral entropy of the pneumonia sample is substantially greater for the majority of the frames. For the three respiratory illnesses stated, other features, such as spectrum flux, MFCC, and feature harmonics, are likewise nonidentical. Using a greater number of MFCCs consistently improves the performance. The study concludes that the machine learning classifiers are extracting the information that is not commonly sensible to human listeners, since the spectral frequency resolution utilized to compute the multidimensional MFCCs exceeds the audible property of the human auditory system, and these internal features are extracted and suitably selected by the time series-based deep learning LSTM model. Fig. 13 shows variation in the frequency domain features for the complete cycle: (a) spectral entropy, (b) spectral flux, (c) MFCC coefficient, and (d) feature harmonics for different cases of cough samples

When compared to previous studies, the work shows encouraging results in the categorization of CT scans into normal, COVID-19, bacterial pneumonia, and viral pneumonia.

Our findings show that analysis based on the spectral components of the cough signal may be utilized to discriminate COVID-19-positive persons and other pneumonia-related cough sound from noninfected people. To enable an effective classification, the collection of features taken from the pictures must be represented and adequate, to avoid producing mistakes in the classification stage. In light of this, a key component of the suggested technique is the use of a GA to choose the most significant traits. The GA and LSTM method used for feature selection improved the classification results and also considerably reduced the dimensionality of the feature used for classification, making the classification process more responsive. Figure 14 shows the comparison of the performance of various ML-based classifiers, and Table 2 gives the details about the comparison of different classifiers.

The suggested architecture had sophisticated capabilities for categorizing CT scans and cough sounds into COVID-19, pneumonia viral, pneumonia bacterial, and normal instances, and it may be utilized as a COVID-19 diagnostic or screening tool.

Fig. 13 Variation in the frequency domain features for the complete cycle: (**a**) spectral entropy, (**b**) spectral flux, (**c**) MFCC coefficient, (**d**) feature harmonics for different cases of cough samples

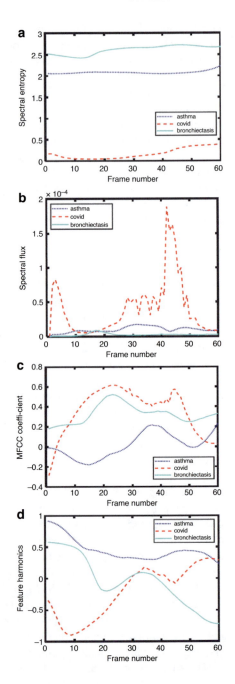

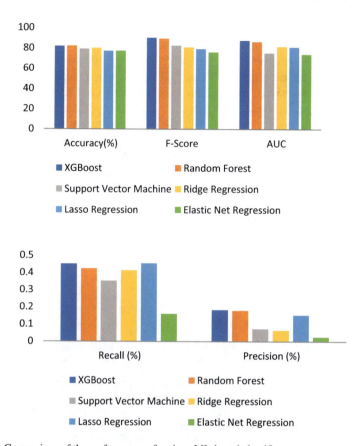

Fig. 14 Comparison of the performance of various ML-based classifiers

Table 2 Comparison of different classifiers

Experiment classifier	Accuracy (%)	Recall (%)	Precision (%)	F-score	AUC
XGBoost	81.9	0.451	0.183	90.2	87.5
Random forest	82.1	0.424	0.179	89.3	86.2
Support vector machine	79.2	0,352	0.073	82.5	75.2
Ridge regression	80.1	0.414	0.065	80.7	81.5
Lasso regression	77.2	0.454	0.153	79.2	81.0
Elastic net regression	97.2	0.26	0.026	0.026	98.7

Conclusion

This article proposes a new method of collecting multi-characteristic dataset of cough and lung images from people diagnosed with COVID-19 and two types of pneumonia along with noninfected individuals. The system studies the main features that contribute to COVID-19 for early results of COVID-19 detection from cough signal and also using the lung images obtained at the later stage, highlighting the importance of using the combined feature of audio signatures and images to detect COVID-19 symptoms. The proposed literature suggests that extracting the features using deep learning algorithms, LSTM, and genetic algorithm for feature selection and machine learning algorithm is suitable for a COVID-19 detection task; also, we go a step further and provide an in-depth analysis of the most useful spatial and spectral characteristics of sound, with the goal of analyzing the phenomena that changes the acoustic characteristics of COVID-19 coughs. Machine learning approaches are useful not just for distinguishing COVID-19 cases from other pneumonia patients but also for assisting doctors in tracking and predicting their patients' prognosis and treatment outcomes. As a result, studies conducted based on the cough sounds; chest x-rays; lung images, along with laboratory data; and other features, like demographic along with usage of deep learning and machine learning algorithms for various process like feature extraction and classification, will result in early diagnosis of the disease.

References

1. E. Soares, P. Angelov, S. Biaso, M.H. Froes, D.K. Abe, SARS-CoV-2 CT-scan dataset: A large dataset of real patients CT scans for SARS-CoV-2 identification. *MedRxiv*. https://doi.org/10.1101/2020.04.24.20078584
2. A.M. Ayalew, A. OlalekanSalau, et al., Detection and classification of COVID-19 disease from X-ray images using convolutional neural networks and histogram of oriented gradients. Biomed. Signal Process. Control **74** (2022). https://doi.org/10.1016/j.bspc.2022.103530
3. S. Aydın, H.M. Saraoğlu, S. Kara, Log energy entropy-based EEG classification with multilayer neural networks in seizure. Ann. Biomed. Eng. **37**(12), 2626 (2009)
4. R. Bachu, S. Kopparthi, B. Adapa, B.D. Barkana, Voiced/unvoiced decision for speech signals based on zero-crossing rate and energy, in *Advanced Techniques in Computing Sciences and Software Engineering*, (Springer, 2010), pp. 279–282
5. K. He, X. Zhang, S. Ren, J. Sun, Deep residual learning for image recognition, in *Proceedings of the IEEE Conference on Computer Vision and Pattern Recognition* (2016), pp. 770–778
6. M. La Salvia, G. Secco, et al., Deep learning and lung ultrasound for Covid-19 pneumonia detection and severity classification. Comput. Biol. Med. **136** (2021). https://doi.org/10.1016/j.compbiomed.2021.104742
7. H. Wright, Genetic algorithms for real parameter optimization, in *Foundations of Genetic Algorithms*, (vol. 1, Elsevier, 1991), pp. 205–218
8. A.E. Eiben, J.E. Smith, et al., *Introduction to Evolutionary Computing*, vol 53 (Springer, 2003)
9. S. Hochreiter, J. Schmidhuber, Long short-term memory. Neural Comput. **9**(8), 1735–1780 (1997). https://doi.org/10.1162/neco.1997.9.8.1735
10. K.E. ArunKumar, V. Dinesh, et al., Comparative analysis of gated recurrent units (GRU), long short-term memory (LSTM) cells, autoregressive integrated moving average (ARIMA), seasonal autoregressive integrated moving average (SARIMA) for forecasting COVID-19 trends. Alex. Eng. J. **61** (2022). https://doi.org/10.1016/j.aej.2022.01.011
11. E.D. Carvalho et al., An approach to the classification of COVID-19 based on CT scans using convolutional features and genetic algorithms. Comput. Biol. Med. **136**, 104744 (2021)
12. P. Anandhanathan, P. Gopalan, Comparison of machine learning algorithm for COVID-19 death risk prediction (2021)

13. R. Islam, E. Abdel-Raheem, M. Tarique, A study of using cough sounds and deep neural networks for the early detection of Covid-19. Adv. Biomed. Eng. **3**, 100025 (2022)
14. V. Despotovic et al., Detection of COVID-19 from voice, cough and breathing patterns: Dataset and preliminary results. Comput. Biol. Med. **138**, 104944 (2021)
15. WHO et al., Summary of probable SARS cases with onset of illness from 1 November 2002 to 31 July 2003. http://www.who. int/csr/sars/ country /table2004_04_21/en/index. html (2003)
16. R. Miyata, N. Tanuma, M. Hayashi, T. Imamura, J.-I. Takanashi, R. Nagata, A. Okumura, H. Kashii, S. Tomita, S. Kumada, et al., Oxidative stress in patients with clinically mild encephalitis/encephalopathy with a reversible splenial lesion (MERS). Brain Dev. **34**(2), 124–127 (2012)
17. F. Pan, T. Ye, P. Sun, S. Gui, B. Liang, L. Li, D. Zheng, J. Wang, R.L. Hesketh, L. Yang, et al., Time course of lung changes on chest ct during recovery from 2019 novel coronavirus (covid-19) pneumonia. Radiology **295**(3) (2020). https://doi.org/10.1148/radiol.2020200370
18. H. Ritchie, E. Mathieu, L. Rodes-Guirao, C. Appel, C. Giattino, E. Ortiz-Ospina, J. Hasell, B. Macdonald, D. Beltekian, M. Roser, Coronavirus pandemic (covid-19), Our World in Data (2020). https://ourworldindata.org/coronavirus
19. A. Halder, B. Datta, Covid-19 detection from lung ct-scan images using transfer learning approach. Mach. Learn. Sci. Technol. **2** (2021). https://doi.org/10.1088/2632-2153/abf22c
20. G. Soldati et al., Proposal for international standardization of the use of lung ultrasound for patients with COVID-19: A simple, quantitative, reproducible method. J. Ultrasound Med. (2020). https://doi.org/10.1002/jum.15285
21. M.J. Fiala, A brief review of lung ultrasonography in COVID-19: Is it useful? Ann. Emerg. Med. (2020). https://doi.org/10.1016/j.annemergmed.2020.03.033
22. T. Ai et al., Correlation of chest CT and RT-PCR testing in coronavirus disease 2019 (COVID-19) in China: A report of 1014 cases. Radiology, 200642 (2020). https://doi.org/10.1148/radiol.2020200642
23. D. Wang, B. Hu, C. Hu, F. Zhu, X. Liu, J. Zhang, B. Wang, H. Xiang, Z. Cheng, Y. Xiong, et al., Clinical characteristics of 138 hospitalized patients with 2019 novel coronavirus–infected pneumonia in Wuhan, China. J. Am. Med. Assoc. **323**(11), 1061–1069 (2020)
24. A. Carfì, R. Bernabei, F. Landi, et al., Persistent symptoms in patients after acute COVID-19. J. Am. Med. Assoc. **324**(6), 603–605 (2020)

The Role of Edge Computing in Pandemic and Epidemic Situations with Its Solutions

A. G. Balamurugan, R. Pushpakumar, S. Selvakumari, and S. Pradeep Kumar

Introduction

Trending technologies that lead the various global technology domains, as related to physical health, the Internet of Things (IoT), and Artificial Intelligence, could have wide-ranging contributions in the monitoring of health care during pandemic and epidemic situations. Globally, the public have lacked access to health care due to traveling restrictions imposed by governments for health measures and facilities are overloaded with high-risk patients. The elderly are highly vulnerable due to the pandemic. Both lay individuals and health care providers are now routinely monitoring health care. Nowadays, the Indian Internet of Medical Things (IIoMT) will help to detect continued behavior, emotional feelings, and all kinds of activity related to vital states through various wearable, off-the-shelf hardware. The Deep Learning technique was specially implemented during the COVID-19 pandemic in public gathering places, identifying the presence of a mask and temperature using the IoT [1]; moreover, Deep Learning with the help of Edge Computing demonstrates the tremendous algorithms that provide high accuracy in interpreting health

---

A. G. Balamurugan
CSE Department, Vel Tech Rangarajan Dr. Sagunthala R&D Institute of Science and Technology, Chennai, Tamil Nadu, India
e-mail: agbm@veltech.edu.in

R. Pushpakumar · S. Pradeep Kumar (✉)
IT Department, Vel Tech Rangarajan Dr. Sagunthala R&D Institute of Science and Technology, Chennai, Tamil Nadu, India
e-mail: pushpakumar@veltech.edu.in; pradeepkumars@veltech.edu.in

S. Selvakumari
Department of ECE, Sri Venkateswara Institute of Science and Technology, Thiruvallur, Tamil Nadu, India

care information [2–4]. With the help of the Deep Learning and Edge Computing algorithms, we can identify, detect, and recognize phenomena from the pi camera or from the sensor obtained data in real time by the IIoMT. This leads us to introduce a new upcoming production of IIoMT – support Edge Computing exertion [5].

Advancements of the emerging hardware devices, among one vital revolution, have led to a transformation of health care known as Edge IIoMT nodes [6]. At present, trend bands of IIoMT nodes can operate self-reliantly at the edge node, for example, health care institutions, homes, and clinics, where the data of the health care system is to be observed. Now the edge nodes have the full operating system (OS) with edge CPU and graphic processing unit (GPU) that permit the nodes to complete compounds from Deep Learning Computations on the edge. To utilize the refined IIoMT edge hubs, DL solicitations have likewise stayed enhanced to help edge knowledge and referring. Information starting from a subject or emergency clinic does not have to go outside the proprietor's area or edge; rather, DL and occasion observing can occur at the edge. This permits information protection, safety, and low-idleness wellbeing solicitations to track on client properties using Deep Learning and the IIoMT. The IIoMT edge has thus introduced new standards of DL, such as united realizing, where learning happens in an appropriated design at the edge, while just the model is disseminated [7, 8]. Modest GPU equipment can uphold IIoMT hubs that go about as unified ignorance hubs.

Moreover, much headway has been made with the DL and IIoMT, as few consumers may be involved in the setting that obliges diverse in-home quality-of-life (QoL) observing situations inside one system. The following original relative study has helped us to introduce basic things.

1. How to implement and recommend a bulk of Edge Computing in IIoMT devices that is used to create the Edge Solutions by Deep Learning.
2. The Edge Deep Learning Edge libraries for creating health applications at each edge, for example, at each house, are established as a result of this. By utilizing the edge computing of the skeleton, our IIoMT nodes assist with Deep Learning (CNN).
3. The developed set of QoL monitoring applications based on IIoMT edge learning. In real time, we can generate alerts using the applications.

The remainder of the article is organized as follows. Section II provides the related works. The outline design and model of the system is shown in Section III, the implementation details are mentioned in Section IV, we discuss the results in Sections V and VI, and finally, we suggest some future work.

Related Works

As the outcome of the excepted work, we have selected the advancements in four main areas as follows:

A. Affective Computing.
B. IIoMT Devices.

C. DL Applications.
D. Edge Computing.

We will have a clear discussion about the above given main areas in this article.

Health Care in Affective Computing

Interpreting the study of human simulations and processes can lead to understanding the study of health care in affective computing, including the process of recognizing the emotions of the human body as well as the temperature, pressure, facial expressions, body posture, and all kinds of gestures, while mice can also lead to recognizing the speech of humans. This magic can be made possible with the help of sensors like emotional cues by updated measures of the physiological data. Many of the algorithms used as classifiers, such as linear discriminant classifiers (LDC), Gaussian mixture model (GMM), K-nearest neighbor (k-NN), artificial neural network (ANN), support vector machine (SVM), hidden Markov models (HMMs), simply improve the enactment of the system.

IIoMT Devices

Information Technology is used to connect the health care and software applications by combining the hardware infrastructure with the Internet-connected medical devices in this network. This process allows the flexible analysis of medical data with medical terms and conditions based on the present state of the patient or is also used to monitor the patient. These safety precautions help to reduce the mortality rate, and lead to providing emergency care. The IIoMT sensors were designed with the intent of patient observation [9]. The 5G and Nano devices can manage the demonstrative Internet of things in health care, can be serviced, and can be portrayed [11]. Another research study was done to design the framework for generating the alerts of social distancing when the distance was violated [12]. Yang et al. [2] used the IIoMT for much of the physical treatment at residences. The IIoMT was studied with regard to versatile edge registering in [8]. An outline of IIoMT sensors was considered with regard to patient checking in [8]. A thorough overview of well-being IoT dependent on the impact of the Internet of Nano Things (INT) and 5G – Technology Material Internet on medical care and the nature of administration was depicted in [9]. Alhussein et al. [10] used the convergence of the IoT and cloud to monitor the patient's wellbeing in a Cognitive Health care IoT (CH-IoT) framework. In [11], an audit of the IIoMT for controlling pandemics, such as COVID-19, was launched. Ahmedet al. [12] devised a system that could track social distancing and sound a warning if it was ignored.

Deep Learning Applications

The term Deep Learning derives from Machine Learning as a part that works on the images, videos, and structured and unstructured data when the Machine Learning cannot easily do the task. Machine Learning leads us to Deep Learning by using the main motivation for the best algorithms structure and related functions of the brain called Artificial Neural Networks. The Applications of Deep Learning are widely becoming a trend among the industries and all kinds of business fields, especially in health care units. With major help from Python, DL plays a vital role worldwide. Overall, DL can work for large data sets. AI was implemented in [6] to combat the COVID-19 pandemic [13]. In order to provide proof and a meaningful explanation, the layers of Deep Learning can get the data as input such as the object classification to identify based on the inputs [14].

Edge Computing

It was presented in [3] that the 5G network is based on the Edge Learning framework, and it was used successfully for patient monitoring during COVID-19. The symptoms of all kinds of patients can be noticed by monitoring [5]. Even though all processes work well, the IIoMT inferences a high level of security for the data and adds extra features for the privacy protection in edge referencing [9]. In addition, the author Hossain [16, 17] contributed to the cloud assisted health monitoring system. The technology also led to support edge learning [6] with federated learning. With more effort, edge computing can be combined with AI [15] to provide a secure medical therapy for patients.

System Design

In this section, we designed a thorough view of the symptom management system. In the designed modular approach, we used the following four dimensions.

Edge Computing Applications

Management Symptom In-Home

In-Home basic support items can be available such as electrocardiogram, thermometer for body temperature detection, and oxygen saturation (SPo2). Our device is well trained to recognize the symptoms of COVID-19 and will provide the raw data to the IIoMT, which may include body temperature, heart rate, and oxygen

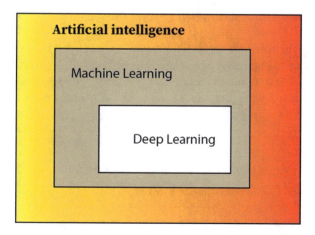

Fig. 1 Combination of learning

saturation level. Drowsiness/tiredness can also be detected by excessive yawning and other classification of symptoms, which are trained with the datasets in the Deep Learning method. Other symptoms of COVID-19 can be identified as speech recognition by the combination of learning methods as mention in the Fig. 1. The major thing is to identify fever temperatures in a non-invasive way by using a camera with thermal specifications.

Safety and Quarantine In-Home

Safety can be easily achieved only by oneself. Especially in the home, safety measures may not be followed, but in the case of people outside the family, we have to follow the safety measures. This can be achieved by the smart edge computing devices implemented in our project. Deep Learning techniques help identify if a mask is worn when someone tries to go indoors. If a mask is not detected, then the door cannot be opened, even by the people inside.

Facial Emotion Detection In-Home

Facial Emotion Detection such as pain that can be seen by facial expression and depression can be identified with the technique in Deep Learning called Computer Vision, which is also called the Third Eye of Computer. We cannot easily see how the vision is viewed by the computer. Deep Learning has n number of inputs, but it helps to find the exact expected output based on the inputs, which models and trains data.

Life Management System with Best Quality In-Home

The basic support of Health Related QoL in the time of COVID-19 is the best metric that can provide the best suggestions about their illness. This can make it possible to provide feedback to human health care providers concerning how they should manage treatment [18]. Figure 2 shows the variety of qualities of each one's present life taken for consideration.

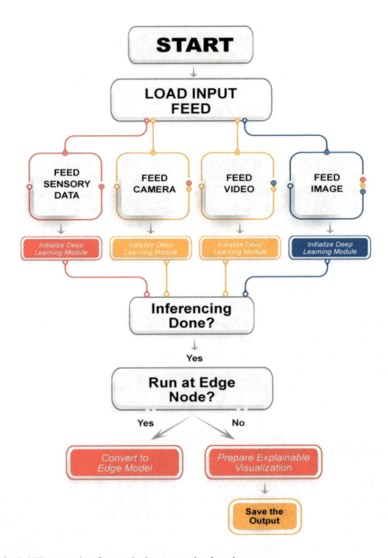

Fig. 2 IIoMT processing flow and edge computing learning

Diagnosis and Treatment In-Home

Smart edge computing also helps to diagnose and provide treatment for patients in their home itself. Based on the dataset we have trained in, the device suggests the Pill Detection and Reminder for the pill without any confusion so the patient can take the pill on time. The smart device also enables the alarm for the health care team who were present near the patient.

Selection of Edge IIoMT Device

Figure 2 shows the IIoMT devices with the corresponding deployment workflow of the entire system. In the initial state, the input can be fed from the pi camera sensor data. The pi camera fetches the data from the image and video whatever may be the input and processes it based on the initializations by Deep Learning. After the inference of the input data, a condition is matched with the trained data, and the next stage can be processed. Once the data is processed in the Run Edge node, the condition is passed if the condition satisfies the Edge Model (EM) and it will prepare the explainable visualization about the input. If the input data is not satisfied with the Run Edge node, it prepares Explainable Visualization, and after this, the output will be saved.

Edge Deep Learning Stack Design

The stack in which the IIoMT edges were developed for the detection of the physiological prospects and emotions of human reactions. Section III describes QoL and continued monitoring of human emotions. As given in Fig. 3, the IIoMT layer contains the sensor data that leads the data collection process of the user's emotions, allowing data to be obtained newly from the edge of the AI layer where the Raspberry pi5 or a Jetson NVIDIA-Nano platform is. The QoL application generates a report based on the programmed written or alert generated based on the input data that is processed with the CPU/GPU.

System Workflow

The system works only for the IIoMT hardware based on all the edge nodes. The system feeds the data from the sensors as input. Inputs can be obtained in various ways: (1) pictures, (2) live camera feed, (3) streaming video, (4) sensory data, etc. For each input feed, appropriate DL libraries were created, including for leveraging the original data set to train the Deep Learning algorithm, improve module accurate output ratio, and execute inferencing. The inferencing process can be done at part of the Edge model such as Tensorflow Lite (tflite). The output of the stimulation can be viewed on an android mobile or the web application.

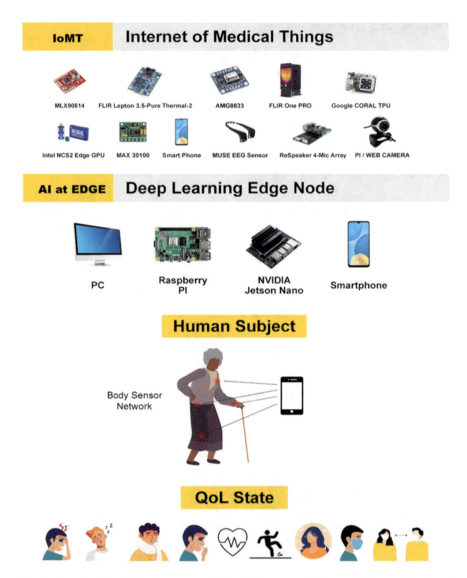

Fig. 3 Emotions detection in-house user QoL data Edge-accomplished IIoMT that are linked with Edge computing hardware

Implementation

The process of implementation is given in Fig. 3. The Internet of Things at the medical level includes the sensors such as MLX90614, FLIR 3.5-pure thermal sensor, AMG8833, FLIR Pro, Google CORAL TPU, Intel NCS Edge GPU, MAX 30100, smart phone, and pi camera. The second layer includes the Edge nodes such as a monitor for viewing the display, the SBC (single board computer) that may be used on any family boards of Raspberry pi, NVIDIA Jetson, Jetson Nano boards or any smart phones for viewing the display. The first layer and the second layer are interconnected with sensors and SBCs with supporting interconnected devices. The human emotions can be captured by the sensors that are interconnected with the human and stored in the smart edge nodes, which will lead to the expected output.

A thermal camera can be used to capture the image of humans and temperature sensor data. The body temperature can be identified. We used the Lepton model for the pure thermal identification 3.5, which was the housed board inter connected with a USB port for interface with the camera. Our created applications use, namely (1) Smartphone, (2) Web Interface, which is left on the surrounding objects, with the people around the expected range of the mask. The process starts with the training data set, including validating and testing and the output can be viewed on smartphone or web applications. Figure 3 indicates the Artificial Intelligence based on the web and smartphone applications that were developed for the research purpose.

For the data set, we gathered all the data for training the device based on Deep Learning, including the Nvidia Docker and Nvidia Jetson Nano with CUDA 10.0 and development of the CuNN in dataset.

A few more software techniques are needed, specifically CUDA 10.0 comfortable version, which may not be accessible and give support from the cloud storage or may be from the server. We have utilized NGROK to safely conceal the information going from own local host Deep Learning server all the way through any organization to deal with interpretation Network Address Translation or firewall. To send the DL application to the cell phone, we changed over the DL model to a tflite model and afterward quantized to help the cell phone GPU/CPU.

Figure 2 shows a smart phone solicitation utilized by an older individual having unstable or helpless visual perception. The solicitations can perceive articles and individuals everywhere around the subject and illuminate humans all the way through text-to-discourse. Figure 2 shows a feeling assortment solicitation that utilizes an internet source for an Edge computing learning customer. Figure 2 shows the actual fever temperature identification utilizing a thermal sensor camera. We additionally fostered a ready framework dependent on IIoMT equipment, displayed in Fig. 2.

To guarantee protection and safety for the IIoMT information, we delivered the value-based information through an Ethereum and Hyper ledger based blockchain structure to help open and secure organizations. The crude wellbeing information was saved off-chain and connected with the blockchain for proof. Figure 2 demonstrates the AI ready age framework in which the basic occasions were caught, perceived, and imparted to the suitable specialists by means of an informing framework. The framework additionally makes the IIoMT-produced proof accessible by means of the blockchain. Notwithstanding, the PC vision-based DL applications, tangible information, such as oxygen immersion and ECG values, were determined utilizing an intermittent NN (RNN).

Test Results

EEG Signal Classification

As per our training, the model we are using here has two kinds of data sets accessible from the Kaggle. The groups of data that offer the psychological and emotional states of all kinds of input from subjects are captured through the wearable biometric control devices (Fig. 2). As displayed in Fig. 2, the prepared irregular timberland classical could characterize whether an individual was feeling good, apathetic, or undesignated. The precision and recalls for three feeling stripes are displayed in Table 1. Because of the unmistakable division of information kinds, we noticed great accuracy and recalls for each type of emotion.

Dissimilar kinds of COVID-19 related symptoms were observed, especially cough such as dry cough, soft cough, and normal cough sounds, drowsiness, mask detection [1], feeling emotions such as positive and negative or neutral. Since the prepared models had satisfactory exactness, accuracy, and recalls, we are presently working with three emergency clinics at Chennai with the goal that the following prepared models may be conveyed at patients' in-home treatment. The genuine test lies in the real information assortment in the home. For that, we are intending to consolidate discrepancy protection, start to finish encryption, and combined training among the edge gadgets. We will likewise research methods of working on the exactness, accuracy, and recalls.

Drowsiness Analysis

The database library is utilized alongside "You only Look once" (YoLo) V4 for facial recognition and facial milestone identification. Resting design was determined using the duration of a shut eye, the recurrence of eyelid closure, and flickering recurrence. These calculations additionally followed head shifting and cavernous. We utilized the UTA sluggishness information set 2 to prepare our calculation. The preparation and approval exactness and misfortune are displayed in Fig. 3.

Table 1 Value of precision & recall with their type of emotions respective activities of daily life

Type of emotions	Value of precision	Value of recall
+Ve data	0.96	0.99
Netural data	0.99	1.00
−Ve data	1.00	0.99

ECG

The Keras design has been used to do a customary CNN design to set up the MIT-BIH-ECG data assortment. The signal from ECG was initially used for pre-handled to deliver a three-dimensional picture spectrogram. After the extension connection, the three dimensional picture was converted to a Convolutional Neural Network design, which is the max pooling of seven layers that are provided by the convolution layers, overall ordinary pooling, a totally related layer, and a softmax layer, with four classes of result. The ensuing precision and survey results through the planning and endorsement system are shown in Table 2.

Fever Detection

The fever identification can be submitted and obtained by the few modules in view of the prepared datasets. The application with a lead to the YoLoV4, face, eyes, and brow gives recognizable proof utilizing the Dlib, and afterward the live feed acquired by the thermal camera readings from the temple was utilized to decide the internal heat level, as displayed in Fig. 3. The software using NVIDIA Jetson Nano was, as far as possible, set at 37.5 °C. We used the data set-4 of Kaggle to set up reference FLIR thermal camera input pictures. The reported exactness and audit potential gains of the planning and endorsement educational assortments are shown in Table 2, and the contrasting chart is shown in Table 3.

Table 2 value of precision & recall with training and validation data

Type of emotions	Value of precision	Value of recall
Trained data	0.95	0.94
Validated data	0.94	0.95

Table 3 Emotions type for precision and recall of emotion classification values

Type of emotions	Value of precision	Value of recall
Sad	0.895	0.893
Neutral	0.889	0.897
Fear	0.801	0.798
Angry	0.971	0.762
Happy	0.965	0.964
Disgust	0.940	0.952
Surprise	0.981	0.962

Face Mask Detection

To set up our facial covering detection estimation, we used a face disclosure computation for the database library. In total, nearly 9046 pictures were used, which contained nearly 4250 pictures with a facial covering and the rest without a facial covering, obtained from a secured-based Google Engine search. Changed trade using the MobieNetV3 plan with a TensorFlow based CNN design was used. We achieved a readiness and endorsement precision of 0.95 and 0.94, separately, which is shown in Fig. 3. As shown in Table 2, the arrangement precision and survey potential gains of the ECG data were reported to be 0.981 and 0.952, correspondingly, for the planning educational assortment; however, the endorsement enlightening assortment conveyed exactness and audit potential gains of 0.98 and 0.96, respectively (Table 3).

Determination of Physiological State Using Excitement Analysis

In our research work, we have included sample pictures up to the pixel level of 1028 inputs for each one of the seven classes in training the data, a hundred pictures for every one of the seven classes in authorization data, and 172 pictures for every one of the seven classes in the testing informational collection, as displayed in Fig. 3. Table 4 shows the disarray framework with the accuracy and recall of seven feeling types. Figure 3 shows the preparation and approval exactness and misfortune, separately. Figure 4 shows the accuracy and recall of six unique kinds of day-to-day exercises, which were recorded through a cell phone.

Residential Cough Sound Analysis from Both Affected and Not Affected

The data library contained 120 dry coughs taken as samples from 30 patients with COVID-19, who were all confirmed by the RT-PCR test. The patients were from different age groups. There are nearly 220 COVID-free, meaning the test result is negative for the cough sounds, which are labeled according to the predefined data reports, in the data set we collected from Google.

Table 4 value of precision and value of recall of ECG data classification values

Data type	Value of precision	Value of recall
Trained data	0.97	0.96
Validation data	0.98	0.97

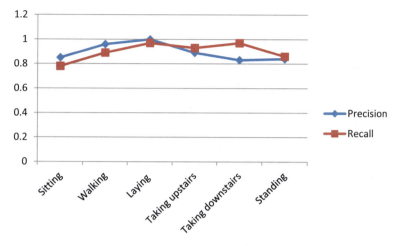

Fig. 4 Classification value of precision and value of recall in activities of daily life

Conclusion and Future Work

We designed a framework that will lead to effective computing advantages in the IIoMT deployment in the user edge environments, which may include the edge nodes such as the home, hospital, and other places. The GPUs help to run the Deep Learning solicitations on each edge node by collecting all kinds of data. By using the collected data, the application can be developed for a variety of symptoms. The data privacy, security, safety, and all kinds of low-latency were obtained by the edge – GPU. The next generation of people from various health care dependencies can get support for essential help for all kinds of symptoms despite the restrictions to traveling in pandemic situations, similar to health care suggestions without doctors.

As a future work, we plan to advance the precision of each kind of application at each edge node to relate to the patients in real time. We are also connected with multiple patients, health care teams, and hospitals to implement our applications in smart Patients Care Systems (SPCs). The application can also help us connect with the AI world of technology in health care systems.

References

1. S. Pradeep Kumar, R. Pushpakumar, S. Selvakuamari, Deep learning- enabled smart safety precautions and Measures in public gathering places for COVID-19 using IoT, in *Machine Learning Paradigm for Internet of Things Applications* (Willey Publication, 2022)
2. S. Pradeep Kumar, K. Jayanthi, S. Selvakuamari, Smart IoT-Enabled Traffic Signs Recognizing with High Accuracy (TSR-HA) using deep learning, in *Machine Learning Paradigm for Internet of Things Applications* (Willey Publication, 2022)

3. Y. Yang, X. Wang, Z. Ning, J.J.P.C. Rodrigues, X. Jiang, Y. Guo, Edge learning for internet of medical things and its COVID-19 applications: A distributed 3C framework, *IEEE Internet Things Magazine*, to be published
4. H. Lin, S. Garg, J. Hu, X. Wang, M.J. Piran, M.S. Hossain, Privacy-enhanced data fusion for COVID-19 applications in intelligent internet of medical things. IEEE Internet Things J. **8**(21), 15683–15693 (2020). https://doi.org/10.1109/JIOT.2020.3033129
5. M.Z. Alom et al., A state-of-the-art survey on deep learning theory and architectures. Electronics **8**(3), 292 (2019). https://doi.org/10.3390/electronics8030292
6. M.S. Hossain, G. Muhammad, Emotion-aware connected healthcare big data towards 5G. IEEE Internet Things J. **5**(4), 2399–2406 (2018)
7. W.Y.B. Lim et al., Federated learning in mobile edge networks: A comprehensive survey. IEEE Commun. Surv. Tutorials **22**(3), 2031–2063 (2020)
8. P. Porambage, J. Okwuibe, M. Liyanage, M. Ylianttila, T. Taleb, Survey on multi-access edge computing for internet of things realization. IEEE Commun. Surv. Tutorials **20**(4), 2961–2991 (2018)
9. M.S. Hossain, G. Muhammad, N. Guizani, Explainable AI and mass surveillance system-based healthcare framework to combat COVID-I9 like pandemics. IEEE Netw. **34**(4), 126–132 (2020)
10. M. Alhussein, G. Muhammad, M.S. Hossain, S.U. Amin, Cognitive IoT-cloud integration for smart healthcare: Case study for epileptic seizure detection and monitoring. Mobile Netw. Appl. **23**(6), 1624–1635 (2018)
11. M.A. Rahman, M.S. Hossain, M.S. Islam, N.A. Alrajeh, G. Muhammad, Secure and provenance enhanced internet of health things framework: A blockchain managed federated learning approach. IEEE Access **8**, 205071–205087 (2020)
12. K. El Asnaoui, Y. Chawki, Using X-ray images and deep learning for automated detection of coronavirus disease. J. Biomol. Struct. Dyn.. https://doi.org/10.1080/07391102.2020.1767212
13. G. Muhammad, M.S. Hossain, N. Kumar, EEG-based pathology detection for home health monitoring. IEEE J. Sel. Areas Commun. **39**(2), 603–610 (2021). https://doi.org/10.1109/JSAC.2020.3020654
14. M.S. Hossain, M. Al-Hammadi, G. Muhammad, Automatic fruit classification using deep learning for industrial applications. IEEE Trans. Ind. Informat. **15**(2), 1027–1034 (2019)
15. M.A. Rahman et al., Blockchain-based mobile edge computing framework for secure therapy applications. IEEE Access **6**, 72469–72478 (2018)
16. M.A. da Cruz, J.J. Rodrigues, P. Lorenz, V.V. Korotaev, V.H.C. de Albuquerque, In IoT–A new middleware for internet of things. IEEE Internet Things J. (2020). https://doi.org/10.1109/JIOT.2020.3041699
17. M.S. Hossain, G. Muhammad, Audio-visual emotion recognition using multi-directional regression and ridgelet transform. J. Multimodal User Interfaces **10**(4), 325–333 (2016)
18. L. Hu, M. Qiu, J. Song, M.S. Hossain, A. Ghoneim, Software defined healthcare networks. IEEE Wirel. Commun. **22**(6), 67–75 (2015)

Advances and Application of Artificial Intelligence and Machine Learning in the Field of Cardiovascular Diseases and Its Role During the Pandemic Condition

Sohini Paul

Introduction

In this present era of digital setting, artificial intelligence (AI) has been documented as a potent device in the marketable industrial setting and a budding automation in the domain of healthcare. AI has shown a widespread potential to influence the various fields of healthcare during the COVID-19 pandemic in a positive way. In the current scenario of data explosion, the implementation of AI in the domain of cardiovascular disorders and imaging is experiencing an exemplary modification toward machine learning (ML) algorithm. Regardless of major advancement in diagnosis and treatment, cardiovascular disease (CVD) is still the chief frequent cause of malaise and death from the global aspect, accounting for roughly one-third of yearly mortalities. Prompt and precise diagnosis is the major route to improve CVD results, and it can be tackled by regular screenings. D'Costa and Zatale [1] have stated that "although screening programmes at present can be cost inefficient for niche diseases, artificial intelligence (AI) has most definitely broken the rules of what our present cardiovascular health monitoring tools can be capable of; from using ECGs for detection of left ventricular systolic dysfunction, to cardiovascular risk prediction with accuracies higher than a mammogram." These multifaceted algorithms can effortlessly evaluate various data and mechanize an array of tasks. The present book chapter explores the role of different AI implementations that includes ML and deep learning and their implementations in cardiovascular medicine. Furthermore, it aims to provide an integrative outline of the modern research in the domain of cardiovascular diseases and AI.

S. Paul (✉)
Faculty of health and wellness, Sri Sri University, Cuttack, Odisha, India

AI and Its Principles

AI may be delineated as the replication of intelligence of human being by the virtue of programming in computers. The computer appears as an ideal tool for replicating interpretation processes. AI in healthcare may help in making faster diagnosis. The system gathers previously available data about the patient and the patient's medical history and current results to form a hypothesis. Another way AI is used is in online computer programs for scheduling appointments, which aids through the billing processes and gathering medical feedbacks. This technology is utilized to endow with progressive technology-based treatment in cardiovascular medicine, because it may help in facilitating the analysis and measurement of the various aspects of human heart functions.

There are various important components of AI, of which ML and DL are essentially included as a part of this book chapter. ML is a task of artificial intelligence that comprises of programs, which analyze records, gain knowledge from the information obtained, and subsequently construct notified conclusions based on the derived interpretations. A more specialized area of ML is identified as DL. DL is more similar to the thought process of humans, operating through a "neural network." In contrast to a ML script, a DL neural network generally consists of manifold stratum, every stratum comprising of a script which in its basic provisions receives an input, runs it via a numerical function, and endows with a pertinent perceptive output. Deep learning, with its capability to gain knowledge by itself, has notably produced novel opportunities in the field of AI studies. In the cardiovascular area, this automation is being employed to identify and categorize arrhythmias and murmurs availing recordings of electrocardiographic and stethoscope, respectively. In case of echocardiography (ECHO), AI image processing may assist in the mechanization of several parameter recognitions, such as ejection fraction, and also in rapid screening assessments.

The utilization of enhanced technology in medical field and diagnostics has been considered from the 1960s. In the domain of cardiovascular medicine, systems based on AI have instituted novel implementations in imaging, risk prediction, and newer drug targets related to cardiology. Prior to the incorporation of artificial intelligence systems in diverse areas of healthcare, the requirement of "training" is essential, and that can happen with the help of the data that are generated from experimental or medical researches and related work, such as screening, diagnosis, proposed mode of treatment etc., so that they can study in comparable groups of patients or volunteers. These data are obtained in various forms like medical notes, electronic recordings of various instruments, images, and so on. Particularly, in the diagnosis stage, a significant percentage of the AI review examines data from diagnosis imaging, genetic experiments, and electrodiagnostic results.

Real-time adjustments of ventilation settings and drug dosage could be done based on monitoring of patients' bodily responses and functions. A single computer can do monitoring on many patients in a unit simultaneously and provide relevant data about further course of action. Rising costs of healthcare could also benefit from AI, since its use improves the quality of care and reduces time in making decisions about treatment prescribed and also diminishes the number of human hours required, effectively reducing the cost. Since part of AI is learning from reasoning, a routine and regular use in clinical aspects would help to better the system. Cardiovascular medicine doctors and scientists at Mayo Clinic are coalescing artificial intelligence with medical practice, viz., with electrocardiogram (ECG) machine learning, to enhance caregiving. AI is employed to recognize innovative drug therapies and ameliorate the effectiveness of the medical practitioner. Explicitly the result of the COVID-19 patient can be predicted from cardiac-based algorithms. In this pandemic scenario, this digital technology was reported to control some processes of treatments.

Applications of AI in the Medical Field Settings

AI has multiple applications in the field of medicine. First of all, AI can help health professional in the analysis and evaluation of the disease and also to delineate an effective treatment protocol. The Application of AI in various medical approaches can diminish the frequency of misdiagnosis and thereby ameliorate diagnostic effectiveness. Secondly, the identification and application of deep learning has augmented the skill of AI to identify healthcare imaging and offer healthcare professionals with additional dependable imaging diagnostic data. Another important application of AI is that by utilizing big data analysis, the algorithms may frequently give additional precise outcomes for patient prediction. AI may also provide assistance for investigations in pharmaceutical industry, which can ameliorate the efficacy of novel drug development. Lastly, the amalgamation of AI and robot-assisted surgery may ameliorate the precision of numerous difficult and complicated procedures. Amidst the advancement of AI, big data analysis, and cloud computing technologies, AI may be capable of offering patients with elevated quality medical services. Furthermore, artificial intelligence will help to lessen patient's time of waiting and charge and get secure, suitable, and elevated standard of therapeutic services. Hence, the accomplishment of DL of AI will be of an added advantage to the field of cardiology.

Application of AI in Cardiovascular Diseases

Presently, AI technologies have been practiced in the area of cardiovascular medicine, which includes "precision medicine, clinical prediction, cardiac imaging analysis and intelligent robots." There are positive promises of the application of AI in the domain of cardiology.

Precision Medicine

At the outset, from the perspective of the patient, AI can be primarily utilized for distant pursuing of the patient, medicine remembrance, real-time ailment analysis, and prior cautions of various signs of diseases. Simultaneously, from the viewpoint of medical professionals, AI can facilitate collection of voice data (e.g., case history), attach electronic health checkup data arrangements, and condense the burden of doctors. It has been reported by researchers that in the subsequent times to come, cognitive computers, which are instruments that are upskilled via ML or DL programming, can decipher certain complications without healthcare professionals support, will assist medical professionals formulate precise assessments, and forecast patient results. Scientists have suggested that there is almost no probability that AI will substitute medical professionals. On the contrary, healthcare professionals should be acquainted with the utilization of AI technology and procure skill in this form of practice through the application of AI for the betterment of CVD diagnosis and management by evaluating the big data.

Clinical Prognosis

By the assistance of ML and analysis of the big data, artificial intelligence can facilitate medical professionals to provide precise prognosis for the patients. It was reported by Dawes et al. [2] that AI may forecast probable time phases of mortality for patients with heart-related disorders. Furthermore, it was also reported by the researchers that AI application documented the reports of cardiac MRI scans and tests of various related blood parameters of 256 patients suffering from heart disorder by various mechanisms. It was observed that AI could guess the possible abnormal circumstances that my lead to the death of the patient. Furthermore, the abovementioned application was capable of estimating the survival rates of patients for the subsequent 5 years, and the precision of the prediction of the succeeding year easily reached 80%. Motwani et al. [3] instituted a predictive model through the lens of DL and evaluated the threat of fatality for the subsequent 5 years for 10,030 patients suspected with coronary heart disease (CHD). The results obtained from their research specified that "the risk assessment based on AI is superior to traditional clinical judgement and coronary computed tomographic angiography."

Cardiac Imaging Analysis

In the current era, for the initiation of DL, cardiac imaging investigations have revealed an immense progress. Deep learning can facilitate the analysis of coronary angiography, ECHO, and ECG. Scientists have predicted that in the near times to come, by using DL, artificial intelligence can recognize coronary atherosclerotic plaques more perfectly than the medical practitioners. Additionally, AI can also be employed for examining the echocardiographic images, encompassing automated evaluation of each chamber dimension and evaluation of left-side ventricular function. Additionally, it can also be utilized to evaluate diseases related to structural aspects, viz., valvular disease, for helping in determining various aspects of the disease. A study by Samad et al. [4] revealed that DL can predict the survival rate of patients with elevated precision after evaluating ECHO of several patients. There are various additional purposes of the application of AI in cardiovascular imaging examination (which is regarded as one of the major important standards for the diagnosis of cardiovascular diseases), such as intravascular ultrasound and optical coherence tomography MRI, to name a few. In the coming days, DL will construct imaging analytics more dependable, simpler, and quicker to achieve results.

Intellectual Robots

The introduction of robots programmed for performing surgeries has helped medical professionals execute surgery for bladder replacement and hysteromyoma resection. In subsequent times to come, the blend of artificial intelligence and modestly invasive surgery technology, such as the Da Vinci Surgical Robot, may formulate the utilization of programmed surgery more pragmatic. This may diminish distress and suffering of the patient, enhance surgical protection, and curtail postsurgical stay in the hospital. It has been suggested by a group of researchers that "with this kind of combination, instead of clinicians, AI can perform cardiac interventional operations, such as percutaneous coronary intervention (PCI) operations and catheter ablations of atrial fibrillation, on patients; which will reduce the radiation exposure for the clinicians from the use of digital subtraction angiography." Therefore, it can be suggested that the integrated use of artificial intelligence and robotic surgeries may encourage the insurgence of conventional medication.

Clinical Decision Support System and Preventive Cardiology: The Application of AI

Yan et al. [5] suggested a fascinating idea by proposing that wherein the conventional model engaged a health professional diagnosing and providing "instructions" to a patient in a straight way, a newer advancement might be relatively that a medical professional will be providing directives to a solution-based AI, thereby acting as a linkage. The programmed application of AI would explore for errors, if any, in the practitioner's analysis and would then ask for assistance from a senior healthcare practitioner prior to ultimately passing the exacted recommendation on to the

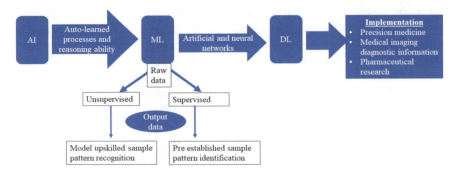

Fig. 1 AI, ML and DL-relationship and its Implementation

patient. These advancements would most certainly aid in declining mistakes in clinical practice, acting as a "redundancy tool." The instance of Google is very apt in this regard, where it has been capable of determining factors leading to cardiovascular risk from retinal fundic images, age, sex, smoking, blood pressure, and key unfavorable measures. This activity allowed the researchers to utilize these records to assess the patient's threat of various cardiovascular diseases, with a precision of 70% (Fig. 1).

Applications of AI During the COVID-19 Pandemic in the Domain of Cardiology

From the above data, we can delineate that digital application can be employed as supervising instruments to construct a considerable quantity of records in cardiology. AI is a smart method that can get accomplishment in the pandemic situation of COVID-19. For these instances, ML is also entailed to build up a smart system as required. This expertise will be able to forecast and treat multifaceted cardiovascular issues of the patient of COVID-19.

AI constructs an affirmative effect on prediction and evaluation of CVDs. A clinician speculates many aspects of a patient suffering from CVD from the provided electronic patient data. AI has been utilized for the evaluation of COVID-19 patients suffering from congenital heart disease. Haleem et al. [6] observed that this tool is helpful in relieving the overload of a cardiologist. The use of AI assists in scrutinizing the collected data and also helps in the decision-making process of the physicians, thus can prove to be beneficial for the patient in certain instances. Therefore, during the pandemic situation, it can be utilized to resolve complex difficulties by using technology-based clinical assessment systems. It assists physicians to give a precise prediction and at the same time also may lead to the enhancement of the human thinking process and cognition. The major noteworthy prospective of this system is to advance the healthcare quality provided to the patients of COVID-19. The physician can virtually verify the information of a patient even without travelling to the hospitals and therefore in the process may circumvent this infection. Expert advice of the cardiologist can be taken by the patient via an application, reducing time by preventing unessential hospital visits during the pandemic scenario.

AI and Cardiology Treatment During the Pandemic Situation

In the exigent circumstances of the pandemic, a critical challenging issue for the cardiologists was to suggest well-timed and suitable advice to the patients. The widened extend of the virus all through the pandemic has provided various obstacles for the patients visiting the healthcare centers, such as clinics, hospitals, medical centers, etc. To provide assistance to both the cardiologists and the patients, specific solicitations of AI have been used, viz., telemedicine, wearable sensors, monitoring devices, robotic implants, intelligent robots, etc. These abovementioned methods also provided aid for patients suffering from angina, fibrillation, strokes, etc., which are regarded to be very difficult conditions to handle with conventional medical care perceptions.

COVID-19 Pandemic and Artificial Intelligence: The Challenges

The distress derived from the devastating impacts of the pandemic is global and it has severely influenced the healthcare system and its correlated areas. In this scenario, it's a necessity to successfully investigate the huge quantity of records obtained at the time of this global emergency, and AI can perform it efficiently. AI processes the unrefined data and then, by the process of data mining, obtains an important conclusion. Further, it utilizes a variety of algorithms for automated data analysis. It has been reported by various studies that it is a useful tool for monitoring the COVID-19 virus and preventing its universal spread. Consequently, AI may also aid in developing a complete perception of certain aspects of COVID-19. The noteworthy proficiencies of artificial intelligence for the pandemic may be enlisted as follows:

- Examining various data related to transport systems in the nation during the spread of the virus
- Tracking and predicting a social evaluation of diverse areas
- Aiding measures in evaluating the effect of the worldwide pandemic
- Investigating the advancement of the enduring COVID-19 condition
- Providing an enhanced resolution for the healthcare management structure during crisis at the universal level

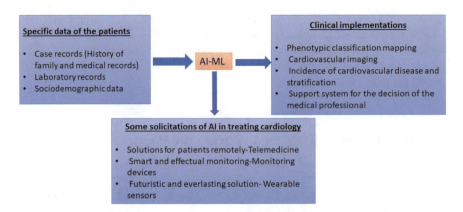

Fig. 2 Application of AI in cardiovascular research and Covid-19 pandemic

- Computing the constant impact by COVID-19
- Suitable supervision of the patient affected by COVID-19
- Automatic and regular tracking of physical condition of the population
- Appropriate investigation of the medical records obtained during the global crisis
- Proficient evaluation of the infection (Fig. 2)

The Future Scope of Artificial Intelligence

The era when AI will substitute a cardiologist is not yet in the future sight. Even though not conventional yet, we are unquestionably in the epoch where artificial intelligence is aiding cardiologists globally routinely in the rapid and enhanced evaluation and image understandings. The prospect rests in utilizing this technology in domains that have not been endeavored owing to some expenditure limitations. Moreover, incorporation of automated evaluation and cardiovascular risk assessment methods into already available electronic medical documentation application would help in developing a comprehensive treatment protocol and also will assist in counseling of patients about amendable risk factors, thus providing a positive impact on morbidity and mortality. In conclusion, AI is a metamorphic technology and has mammoth prospective in the healthcare settings.

References

1. A. D'Costa, A. Zatale, AI and the cardiologist: When mind, heart and machine unite. Open Heart **8**, e001874 (2021). https://doi.org/10.1136/openhrt-2021-001874
2. T.J.W. Dawes, A. de Marvao, W. Shi, et al., Machine learning of three-dimensional right ventricular motion enables outcome prediction in pulmonary hypertension: A cardiac MR imaging study. Radiology **283**, 381–390 (2017)

3. M. Motwani, D. Dey, D.S. Berman, et al., Machine learning for prediction of all-cause mortality in patients with suspected coronary artery disease: A 5-year multicentre prospective registry analysis. Eur. Heart J. **38**, 500–507 (2017)
4. M.D. Samad, A. Ulloa, G.J. Wehner, et al., Predicting survival from large echocardiography and electronic health record datasets: Optimization with machine learning. JACC Cardiovasc. Imaging **12**, 681–689 (2019)
5. J. Yan, Z. Wang, L.J. Xu, et al., Effects of new regional cooperative rescue model on patients with ST-elevation myocardial infarction. Int. J. Cardiol. **177**, 494–496 (2014)
6. A. Haleem, M. Javaid, R.P. Singh, et al., Applications of artificial intelligence (AI) for cardiology during COVID-19 pandemic. Sustain. Oper. Comput. **2**, 71–78 (2021)

Effective Health Screening and Prompt Vaccination to Counter the Spread of COVID-19 and Minimize Its Adverse Effects

Sandip Bag and Swati Sikdar

Introduction

In the month of November 2019, an epidemic of relentless intense respiratory ailment was detected as a source of bunch of pneumonia patients in city of Wuhan, China, in the name of novel coronavirus perceived as SARS-CoV-2 [1–3]. At the end of February, 2020, i.e., 10–12 weeks after such outbreak, the World Health Organization (WHO) named this disease as the novel coronavirus and considered as the biggest threatening epidemic of the earth in the twenty-first century [4, 5].

People are affected with the COVID-19 virus by many different ways, and in major cases, contaminated person will grow mild to moderate illness and also salvage without admission in hospital [6]. The clinical malady of such coronavirus ranges from mild delirium, cold, fatigue, distaste, absence of smell, hurting throat, diarrhea, etc. to difficulty in breathing or shortness of breath with very severe pneumonia, loss of speech or mobility, chest pain, infected trauma, and multi-organ breakdown that may lead to loss of life [7, 8]. Due to the severity of such infectious disease, the WHO announced such pandemic disease as community health exigency of universal burden and plead to all countries for taking necessary measurable action to detect and prevent such contagious virus and take appropriate steps against the spreading of this pandemic outbreak [9].

Infectious COVID-19 antigen is primarily spread explicit from one to other, through nasal droplets formed from coughing or sneezing of an infected person, and that soggy aerosol can transfer in the entrance of the respiratory tract of people who

---

S. Bag (✉) · S. Sikdar
JIS College of Engineering, Kalyani, West Bengal, India

© The Author(s), under exclusive license to Springer Nature Switzerland AG 2023
G. R. Kanagachidambaresan et al. (eds.), *System Design for Epidemics Using Machine Learning and Deep Learning*, Signals and Communication Technology, https://doi.org/10.1007/978-3-031-19752-9_14

are in adjacent proximity of the contaminated individual and probably inhaled into the lungs [10, 11]. Other feasible avenues include unambiguous meeting with attenuated fomites and penetration of droplets as well as probable transportation of SARS-CoV-2 from an individual of asymptomatic nature (or persons within the incubation phase) to others [12, 13].

When COVID-19 outbreak was first experienced, there is neither FDA-approved medication nor vaccines in the market, which is able to intercept the outspread of infectious virus as well as to restrict the world's most critical situation [14]. Therefore, the WHO recommended guidelines and protocols are the only option to stop the spreading of coronavirus (Fig. 1) [15]. Furthermore, most of the countries try to prevent such infection by forceful lockdown to break the transmission chain of the COVID-19 virus [16].

Before vaccination of people to preclude SARS-CoV-2 bug, effective screening is the most potent tools against such pandemic outbreak [17]. After a successful three-phase clinical trial, COVID-19 vaccines are considered as the best encouraging path for curbing the pandemic and are being vigorously pursued to restrict coronavirus. At the end of November or early December, 2020, quite a large number of COVID vaccines are validated and approved by the WHO for application on emergency basis in different parts of the world [18].

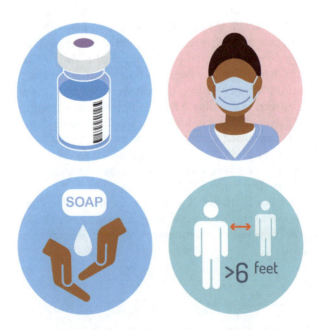

Fig. 1 The WHO recommended guidelines and protocol against COVID-19

Screening

Screening is an important process of identifying or examining within an allegedly healthy population in order to diagnose individuals, who may be at elevated risk of disease or plight but do not yet have symptoms, and also contributing to support individuals to make better informed options about their health [19]. The healthcare provider then offers information about advanced tests and medication that reduces the associated complications or dangers. Although diagnosis is a potential tool and effective process to recover lives and/or to revamp the quality of life through an early clinical testing of severe conditions, this is not an ideal practice, and it cannot offer a guaranteed protection, because there is a chance of false-positive results and erroneous negative results [20].

COVID-19 Screening Tools and Procedure

Screening analysis aims to disclose the risk factors for certain diseases at the preliminary stage, before any symptoms become noticeable, and it is advantageous to cure the disease much earlier before spreading into the population [21, 22]. Therefore, treating a disease at the very first phase will accelerate a better health outcome over correcting it at a final stage after the development of symptoms. There are several COVID-19 screening tools and procedure available to identify the people affected by coronavirus disease 2019 [23].

List of the easier and decisive screening procedures are as the following:

(a) **Temperature Measurement using IR Thermal Gun.**

An infrared thermometer is one of the screening devices that are used most of the places to measure the body temperature or skin surface temperature of any subject within seconds [24].

This device is also known as thermal gun due to its gun shape. This IR thermometer is accurate and reliable and can be used safely to measure the body heat from a certain length in the absence of direct body contact with the subject. That's why this apparatus is further referred as a contactless temperature-measuring device that calculates the temperature from a portion of thermal irradiation often called blackbody radiation emitted by the object being measured [25]. These thermic gadgets have the ability to determine the actual temperature of the human body within a predefine range by calculating the extent of IR energy emitted by the person w.r.t the emissivity of the thermometer.

During the pandemic, it was observed that there is a tremendous application of such machineries at various entryway and key points of airfield campuses, railway premises, healthcare facilities, market place, and other areas with the growing COVID-19 (coronavirus) outbreak to confine the widening of virulent disease in the

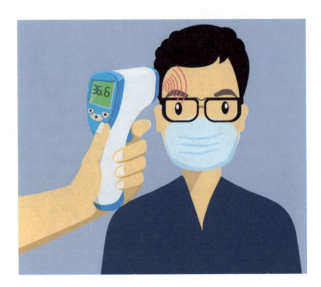

Fig. 2 Body temperature measurement during the COVID-19 outbreak using thermal gun

society by comfortably revealing the COVID-19 patient and confine them through a dynamic manner (Fig. 2) [26].

The basic intent of these devices is to examine the subject's body temperature from a specified length, without placing the thermometer in everybody's mouths or rear ends that would be inapplicable, infeasible, and potentially a bit disappointing.

This form of touchless IR thermal gun can check and measure the subject skin heat within a fraction of second. So, tons of crowd can be investigated individually at checkpoints without any trouble, which may support to dwindle the chance of increasing COVID-19 infections.

(b) **RT-PCR Test.**

Presently, reverse transcription-polymerase chain reaction or RT-PCR assay, also known as molecular test, is the most popular diagnostic test for the deadly disease COVID-19 and provides the maximum COVID-19 analysis outcomes that have been recorded [27]. This test is performed using swab obtained from the nasal or mouth of the patient to detect the genetic material of the virus. RT-PCR test specimen is collected by entering a long nasopharyngeal mop into snout and drawing fluid from the rear of our nose or by using a concise nasal swab to bring a sample (Fig. 3). Alternatively, a long oropharyngeal daub is infused in the posterior of our larynx, or we may spit into a test tube to produce a saliva sample.

RT-PCR examination principally recognizes the abiogenic message of the RNA virus, and it is possible if the virus is present within the ardently infected subjects. So, PCR assessments are ordinarily accomplished to precisely reveal the existence of a ragweed, rather presence of the body's immune response in the form of

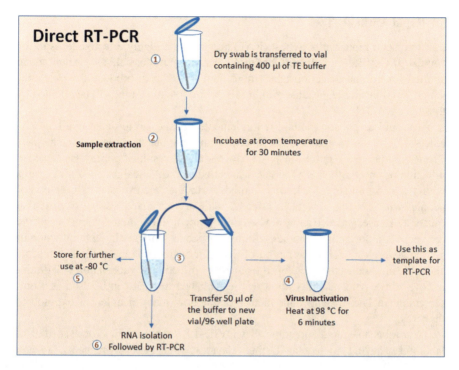

Fig. 3 Procedure of RT-PCR test

antibodies. This arrangement can only persuade the presence of viral RNA within the system before the production of antibodies or ailments of the disease present [28]. As a result, this diagnostic procedure is also referred as SARS-CoV-2 test or COVID diagnostic test. Furthermore, an RT-PCR test is cost-effective and reasonable to afford.

This investigation provides a better expression of the people's physical condition to indicate whether they are affected or not. Therefore, an affected person can be easily isolated and quarantined the crowd who get in contact with infected people. By allotment PCR analysis to screen enormous swaddle of nasopharyngeal swab samples from heavy populace, public health committee get a clear image of the spreading of such infectious disease within a community [29].

The analytic test is hypersensitive and very definitive to the COVID-19 virus. This testing procedure can provide a decisive investigation result within a very short time, i.e., 2–3 h, although laboratories take ordinarily 6–8 h to deliver the result. In contrast with other anticipated approach for virus recognition, RT-PCR test is really faster and presented more authenticate results with fewer chances for contagion or interference, as whole operation is performed within a sealed duct [30]. Thus, it is considered as the most authentic and impressive process convenient for the detection of the COVID-19 virus.

(c) **Rapid Antibody Test.**

At present, rapid antibody test (RAT) is one of the highly effective tools in the context of COVID-19 outbreak, because the maximum possible assessment mode applied for corona detection takes more than 48–72 h to produce the outcomes which is not desirable, because within this period lots of people will be affected by those people [31].

Aforesaid diagnostic method is implemented in the lab to determine the existence of coronavirus genomic sequence within the mucous and/or saliva samples. The testing process requires only 1–2 days to furnish results if patient has an active infection or not. Further, RAT assay, also called as serological test, can give results within 10–15 min (Fig. 4). In this method, antibodies are exposed in the blood of people, who have already been infected with or vaccinated against a virus that causes a disease, and also show the body's attempt or intention to fight off a specific antigen. Once formed, antibodies will protect people from getting that infection or getting severely ill for some period of time afterward. This test will also indicate about the antibodies that developed from either infection or vaccination will diminish over time. After all, it is not a well-established test but can be used as a prescreening analysis to engender picture about how many people got exposed to the virus.

To combat the rapid spreading of COVID-19 pandemic situation, shortfall of laboratory having molecular testing capacity, and lack of reagents, several

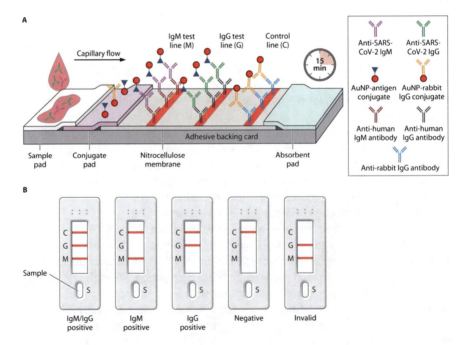

Fig. 4 Mechanism of SARS-CoV-2 rapid antibody test

diagnostic kit manufacturers have developed an expeditious and user-friendly device to promote analyzing procedure outside the laboratory settings. These transparent, safe, and reliable test kits are proficient of detecting antibody strength in the blood of the patient infected with COVID-19.

(d) **SARS-CoV-2 Rapid Antigen Test.**

The analytical evaluation is a faster chromatographic immunoassay for the qualitative scrutiny of explicit antigens of SARS-CoV-2 existence in human nasopharynx [32].

This assessment is highly precise to identify unique antigens from the SARS-CoV-2 virus in a person who imagined for COVID-19 infection. This special diagnostic examination is convenient for both symptomatic and asymptomatic people (Fig. 5); and it may provide backing the healthcare specialists to find out SARS-CoV-2-infected people who are suspected to carry the virus, with results typically ready within 15 minutes. Accordingly, such assay accurately screens individuals with known exposure to infected SARS-CoV-2 patients, providing rapid answers regarding their infection status and also allowing informed treatment decisions. The available test kit for COVID-19 is portable, reliable, and instrument-less testing tool that facilitates acceptable use for medical experts at different point of healthcare locations or in resource-limited settings. Considering various laboratory testing approach and/or patient mobility, the rapid antigen testing increases the access of high-quality diagnostics solutions for the detection of a present SARS-CoV-2

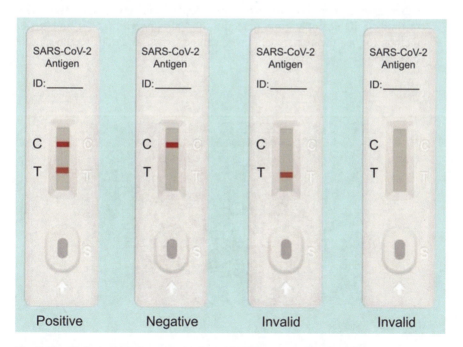

Fig. 5 Test kit for rapid antigen examination of SARS-CoV-2 (colloidal gold)

infection in a best possible way and, additionally, maintains a beneficial early screening result for every individual who have been exposed with SARS-CoV-2-infected patients or high-risk environment.

This type of unambiguous test procedure will reveal results of person who is presently infected with the SARS-CoV-2 virus or not. The antigen diminishes immediately after the recovery from COVID-19 infection. Unlike RT-PCR test, RAT techniques are of low cost and profitable, as it lends the test results to also distinguish glycan's like spike proteins availability on the surface of the SARS-CoV-2 immediately. Furthermore, such diagnostic procedure can be more susceptible to point-of-care use, which could make them more relevant for testing in the community or even in remote locations.

In addition to the abovementioned screening procedure, some different pathways for diagnosing new test samples are available with added benefits.

(i) For fast, point-of-care diagnostic test procedure, a mucus sample obtained from the nose or throat is used for analysis at the doctor's chamber or clinic, and results may be available within a few minutes. This method may be either molecular or antigen test.
(ii) Internal collection test measure is feasible only by the instruction from a medical practitioner that allows the patient to collect the sample from home and deliver it precisely to the pathological laboratory for investigation.
(iii) Apart from collecting mucus from the nose and throat, saliva tests are also accomplished in which patient is endorsed to spit inside a test tube. This experiment is comfortable for some people than any other assessment method available for corona detection and also provides safer and easier method for healthcare personnel who can be farther away during the sample collection.

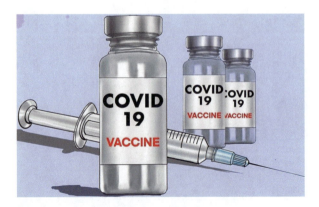

Fig. 6 COVID-19 vaccine

Vaccine

Vaccine is a biological preparation that typically contains a bioactive element that stimulates any disease-causing microorganism and is often prepared from deactivated forms of pathogen and its toxins, or one of its surface proteins that provides active acquired immunity to a particular infectious disease (Fig. 6) [33].

This biological element triggers the immune response of our body to remember the agent as a hazards and sabotage and to further recognize and destroy any of the microorganisms associated with that agent that it may confront in the near future. Once administered with the vaccine, the body is able to produce antibodies as the initial response against an antigen. It also initiates to create antibody-generating memory cells, which stand active after defeat of foreign bodies through by the antibodies. If the host tissues again are exposed to the similar nature of pathogen more than once, the antibody reaction is much faster and more impressive than first-time action, because the memory cells are ready to release antibodies against those antigens. Vaccines may be prophylactic to intercept the facets of upcoming disease by an instinctive pathogen and/or therapeutic agent to combat an infection that has already entered into the system. Some vaccines provide full castrate immunity against the disease as it interrupts the pathogen comprehensively.

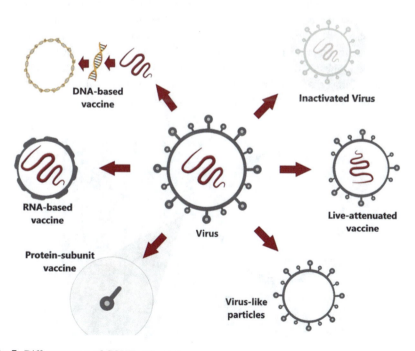

Fig. 7 Different types of COVID-19 vaccine

COVID-19 Vaccine

All over the universe, scientists are advancing to develop many potential vaccines for COVID-19 (Fig. 7) [34–36]. There are almost 12 different vaccines developed to counter COVID-19 disease that have been approved by the WHO for use in various locations around the world, although a number of potential vaccines to prevent COVID-19 disease have been developed [37, 38].

These types of vaccines are broadly classified into four categories such as:

(i) **RNA and DNA vaccines** are the most modern and updated vaccines that apply genetically constructed RNA or DNA-created protein that itself cautiously encourages our immunity [39, 40].

 The first authorized mRNA vaccines for COVID-19 developed by BioNTech-Pfizer and Moderna are used in humans after successful clinical trials. This antiserum does not consist of any specimen of the SARS-CoV-2 virus, but it carries a chemically synthesized messenger (m)RNA obtained from the COVID-19 virus itself that gives the necessary instruction to host cells about the making of harmless spike protein unique to virus (Fig. 8) [41].

 After making imprint of that protein, they kill the genetic material from the vaccine. When our immune system recognizes the undesired protein, they build long-serving immunity in the name of T-lymphocytes, immediately followed by B-lymphocytes that will commemorate how to fight against the virus that is responsible for COVID-19 if we are infected in near future. It is impossible to evolve coronavirus against mRNA vaccine, as it does not bring any necessary information to generate the integrated coronavirus [42].

 Like any other available vaccines against coronavirus, mRNA vaccines will provide highest satisfaction to the vaccinated subject by providing them safeguard against diseases like COVID-19 without any risk of the potentially dangerous consequences of capturing sick. mRNA vaccines are freshly available

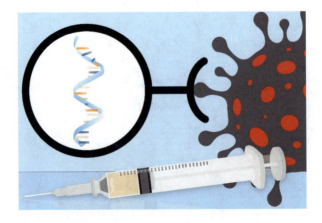

Fig. 8 The COVID-19 mRNA vaccine

in the market for the common people. Identical composition of such vaccine is applied as double shots of elementary series.

(ii) **Protein subunit vaccines** utilize harmless fragments of proteins or protein shells of the SARS-CoV-2 virus that mimic the nature of the COVID-19 virus instead of the entire germ to harmlessly achieve an immune response [43]. This type of vaccines delivers the protein directly to our cell instead of providing necessary genetic code to make a viral protein. Once vaccinated, our bodies easily recognize the disease-causing protein and build T-lymphocytes followed by antibodies accordingly, which will remember how to fight against such virus that is responsible for COVID-19 disease if we are infected in the future [44].

The Novavax COVID-19 vaccine is an example of this type of vaccine. Scientists are trying to produce enormous numbers of the SARS-CoV-2 spike protein in laboratory for this empirical vaccine using insect cells to cultivate proteins before purification. The purified proteins then are converted to nanoparticles. Individually, such nanoparticles are not strongly sufficient to produce the adequate immune reaction through antibody production, so Novavax addition acts as a catalyst to stimulate the immune system. Subunit vaccines does not produce any COVID-19 symptoms, because they do not import adequate viral component to make integrated SARS-CoV-2 virus.

This vaccine incorporates only a part of the virus, i.e., harmless S proteins that best stimulate our immune system. Once our body's resistance system remembers these components, it builds antibodies and white blood cells for defensive mechanism. If we are infected with coronavirus in the near future, the antibodies will fight against that virus.

(iii) **Viral vector vaccines** contain a safe, altered variant of a virus that is different from the original one being targeted to deliver imperative lessons to host cells to make spike protein, which doesn't create disease but provides as base to generate coronavirus proteins to produce resistance power [45]. Inside exoskeleton/cover of the mutated virus, there is a substance available within the virus to make COVID-19. Once viral vector invades the owner's cells, the

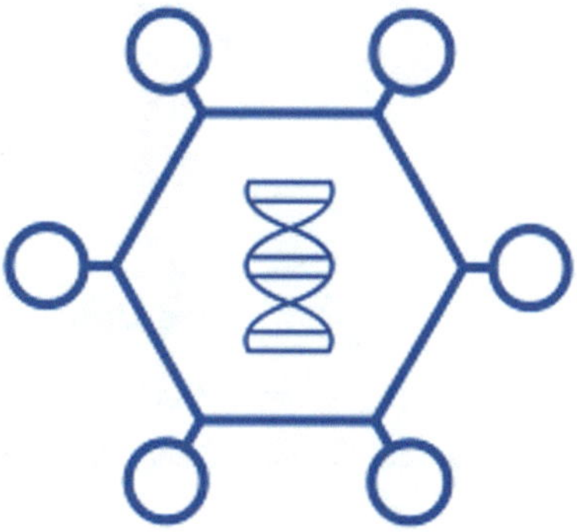

Fig. 9 Viral vector vaccine to coronavirus

ancestral material gives directions to the cells for formation of protein that is exclusive to the virus that causes COVID-19 [46].

Following these guidance's, our cells form imprint of such protein, which stimulates our immune system to evolve T-lymphocytes and B-lymphocytes that memorize how to battle with virus if we are infected in the upcoming days (Fig. 9).

Like mRNA vaccines, these types of vaccines don't bring indispensable message for presenter cells to compose the entire SARS-CoV-2 virus, because they are not incorporated in the full SARS-CoV-2 virus. Accordingly, they are unable to cause COVID-19 disease [47].

Three types of viral vector vaccines, named Oxford-AstraZeneca, Sputnik V, and Johnson & Johnson vaccines, utilizes different adenoviruses as the delivery system. Chimpanzee adenovirus vector ChAdOx1 is used in the Oxford-AstraZeneca vaccine, but two different human adenoviruses, i.e., Ad26 and Ad5, are incorporated in Russian Sputnik V vaccine. Further, Johnson & Johnson uses only one virus, i.e., Ad26, in such product. All three vaccines incorporate the gene for the spike protein and deliver into cells after injection. After that, this cell makes such protein and available within our immune system.

(iv) **Inactivated or weakened virus vaccine normally** uses the killed version of germ that doesn't motivate the disease but develops a strong immune response like live vaccines (Fig. 10). Therefore, we need a number of same doses over time (booster dose/precaution dose) in order to maintain the ongoing protection against diseases. Unlike the abovementioned three different classes of vaccines (i.e., mRNA, viral vector, and subunit), inactivated vaccines consist of the unified SARS-CoV-2 virus, but this virus is synthetically mutated to appease or weakened that is incapable to induce disease [48–50]. For the inactivation of SARS-CoV-2 virus in their vaccines, Sinovac, Sinopharm, and Bharat Biotech apply beta-propiolactone, which modifies the genetic material as well as nature of viruses. This form of vaccines is impotent to originate

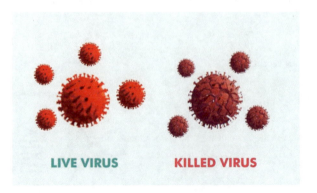

Fig. 10 Inactivated virus vaccine for COVID-19 disease

COVID-19 disease, because the virus is unable to reprint itself. Additionally, such antibody generated element does not induce sufficient immune response; as a result, immunity may not be long-lasting like the others. All the above-mentioned manufacturers are practiced with different adjuvants in their corona vaccines to achieve an improved and stronger immune response.

Working Mechanism of COVID-19 Vaccine

Although all the available vaccines offer protection by working in different ways, all types of vaccines are effective to generate sufficient number of "memory" T-lymphocytes and B-lymphocytes that may recall how to combat with this virus in the upcoming days (Fig. 11). In general, after 2–3 weeks of vaccination, our immune system is able to produce antibody generating T-lymphocytes as well as B-lymphocytes [51].

Therefore, it is impossible to protect a person from the infection of coronavirus just before or after vaccination and getting sick, because the vaccine did not have adequate time to develop immunity power for protection.

Occasionally just after vaccination, the mechanism of building immunity can cause mild to moderate symptoms in the form of fever, tiredness, muscle pain, headache, etc. These ailments are quite familiar and are normal signs, indicating that our body is developing immunity. To combat such symptoms, our doctors mainly prescribed pain-relieving medicine paracetamol, such as ibuprofen, acetaminophen, and aspirin (applicable for people age 18 years or above), or antihistaminic drug for any pain and/or discomfort experienced after vaccination.

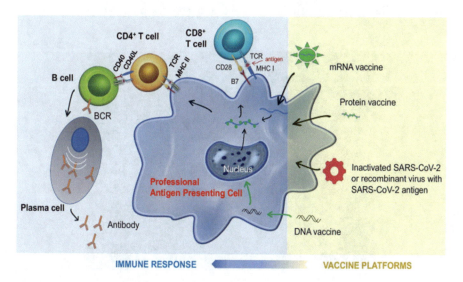

Fig. 11 Working mechanism of COVID-19 vaccine

Therefore, COVID-19 vaccines start working after administering into the immune system as mitigated form of the SARS-CoV-2 coronavirus or a part which is not responsible for COVID-19 but prepare hosts to confront against impending disease with same type of antigen [52].

The vaccines teach our body's resistance system about the recognition principle and how to wipe out the virus, before it causes us to be seriously ill. Our body's immune system builds such safeguard over time against such virus. We are fully secured within 7–14 days after the second dose of vaccination.

The vaccines help the body to:

- Confess these spike proteins as a threat
- Fight against coronavirus that has similar proteins

Vaccination

Vaccination is the process of a straightforward, secure, and successful approach of protecting people from detrimental pathogens by introducing a chemical compound into the body, before we come into contact with affected people (Fig. 12). It enhances our body's inherent defense mechanism to frame resistance toward distinct infections and builds our immune system stronger and stronger [53].

Vaccines to counter the COVID-19 disease are the most supreme tool to break the pandemic condition, but they are unable to do it individually. Public health and social measures including surveillance, contact tracing, isolation, and individual protective behaviors, such as social distancing (staying minimum 6 ft away from others), wearing the WHO recommended N95 or surgical mask over nose and mouth, avoiding poorly ventilated places and staying home if feeling unwell,

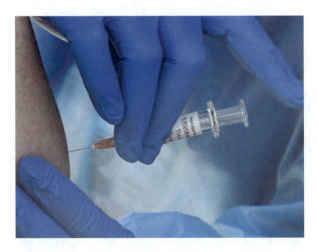

Fig. 12 Vaccination drive to stop the COVID-19 outbreak

covering coughs and sneezes, and cleaning our hands frequently with soap, remain crucial to breaking the chain of transmission [54, 55].

The impact of aforesaid vaccines over the pandemic situation depends on various factors, such as the effectiveness of the vaccines; how fast they are approved; how many people get vaccinated, produced, and delivered; the possible development of other variants; etc. [56].

Vaccination preserves us from serious danger and possible death of COVID-19 disease. After inoculation, for the first 14 days, we do not have satisfactory levels of protection as sufficient number of antibodies, but afterward, antibodies increased progressively. For the single-dose vaccine, prerogative will typically grow after 15 days of vaccination, but for double-shot vaccines, two doses, maintaining the prescribed interval between both shots, are essential to achieve the highest degree of immunity possible.

Although all of us know that any type of COVID-19 vaccine will defend us from serious disturbances and death, we still be studying and collecting information about the scope to which it keeps us from being infected and transmitting the virus to the others [57]. Statistical report obtained from other countries proclaiming that currently use vaccines are protecting us from severity of coronavirus disease and hospitalization. However, it is true that no vaccine is 100% proficient and breakthrough infections are regrettable, but to be expected up to that.

Present analytical data concede that vaccines provide some shelter from corona infection and spreading, but that safeguard is not up to the mark to counter serious illness and death. We are still researching about the latest variants of concern and also investigating whether the vaccines provide sufficient protection against those strains as non-variant virus. For these testaments, if most of the peoples of society may not be vaccinated, then maintaining other preventive measures is of paramount importance, especially in communities having notable SARS-CoV-2 transmission [58].

Service to keep us and others safe, and while efforts continue to reduce viral transmission and ramp up vaccine coverage, we should continue to maintain the WHO specified social distancing from others, cover a cough or sneeze in our elbow, clean our hands frequently, and wear an appropriate mask, particularly in enclosed, crowded, or poorly ventilated spaces or areas. Therefore, it is recommended to always pursue guidelines from the local authorities based on the situation and risk where we survive.

The COVID-19 vaccines available in the emergency use listing (EUL) of the WHO recommendation furnished different levels of protection toward mild infection, serious problems like respiratory syndrome, hospitalization, and possible death. Ongoing research investigation is carried out by thousands of scientists around the globe to understand how new virus mutations and variants will affect the effectiveness of different COVID-19 vaccines. In general, the COVID-19 vaccines are highly trustworthy against serious illness, hospitalization, and death from all current virus variants, but they are less active for protection to infection and mild disease than they were for earlier virus variants. If we do get ill after being vaccinated, our symptoms are more likely to be mild.

However, it is proven that the WHO-recommended COVID-19 vaccines are incredibly effective at reducing our risk of developing serious illness and death, but no vaccine is 100% potent. A small percentage of people will still get affected with COVID-19 disease even though they have been vaccinated. Presently, there is very limited information about the risk of vaccinated people who are passing the virus to another infected person. Thus, it is very relevant to continue to practice public health and social measures, even after we have been fully vaccinated.

The commonly used COVID-19 vaccines are:

(a) **Covaxin vaccine** – India's first indigenous, inactivated virus-based COVID-19 vaccine is Covaxin, developed by Bharat Biotech in collaboration with the Indian Council of Medical Research (ICMR) and National Institute of Virology (NIV) (Fig. 13). Whole-Virion Inactivated Vero Cell-derived platform technology is implemented for the evolution of this vaccine. It is a two-dose vaccination system given 4 weeks apart that received approval from Drugs Controller General of India (DCGI) for Phase I and II clinical trials, and the trials began all over India from July, 2020. It is proved and well-documented that this vaccine is able to neutralize the variants: B.1.1.7 (Alpha), first isolated in the UK; P.1 – B.1.1.28 (Gamma) and P.2 – B.1.1.28 (Zeta), primarily confined in Brazil; B.1.617 (Kappa), initially segregated in India; B.1.351 and B.1.617.2 (Beta and Delta), mainly outlined in RSA and India. According to analysis and subsequent findings of clinical trial, Bharat Biotech confirms that this vaccine is 65.2% effective against the SARS-CoV-2, B.1.617.2 Delta variant.

(b) **Covishield vaccine** – The Covishield vaccine, formerly known as ChAdOx1 nCoV-19 vaccine, is formulated from a deactivated variant of a common cold virus ChAdOx1, i.e., adenovirus (Fig. 14). A hereditary substance has been added to the adenovirus to build the spike (S) glycoprotein from the SARS-CoV-2 coronavirus. It is a recombinant, reproduction-impaired chimpanzee

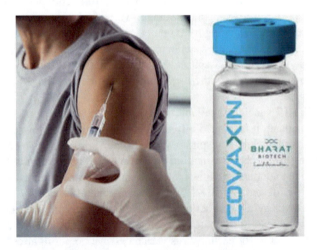

Fig. 13 Covaxin – India's first indigenous vaccine against COVID-19

Fig. 14 The Covishield COVID-19 vaccine

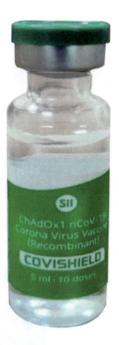

adenovirus vector encoding the SARS-CoV-2 spike (S) glycoprotein. After vaccine is administered, the genetic material from a part of the coronavirus is exposed, which stimulates an immune response.

On emergency basis, drug regulators in India approved this coronavirus vaccine for public uses that is developed by AstraZeneca Plc, along with the University of Oxford on January 1, 2021. The World Health Organization (WHO) recommended Serum Institute of India Pvt. Ltd. COVID-19 to produce Covishield on February 15, 2021. On March 19, 2021, the regulatory organization also confirmed that the AstraZeneca COVID-19 vaccine (Covishield) has a favorable benefit-risk profile, with an exceptional potential to prohibit infections and reduce deaths worldwide.

AstraZeneca announced on December 23, 2021, about Vaxzevria (ChAdOx1-S) that it substantially endorsed the levels of antibodies against the Omicron SARS-CoV-2 variant (B.1.1.529), following a third booster dose, according to the report obtained from a new laboratory study. The neutralizing antibody levels against Omicron following a third booster dose of Covishield was predominantly similar to levels accomplished after two doses to counter the Delta variant.

(c) **Johnson & Johnson vaccine** – COVID-19 vaccine formulated and developed by Johnson & Johnson contains a fragment of a modified virus, known as vector virus that is not the microbes that is responsible for corona, as they are unable to reproduce itself (Fig. 15). The composition used gives instructions to host cells to constitute an immune response which cooperates to insulate us from

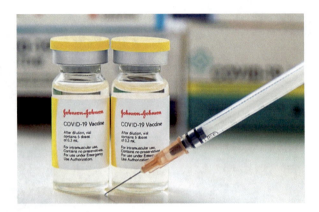

Fig. 15 Johnson & Johnson-developed COVID-19 vaccine

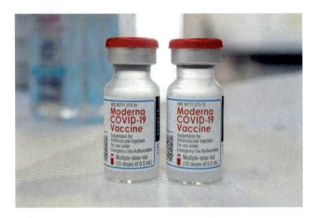

Fig. 16 Moderna COVID-19 vaccine

getting ill with COVID-19 in the forthcoming days. After the host develops sufficient immunity, it gets rid of all of the vaccine ingredients, just as it would discard any information that cells no longer need. Based on the investigation and results obtained from the clinical trial by the manufacturer, this vaccine has shown to be 66.9% effective on Delta and other variants.

(d) **Moderna vaccine** – The COVID-19 vaccine developed by Moderna is available under the EUA category of the WHO as a two-dose primary course, for individuals of 18 years or more; as a third dose, as precaution dose for individuals of the same age group who have been determined to have certain kinds of immune compromise; and as a single booster dose for individuals at least 6 months after completing an elementary series of the vaccine. The Moderna COVID-19 vaccine consists of a harmless piece of messenger RNA (mRNA) (Fig. 16). Based on the evidence and data obtained from clinical trials of people in the age group of 18 years or more, this vaccine was 94.1% effective against COVID-19 disease.

(e) **Sputnik V vaccine** – The Russian COVID-19 vaccine named as Sputnik V (Gam-COVID-Vac) is a viral vector vaccine based on adenovirus DNA, in which the SARS-CoV-2 coronavirus gene is unified. It is a twofold vaccine against the SARS-CoV-2 coronavirus, in which a weakened virus is to deliver small parts of a pathogen and stimulate an immune response to body. The host cell will utilize the gene of deactivated virus to grow the spike protein. The owner's immune system will determine this spike protein as foreign substances and cultivate a natural defense mechanism by developing antibodies and T cells against this protein. Unlike other vaccines, the Sputnik V vaccine minimizes the time required for the actual development of immunity to SARS-CoV-2, i.e., the Beta variants of COVID-19 pandemic. Gam-COVID-Vac is one of three corona vaccines in the world whose potency is more than 90% and became the world's first registered vaccine against coronavirus (Fig. 17).

(f) **Zydus Cadila vaccine** – On August 20, 2021, DCGI recommended Zydus Cadila-manufactured ZyCoV-D vaccine for emergency use authorization (EUA). This is the first DNA-based vaccine for COVID-19 in the world, indigenously developed by India, and has been administered in human beings, including youngster of 12 years and above and adults (Fig. 18). In association with DBT, the Government of India, Zydus Cadila developed this vaccine under "Mission COVID Suraksha" scheme implemented by Biotechnology Industry Research Assistance Council (BIRAC). ZyCoV-D has been financed through the National Biopharma Mission for preclinical studies, Phase I and Phase II clinical trials under COVID-19 Research Consortia, and subsequently the Mission COVID Suraksha for Phase III clinical exploration. The three-dose vaccine in injected form produces the spike protein of SARS-CoV-2 virus and extorts an immunity, which plays an indispensable role in security from disease as well as viral removal.

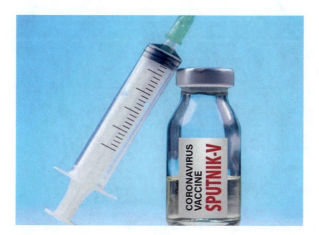

Fig. 17 Russian Sputnik V vaccine against COVID-19

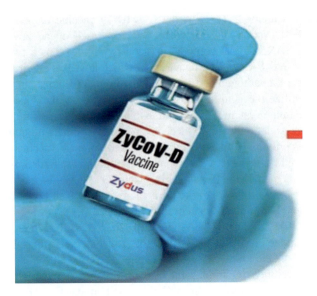

Fig. 18 ZyCoV-D vaccine manufactured by Zydus Cadilla

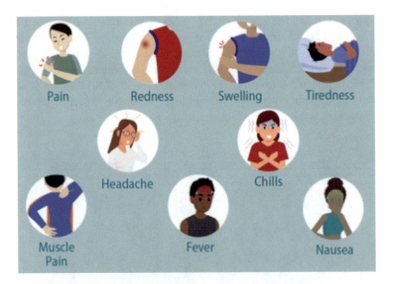

Fig. 19 Various side effects of COVID-19 vaccine

Side Effects of COVID-19 Vaccine

Just like other vaccines, few people experience mild to moderate reaction after being vaccinated against COVID-19, because this is a normal signal which indicate that our body is developing shelter (Fig. 19). Aftereffects to COVID-19 vaccines are not common for all, as well as it differed according to the specific vaccine, including delirium, fatigue, headache, muscle spasm, cold, diarrhea, and pain or redness at the injection spot. Most of the side effects disappear within a few days without medication by their own healing mechanism. We can subside the syndrome with rest, plenty of nonalcoholic liquids, and taking anti-inflammatory medication to manage pain and fever, if required.

More dangerous or lifelong side effects to COVID-19 vaccines are possible but exceptionally scarce and uncommon. In case of anyone struggling with any difficulty in respiration, chest spasm, distraction, speech loss, or impaired mobility after vaccination, it is advised to contact his/her healthcare provider immediately. The side effects of COVID-19 vaccines are under microscope for a long time since their use to detect and respond to rare adverse effects.

Importance of COVID-19 Vaccination

The inception of COVID-19 vaccine is the most important and massive step toward diminishing the acceleration of pandemic situation and further reducing the identical disease and deaths. The introduction of COVID-19 vaccine is the largest injection drive of globe and roll out that requires effective planning at various levels for proper execution. The major advantages of getting COVID-19 vaccines includes the following:

(i) **The vaccine reduces our risk of infection.**

Once we reap our maiden dosage of COVID-19 vaccine, our system starts to produce antiserum against coronavirus and support the resistance system to prevent such virus. If we were exposed to the infection, it lowers the chance of catching the disease. All types of available vaccines used worldwide are 70% or more effective toward infection.

It's true that some peoples are still affected after the full course of vaccination, but when a maximum number of people are vaccinated, those risks are progressively decreased. This adoption is known as herd immunity. So, fully vaccinated people will not only diminish their chance of getting infected but also devote to neighborhood protection, shortening the tendency of virus transmission.

(ii) **The vaccine can help the unborn or newborn baby.**

Researches admit that pregnant women who received COVID-19 vaccine create antibodies to counter the virus and transmit serum to their awaited baby through the placenta. Mothers were also shown to transfer immunity to newborn offspring through breast milk. The aforementioned study suggests that if mothers were fully vaccinated, then their newborn babies have some sort of immunity toward the virus, which is so crucial as budding children up to 12 years of age cannot get the vaccine till now.

(iii) **The vaccine protects against severe illness.**

During investigation, it was confirmed that all available vaccines are powerful against coronavirus and prevent severe illness from COVID-19. Thus, by any means, if we were infected after vaccination, chances of serious illness and possible death are reduced further. The clinical studies reveal that Pfizer-BioNTech- and Moderna-manufactured vaccines were 100% successful to prevent serious collapse, whereas Johnson & Johnson products exhibit 85% success rate to counter severe illness. Others offered more than 75% effectiveness for such infectious disease. These vaccines are also effective against different variants of the COVID-19 virus. As a result, all the vaccines will defend us from serious illness and scale down the possibility for hospitalization against COVID-19 disease.

As per the statistical report received from different studies, it is clear that the vaccinated people have less fierce effect of corona disease than the mass who aren't vaccinated if they were infected. Thus, our prospect toward hospitalization and the likelihood of death due to COVID-19 is almost dissipated once we are fully vaccinated.

(iv) **The vaccine helped us ditch the mask.**

Vaccine is the utmost solution in our attempt to recoup with the new normal of life, along with communal health screening, like skin temperature monitoring, face covering, social distancing, avoid gathering, hand-cleaning, sanitization, etc., executed properly to ease down the spread of the virus, and that has proven to work effectively. Although masks are still recommended in indoor areas, with high infection rates, as well as in public places, vaccine is our avenue toward the final destination beyond them.

Research data reveals that fully vaccinated people, if infected with such novel virus, have contain lesser virus particles in their body, especially in the respiratory path and mouth, and are less possible roll out to others. This statement is so salient that getting vaccinated now not only preserves us but also restricts the transmission of virus to our loved ones and friends.

Till now, people continue to receive their vaccine in time, we might reach herd immunity that clearly impede the spreading of virus becomes unlikely. Therefore, it is of paramount importance that all should receive vaccine in time to helps us accomplish this public health goal.

(v) **The vaccine will help us to reconnect with friends and family.**

After receiving the double dose of vaccine and waiting for the approved period for our body to develop the immunity, we can talk in person with other vaccinated people without wearing a mask. Moreover, if we've been near someone who has tested positive for COVID-19, we don't need any quarantine period to segregate ourselves.

Almost 1 year of anxiety, the vaccine has finally boomed and has clear benefits that should make everyone strongly believe for getting the shot. By selecting every individual to be vaccinated, we can't only protect ourselves but also provide safeguard to our family and community.

Conclusion

From the various literature and evidence collected from different incident and research, we know that proper health screening and vaccination against COVID-19 will minimize the chances of spreading coronavirus in the community. Through different health screening practices, we can quickly find out a COVID-19 victim at the initial phase and isolate them from their family and common people. All the above-mentioned examination and analysis steps will support the medical personnel to segregate affected people from others and outset medication to sufferer at the primary step of such infection. If the picture of screenings raises successfully for every individual, we can prohibit the growing of coronavirus to the society. Furthermore, vaccination against coronavirus disease may be the best hope in the world for the denouement of current pandemic situation. Available COVID 19-vaccines, such as Covishield, Covaxin, Sputnik V, etc., are highly impressive and competent and can easily weaken the endanger of getting and spreading the virus that causes COVID-19. Accelerated vaccination will not only protect us from getting mild to moderate symptoms, being more seriously ill, or dying due to coronavirus but also restrict us from spreading the pathogen that is responsible for COVID-19 disorder to a number of people in the community. Intercepting from thriving and reproducing the virus concedes it to mutate into less threatening genomic sequences that are least resistant to vaccines. Additionally, continuous awareness program also enforced to restrict the COVID-19 virus transmission within the population and efficiency of vaccines to curb the virus. Therefore, effective health screening and prompt vaccination will prevent the spreading of virus that causes COVID-19 disease and also minimize its adverse effects.

References

1. S. Bag, S. Sikdar, K. Ganguly, S. Banerjee, P. Lahiri, Effective health screening to prevent infection and control the spreading of COVID-19. J. Phys. Conf. Ser. **1797**(1), 012040 (2021)
2. H. Zhu, L. Wei, P. Niu, The novel coronavirus outbreak in Wuhan, China. Glob. Health Res. Policy **5**, 6 (2020)
3. A. Sharma, S. Tiwari, M.K. Deb, J.L. Marty, Severe acute respiratory syndrome coronavirus-2 (SARS-CoV-2): A global pandemic and treatment strategies. Int. J. Antimicrob. Agents **56**(2), 106054 (2020)
4. C.-C. Lai, T.-P. Shih, W.-C. Ko, H.-J. Tang, P.-R. Hsuehe, Severe acute respiratory syndrome coronavirus 2 (SARS-CoV-2) and coronavirus disease-2019 (COVID-19): The epidemic and the challenges. Int. J. Antimicrob. Agents **55**(3), 105924 (2020)
5. Y.-C. Wu, C.-S. Chen, Y.-J. Chan, The outbreak of COVID-19: An overview. J. Chin. Med. Assoc. **83**(3), 217–220 (2020)
6. D. Wu, T. Wu, Q. Liu, Z. Yang, The SARS-CoV-2 outbreak: What we know. Int. J. Infect. Dis. **94**, 44–48 (2020)
7. W. Guan, Z. Ni, Y. Hu, W. Liang, C. Ou, J. He, L. Liu, H. Shan, C. Lei, D.S.C. Hui, B. Du, L. Li, G. Zeng, K.Y. Yuen, R. Chen, C. Tang, T. Wang, P. Chen, J. Xiang, S. Li, J.-l. Wang, Z. Liang, Y. Peng, L. Wei, Y. Liu, Y.-h. Hu, P. Peng, J.-m. Wang, J. Liu, Z. Chen, G. Li, Z. Zheng, S. Qiu,

J. Luo, C. Ye, S. Zhu, N. Zhong, Clinical characteristics of coronavirus disease 2019 in China. N. Engl. J. Med. **2020**, 1708–1720 (2020)
8. S. Zaim, J.H. Chong, V. Sankaranarayanan, A. Harky, COVID-19 and multiorgan response. Curr. Probl. Cardiol. **45**(8), 100618 (2020)
9. S. Mandal, T. Bhatnagar, N. Arinaminpathy, A. Agarwal, A. Chowdhury, M. Murhekar, R.R. Gangakhedkar, S. Sarkar, Prudent public health intervention strategies to control the coronavirus disease 2019 transmission in India: A mathematical model-based approach. Indian J. Med. Res. **151**(2 & 3), 190–199 (2020)
10. M. Jayaweera, H. Perera, B. Gunawardana, J. Manatungea, Transmission of COVID-19 virus by droplets and aerosols: A critical review on the unresolved dichotomy. Environ. Res. **188**, 109819 (2020)
11. S. Sanche, Y.T. Lin, C. Xu, E. Romero-Severson, N. Hengartner, R. Ke, High contagiousness and rapid spread of severe acute respiratory syndrome coronavirus 2. Emerg. Infect. Dis. **26**, 1470–1477 (2020)
12. W.E. Wei, Z. Li, C.J. Chiew, S.E. Yong, M.P. Toh, V.J. Lee, Singapore presymptomatic transmission of SARS-CoV-2. MMWR Morb. Mortal. Wkly Rep. **69**, 411–415 (2020)
13. J. Chen, Pathogenicity and transmissibility of 2019-nCoV – a quick overview and comparison with other emerging viruses. Microbes Infect. **22**, 69–71 (2020)
14. R. Guner, İ. Hasanoğlu, F. Aktas, COVID-19: prevention and control measures in community. Turk. J. Med. Sci. **50**(SI-1), 571–577 (2020)
15. M. Lotfi, M.R. Hamblin, N. Rezaei, COVID-19: Transmission, prevention, and potential therapeutic opportunities. Clin. Chim. Acta **508**, 254–266 (2020)
16. R. Keni, A. Alexander, P.G. Nayak, J. Mudgal, K. Nandakumar, COVID-19: emergence, spread, possible treatments, and global burden. Front. Public Health **8**, 216 (2020)
17. F. Krammer, SARS-CoV-2 vaccines in development. Nature **586**, 516–527 (2020)
18. J.P. Moore, P.A. Offit, SARS-CoV-2 vaccines and the growing threat of viral variants. JAMA **325**(9), 821–822 (2021)
19. J.M.G. Wilson, G. Jungner, *Principles and Practice of Screening for Disease*, Public Health Papers Number 34 (Geneva, WHO, 1968)
20. L.D. Maxim, R. Niebo, M.J. Utell, Screening tests: a review with examples. Inhal. Toxicol. **26**(13), 811–828 (2014)
21. A.N. Desai, P. Patel, Stopping the spread of COVID-19. JAMA **323**, 1516 (2020)
22. B. Nussbaumer-Streit, V. Mayr, A.I. Dobrescu, A. Chapman, E. Persad, Quarantine alone or in combination with other public health measures to control COVID-19: A rapid review. Cochrane Database Syst. Rev. **4**(4), CD013574 (2020)
23. S.H.S. Tali, J.J. LeBlanc, Z. Sadiq, O.D. Oyewunmi, C. Camargo, B. Nikpour, N. Armanfard, S.M. Sagan, S. Jahanshahi-Anbuhi, Tools and techniques for severe acute respiratory syndrome coronavirus 2 (SARS-CoV-2)/COVID-19 detection. Clin. Microbiol. Rev. **34**(3), e00228-20 (2021)
24. R.S. Burnham, R.S. McKinley, D.D. Vincent, Three types of skin-surface thermometers: a comparison of reliability, validity, and responsiveness. Am. J. Phys. Med. Rehabil. **85**(7), 553–558 (2006)
25. G.B. Dell'Isola, E. Cosentini, L. Canale, G. Ficco, M. Dell'Isola, Noncontact body temperature measurement: uncertainty evaluation and screening decision rule to prevent the spread of COVID-19. Sensors **21**, 346 (2021)
26. P. Ghassemi, T. Joshua Pfefer, J.P. Casamento, R. Simpson, Q. Wang, Best practices for standardized performance testing of infrared thermographs intended for fever screening. PLOS ONE **13**, e0203302 (2018)
27. R. Wölfel, V.M. Corman, W. Guggemos, M. Seilmaier, S. Zange, M.A. Müller, D. Niemeyer, T.C. Jones, P. Vollmar, C. Rothe, M. Hoelscher, T. Bleicker, S. Brünink, J. Schneider, R. Ehmann, K. Zwirglmaier, C. Drosten, C. Wendtner, Virological assessment of hospitalized patients with COVID-2019. Nature **581**, 465–469 (2020)

28. B.D. Kevadiya, J. Machhi, J. Herskovitz, M.D. Oleynikov, W.R. Blomberg, N. Bajwa, D. Soni, S. Das, M. Hasan, M. Patel, A.M. Senan, S. Gorantla, J.E. McMillan, B. Edagwa, R. Eisenberg, C.B. Gurumurthy, S.P.M. Reid, C. Punyadeera, L. Chang, H.E. Gendelman, Diagnostics for SARS-CoV-2 infections. Nat. Mater. **20**, 593–605 (2021)
29. W. Joost Wiersinga, A. Rhodes, A.C. Cheng, S.J. Peacock, H.C. Prescott, Pathophysiology, transmission, diagnosis, and treatment of coronavirus disease 2019 (COVID-19): A review. JAMA **324**(8), 782–793 (2020)
30. K.C. Coffey, D.J. Diekema, D.J. Morgan, Interpreting SARS-CoV-2 test results. JAMA **326**(15), 1528–1529 (2021)
31. B. Udugama, P. Kadhiresan, H.N. Kozlowski, A. Malekjahani, M. Osborne, V.Y.C. Li, H. Chen, S. Mubareka, J.B. Gubbay, W.C.W. Chan, Diagnosing COVID-19: the disease and tools for detection. ACS Nano **14**(4), 3822–3835 (2020)
32. L.E. Brümmer, S. Katzenschlager, M. Gaeddert, C. Erdmann, S. Schmitz, M. Bota, M. Grilli, J. Larmann, M.A. Weigand, N.R. Pollock, A. Macé, S. Carmona, S. Ongarello, J.A. Sacks, C.M. Denkinger, Accuracy of novel antigen rapid diagnostics for SARS-CoV-2: a living systematic review and meta-analysis. PLOS Med. **18**(10), e1003825 (2021)
33. A.E. Fiore, C.B. Bridges, N.J. Cox, "Seasonal influenza vaccines". Vaccines for pandemic influenza. Curr. Top. Microbiol. Immunol. **333**, 43–82 (2009)
34. K.M. Edwards, W.A. Orenstein, *COVID-19: Vaccines* (UpToDate – Literature Review Current Through, 2022)
35. F. Krammer, SARS-CoV-2 vaccines in development. Nature **586**, 516 (2020)
36. B.S. Graham, Rapid COVID-19 vaccine development. Science **368**, 945 (2020)
37. M.K. Andrew, J.E. McElhaney, Age and frailty in COVID-19 vaccine development. Lancet **396**(10267), 1942–1944 (2020)
38. G. Dagotto, J. Yu, D.H. Barouch, Approaches and challenges in SARS-CoV-2 vaccine development. Cell Host Microbe **28**(3), 364–370 (2020)
39. S. Jain, H. Batra, P. Yadav, S. Chand, COVID-19 vaccines currently under preclinical and clinical studies, and associated antiviral immune response. Vaccine **8**(4), 649 (2020)
40. N. Pardi, M.J. Hogan, F.W. Porter, D. Weissman, mRNA vaccines—a new era in vaccinology. Nat. Rev. Drug Discov. **17**(4), 261–279 (2018)
41. J. Abbasi, COVID-19 and mRNA vaccines—first large test for a new approach. JAMA **324**(12), 1125–1127 (2020)
42. B. Pulendran, P.S. Arunachalam, D.T. O'Hagan, Emerging concepts in the science of vaccine adjuvants. Nat. Rev. Drug Discov. **20**, 454–475 (2021)
43. S.P. Kaur, V. Gupta, COVID-19 vaccine: a comprehensive status report. Virus Res. **288**, 198114 (2020)
44. V. Bajaj, N. Gadi, A.P. Spihlman, S.C. Wu, C.H. Choi, V.R. Moulton, Aging, immunity, and COVID-19: How age influences the host immune response to coronavirus infections? Front. Physiol. (2021). https://doi.org/10.3389/fphys.2020.571416
45. T. Ura, K. Okuda, M. Shimada, Developments in viral vector-based vaccines. Vaccines (Basel) **2**(3), 624–641 (2014)
46. Y. Lazebnik, Cell fusion as a link between the SARS-CoV-2 spike protein, COVID-19 complications, and vaccine side effects. Oncotarget **12**(25), 2476–2488 (2021)
47. Z. Matić, M. Šantak, Current view on novel vaccine technologies to combat human infectious diseases. Appl. Microbiol. Biotechnol. **106**, 25–56 (2022)
48. A. Jara, E.A. Undurraga, C. González, P. Paredes, T. Fontecilla, G. Jara, A. Pizarro, J. Acevedo, K. Leo, F. Leon, C. Sans, P. Leighton, P. Suárez, H. García-Escorza, R. Araos, Effectiveness of an inactivated SARS-CoV-2 vaccine in Chile. N. Engl. J. Med. **385**, 875 (2021)
49. N. Al Kaabi, Y. Zhang, S. Xia, Y. Yang, M.M. Al Qahtani, N. Abdulrazzaq, M. Al Nusair, M. Hassany, J.S. Jawad, J. Abdalla, S.E. Hussein, S.K. Al Mazrouei, M. Al Karam, X. Li, X. Yang, W. Wang, B. Lai, W. Chen, S. Huang, Q. Wang, T. Yang, Y. Liu, R. Ma, Z.M. Hussain, T. Khan, M.S. Fasihuddin, W. You, Z. Xie, Y. Zhao, Z. Jiang, G. Zhao, Y. Zhang, S. Mahmoud, I. ElTantawy, P. Xiao, A. Koshy, W.A. Zaher, H. Wang, K. Duan, A. Pan, X. Yang, Effect of 2

inactivated SARS-CoV-2 vaccines on symptomatic COVID-19 infection in adults: a randomized clinical trial. JAMA **326**, 35 (2021)
50. S.L. Xia, Y.T. Zhang, Y.X. Wang, H. Wang, Y.K. Yang, G.F. Gao, W.J. Tan, G.Z. Wu, M. Xu, Z.Y. Lou, W.J. Huang, W.B. Xu, B.Y. Huang, W. Wang, W. Zhang, N. Li, Z.Q. Xie, X. Zhu, L. Ding, W.Y. You, Y.X. Zhao, J. Zhao, L.L. Huang, X.Z. Shi, Y.L. Yang, G.X. Xu, W.L. Wang, P.P. Liu, M. Ma, Y.L. Qiao, S.H. Zhao, J.J. Chai, Q.Q. Li, F. Hui, Y. Xu, X.T. Zheng, W.S. Guo, X.M. Yang, Safety and immunogenicity of an inactivated COVID-19 vaccine, BBIBP-CorV, in people younger than 18 years: a randomised, double-blind, controlled, phase 1/2 trial. Lancet Infect. Dis. **22**(2), 196–208 (2022)
51. M. Sadarangani, A. Marchant, T.R. Kollmann, Immunological mechanisms of vaccine-induced protection against COVID-19 in humans. Nat. Rev. Immunol. **21**, 475–484 (2021)
52. M.T. Mascellino, F. Di Timoteo, M. De Angelis, A. Oliva, Overview of the main anti-SARS-CoV-2 vaccines: mechanism of action, efficacy and safety. Infect. Drug Resist. **14**, 3459–3476 (2021)
53. H.F. Florindo, R. Kleiner, D. Vaskovich-Koubi, R.C. Acúrcio, B. Carreira, E. Yeini, G. Tiram, Y. Liubomirski, R. Satchi-Fainaro, Immune-mediated approaches against COVID-19. Nat. Nanotechnol. **15**, 630–645 (2020)
54. E.N. Perencevich, D.J. Diekema, M.B. Edmond, Moving personal protective equipment into the community: face shields and containment of COVID-19. JAMA **323**(22), 2252–2253 (2020)
55. L. Martinelli, V. Kopilaš, M. Vidmar, C. Heavin, H. Machado, Z. Todorović, N. Buzas, M. Pot, B. Prainsack, S. Gajović, Face masks during the COVID-19 pandemic: a simple protection tool with many meanings. Front. Public Health **8**, 606635 (2021)
56. T. Hasan, J. Beardsley, B.J. Marais, T.A. Nguyen, G.J. Fox, The implementation of mass-vaccination against SARS-CoV-2: a systematic review of existing strategies and guidelines. Vaccines (Basel) **9**, 326 (2021)
57. E.J. Haas, F.J. Angulo, J.M. McLaughlin, E. Anis, S.R. Singer, F. Khan, N. Brooks, M. Smaja, G. Mircus, K. Pan, J. Southern, D.L. Swerdlow, L. Jodar, Y. Levy, S. Alroy-Preis, Impact and effectiveness of mRNA BNT162b2 vaccine against SARS-CoV-2 infections and COVID-19 cases, hospitalisations, and deaths following a nationwide vaccination campaign in Israel: an observational study using national surveillance data. Lancet **397**, 1819–1819 (2021)
58. A. Singanayagam, S. Hakki, J. Dunning, K.J. Madon, M.A. Crone, A. Koycheva, N. Derqui-Fernandez, J.L. Barnett, M.G. Whitfield, R. Varro, A. Charlett, R. Kundu, J. Fenn, J. Cutajar, V. Quinn, E. Conibear, P.W. Barclay, P.S. Freemont, G.P. Taylor, S. Ahmad, M. Zambon, N.M. Ferguson, P.A. Lalvani, Community transmission and viral load kinetics of the SARS-CoV-2 delta (B.1.617.2) variant in vaccinated and unvaccinated individuals in the UK: a prospective, longitudinal, cohort study. Lancet **22**(2), 183–195 (2022)

Crowd Density Estimation Using Neural Network for COVID-19 and Future Pandemics

S. U. Muthunagai, M. S. Girija, R. Iyswarya, S. Poorani, and R. Anitha

Introduction

COVID'19 is a corona virus-related disease that was first discovered in Wuhan, China, in late December 2020. Several healthcare organizations struggled a lot to combat this deadly virus, but no solution is obtained to get rid of this disease. Many nations have implemented new laws regarding the use of face masks for corona virus epidemic. Governments have begun to develop new techniques for managing space, social distance [1], and supplies for medical personnel and ordinary citizens. But still, it spreads quickly in crowded places and through close touch. In many nations, governments face enormous obstacles and hazards in protecting people from the corona virus. To combat and win the COVID'19 pandemic, governments will need advice and surveillance of people in public places, particularly those that are packed, to ensure that laws prohibiting the use of face masks are followed. This might be accomplished by combining surveillance technologies with artificial intelligence models.

Moving object tracking [2–4] in videos is an actively researched area for the last two decades due to its practical applications in many areas, such as event analysis, human-computer interaction, crowd analysis, etc. Although extensive research has revealed some successful applications in highly confined environments, there are still numerous obstacles to overcome, such as sudden object motion, changes in object appearance, nonrigid objects, occlusion, illumination, and other issues. Many researchers are working on computer vision systems that try to simulate the

---

S. U. Muthunagai (✉) · M. S. Girija · R. Iyswarya · S. Poorani · R. Anitha
Department of Computer Science and Engineering, Sri Venkateswara College of Engineering, Sriperumbudur, India
e-mail: muthunagai@svce.ac.in; girijamagesh@svce.ac.in; iyswarya@svce.ac.in; spoorani@svce.ac.in; ranitha@svce.ac.in

© The Author(s), under exclusive license to Springer Nature Switzerland AG 2023
G. R. Kanagachidambaresan et al. (eds.), *System Design for Epidemics Using Machine Learning and Deep Learning*, Signals and Communication Technology, https://doi.org/10.1007/978-3-031-19752-9_15

biological systems' basic abilities, such as the ability to understand scenes, detect objects (static or moving), understand the environment, recognize events, analyze crowds, count people, detect people and vehicles, and so on. Object detection is the process of detecting an object of interest in a scene, such as people, automobiles, and other objects. Tracking of object is defined as the determination of a moving object's trajectory, such as following a moving car's trajectory to detect lane violations. Videos are made from either static cameras, such as surveillance cameras, or moving cameras, such as cameras installed on a mobile robot, for tracking objects. The background is constantly static, and objects move in a static camera, but things move in a dynamic background with a moving camera.

Tracking Framework for Objects

In the realm of computer vision, object tracking is a critical problem. Object tracking algorithms have attracted a lot of researchers with highly available and low-cost multimedia data. Detection, tracking, and analyzing the activity-based objects are the three main phases involved in the multimedia domain. Among the three phases, tracking is one of the tedious processes, as it involves determination of time-sensitive data in the scene. It also provides object-related information, such as direction of object, object's region, and object's form. It has been approached in a variety of ways. These mainly differ from one another in terms of how they tackle the following issues: Which representation of an object is best for tracking? What image attributes should you employ? How should the object's motion, look, and shape be modeled? The extracted data that contains the tracking information answers all the above questions.

Object Detection

Object detection refers to locating the entity in each frame of a video, which is a prerequisite for starting a tracking procedure. There are two types of object detection algorithms: (1) to examine the corners of an object in the frame and (2) self-acted object detection using predetermined features, such as color. A variety of methods for detecting moving objects, including background subtraction, Kalman filter, and particle filter, are some of the techniques used. In video sequences with a static background, background subtraction is commonly employed. The image is divided into foreground and background using this method. The objects that are in motion, such as human and vehicles, are in foreground, while immobile elements, such as roads, buildings, trees, and motionless cars, are in the background.

If there are no objects in the scene, a reference background image is acquired first. By removing the existing picture frame from the base picture, the moving object is detected. Except for the area occupied by the object, the generated gap has a range within the threshold limit. Foreground pixels are those with a difference greater than the threshold, because the background picture has to be updated periodically.

Temporal differencing is a technique that works well in situations when the camera moves. It detects objects using pixel-by-pixel comparisons of two or three successive frames. The moving camera and moving object are jumbled up in a moving camera situation. As a result, several researchers advocated that the camera motion be measured and adjusted first, followed by the backdrop subtraction method. For a fast-moving object, this approach does not work for the overlapping regions of the entities, which are in motion, because it does not detect the trailing portion.

Another method that detects motion objects in video is the optical flow. It produces a 2D vector field in which each point direction and velocities in a series of images are detected. Images can be segmented into sections that correspond to various objects, thanks to discontinuities in the optical flow. Despite its processing cost, the approach has the advantage of being able to detect movement in the series of frames in video.

Identifying entities in a video can be accomplished by using supervised learning approaches to build a classification model that understands the views of multiple objects and appearances. Following the training of a classifier, the test region of the target object can be concluded.

Object Modeling

The object of interest in a scene is represented via object modeling. To represent an object, features that define it uniquely are extracted. These characteristics, or descriptors, are utilized to trail the object. A feature is a visual design, which distinguishes an object from its surroundings. Using some procedures around the features, items are turned into descriptors, also known as appearance features.

Object Representation

The way an object is exhibited for tracking is referred to as object representation. In general, the type of object representation to use is determined by the application domain. Point representation means one point or a series of points used to represent an object. Points are calculated based on the object of statistics. The key benefit of adopting the point representation is how quickly it can be processed and manipulated.

- Primitive geometric shapes
  Rectangle, square, ellipse, circle, and other primitive geometric forms are used to depict the item. The most common shape for tracking people and vehicles is the rectangle.

- Articulated shape models
  Articulated objects – human body made up of body parts connected by joints. Rectangles, cylinders, and ellipses are among the primordial geometric shapes that make up the body parts. Kinematic motion models manage the connection between the pieces.
- Skeletal models
  Both articulated and rigid objects are modeled using skeleton representation. The skeleton is a set of articulations within an entity that terms dependencies and restrictions amid part illustrations. The authors used the skeletal model to detect a large number of persons.
- Contour
  The boundary of an item is defined by contour. It just describes the object's edges, which is an acceptable representation for nonrigid objects. The silhouette is expressed either explicitly or implicitly in contour-based approaches.

Appearance Features

The appearance features of an item, also known as descriptors, can be represented in a variety of ways, and color histogram is used for estimating the density of an object's appearance. The main disadvantage of using histograms is that two things with very similar color histograms can appear to be completely different. Simple geometric forms or silhouettes are used to create templates, which are only useful for tracking objects whose stances do not change much throughout monitoring. It contains both geographical and appearance information. Templates, on the other hand, simply save the appearance of an object generated by a single view.

Object Tracking

It is a process of calculating a moving object's trajectory in a video. To produce the trajectory for tracking, identify the positions of the object in two successive frames, and continue this step for the whole video series. Occasionally, the object is obscured by another object for a few frames before reappearing. As a result, the tracker must be capable of handling partial or complete occlusion. A comprehensive visual tracker must address a number of difficulties, including sudden object movements, noise in image sequences, changes in the appearance of the item and the scene, illumination, and so on.

The surveys have been published on object tracking, as well as their limitations and applications. Before 2006, Yilmaz et al. evaluated object tracking systems, providing classification and analysis.

In the literature, the methods for simplifying visual tracking have been presented. This section provides an overview of object tracking strategies and recommends a classification based on the approaches used to track things.

Feature-Based Methods

In feature-based methods – attributes are extracted, viz., texture, gradient, color, etc., that are priorly defined during object tracking. It is ensured that the defined attributes are unique in nature in order to distinguish from others. The objects, which are similar in the upcoming frames, are extracted using the above information as reference. There are color-based models, interest point operator, texture-based models, and optical flow-based methods.

Estimation-Based Methods

The tracking of entities in video is formulated as a state computation problem, in which an entity is denoted as a vector. Estimation or filtering-based methods express the tracking problem as a state estimation problem. The state vector depicts the system's dynamic behavior and contains motion properties of the object in question, such as position, velocity, and acceleration. Bayesian approaches provide a generic framework for dynamic state estimation problems. The probability density function of the state vector is constructed utilizing all available data at the time in this method. The posterior probability density function contains all of the information about the object's state, making it a full solution to the state estimation problem. Two models are employed to compute the posterior probability density functions of the states, which are based on state and observation.

Observation model depicts the relationship between observation and state, whereas the state model describes the system's evolution. The Kalman filter and the particle filter are the two common Bayesian algorithms for estimating object trajectories. It provides a full discussion of these two filters. There are two steps to the filters: prediction and correction. The representation, which is based on the state, is used for prediction and also for estimating new set of attributes at the next step. Whereas the observation model enables to perform the correction step to update the object's state. Each image frame in the movie is used to perform the prediction and correction stages which is done using the Kalman and particle filter.

Segmentation-Based Methods

The most basic and crucial stage in visual tracking will be a focus on nearby objects from a given video frame, to distinguish focused objects from the background image, using a foreground segmentation. Typically, the foreground objects in a scene are those that move. These objects must be segregated from the backdrop scene in order to be tracked. The methodologies for tracking moving objects using segmentation algorithms are discussed in the next section.

Learning-Based Methods

The visual tracking problem can also be thought of as a decision-making process, in which a classifier is well trained, and they can be able to obtain the object similarity between the target and background object. A classification function learns the different viewpoints and appearances of the object [6] first and then decides whether it is the target object or not on the test region. To extract features from various view, different supervised algorithm is used here, mainly boosting, decision trees, neural networks, and support vector machines (SVM). The maximum marginal hyperplane in a multidimensional space is used to classify data into two separable classes using SVM. The margin is obtained by calculating the difference between the hyperplane and the nearest data points. The support vectors is calculated by the data points that fall on the edge of the hyperplane's margin.

The SVM [8, 9] was combined with an optic-flow tracker to detect the vehicles' rear end. By maximizing the SVM classification score, the SVM was trained offline to distinguish between vehicles and non-vehicles. To address huge image motions, a Gaussian pyramid was built from each support vector. Tian presented an ensemble classifier, the linear SVM with online learning process, that uses history information to automatically choose useful key frames of the target. The ensemble SVM classifier is made up of many classifiers that aid in the classifier's online updating, allowing it to better manage target appearance variation. Exemplar-SVM is a system proposed by Tomasz Malisiewicz that trains a separate classifier for each exemplar, resulting in a collection of simpler exemplar-SVM. A single positive example and millions of negatives are used to train each exemplar-SVM. This SVM ensemble produces good results. Zhang recommended using multi-view to obtain more accurate findings.

Another learning-based method for tracking objects is boosting. It is used to reduce the error of any weak learning algorithm and to find an accurate classifier by integrating a large number of base classifiers. It performs a weak learning algorithm over the training data several times before combining the weak learner's classifiers into an accurate classifier. Kim presented a multi-classifier boosting technique that softly splits the input space for each classifier and learns numerous object appearances.

Proposed Model

The crowd density estimator detects the amount to which social distancing protocols are observed in the region automatically. Its usage on existing surveillance systems and drones used by the police to monitor broad regions can aid in the prevention of coronavirus, by allowing for automatic and better tracking of activities in the area. It displays real-time analytics of the area. It can also be used to warn the police in the event of a significant breach of social distancing standards in a specific area. Figure 1 represents the flow diagram of the proposed framework.

Controlling the transmission of COVID-19 has relied heavily on social distance. Monitoring social distance between people in public places is a time-consuming operation, but it is an important aspect in the propagation of COVID-19. While there are many different ways for detecting crowd density in a given region in real time, the key feature of the crowd density estimation cum social distance analyzer is that the distance between any two items categorized as "person" should be higher than

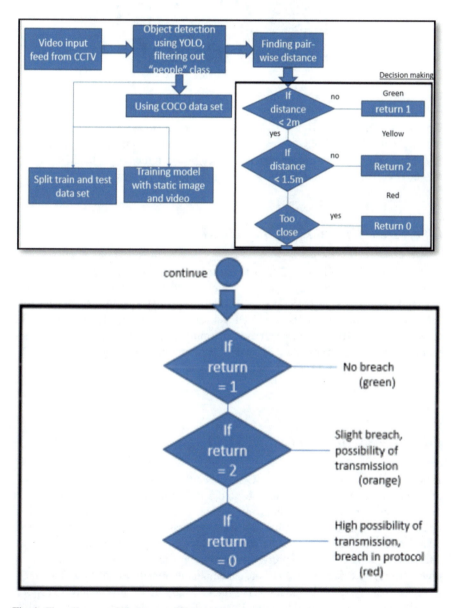

Fig. 1 Flow diagram of the proposed framework

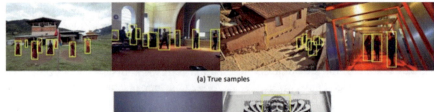
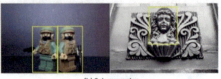

Fig. 2 Dataset containing (**a**) true samples and (**b**) false samples

2 m or 6 ft. The proposed model extracts the "people" object from the video input feed and calculates not only the overall number of people in the region as shown in Fig. 2 but also the pairwise Euclidean distance between the two individuals, allowing the social distance protocol to be maintained to its maximum.

Object Detection and Tracking Model

On the PASCAL-VOC and MS-COCO datasets, many object detection models are used to find speed, accuracy based on region-based convolutional neural network (RCNN), fast RCNN, faster RCNN, SSD, YOLO ver1 [3], YOLO ver2 [4], and Yolo [5], which is influenced by factors such as backbone architecture, *i/p* sizes, model depth, and the software and hardware environment. A feature separator converts input into a feature representation, used to learn and identify patterns related to the desired objects. YOLO employs the Darknet-53 architecture described by Redmon et al.

YOLO Object Detection

By just looking at an image once, YOLO [7] can determine the nature and location of an object. To give class probabilities to the anchor boxes, YOLO treats the object detection as a regression process rather than a classification process. Multiple bounding boxes and class probabilities are predicted simultaneously by a single neural network. YOLO [2] is divided into three versions: ver1, ver2, and ver3. YOLO ver1 is based on GoogLeNet (Inception network), which is used to classify objects in images. Figure 3 shows the schematic demonstration of YOLO architecture. There are 24 convolutional layers [9] and 2 fully linked layers in this network. The Inception modules used by GoogLeNet has been replaced with YOLO ver1. It used reduction layer, followed by convolutional layers.

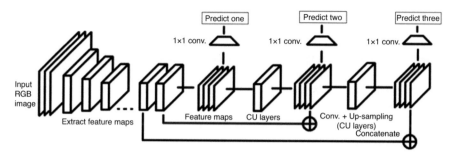

Fig. 3 Schematic representation of YOLO architecture

Later, YOLO v2 [8] was presented with the goal of considerably enhancing accuracy while also making it faster. Darknet-19, consists of 19 convolution layers, 5 max pooling layers, and an output softmax layer for object categorization, is used in YOLO ver2. With considerable increases in mAP, FPS, and object categorization score, YOLO v2 surpassed its predecessor (YOLO ver1). In contrast to YOLO ver1 and ver2, YOLO does multi-label classification using logistic classifiers rather than softmax, like in YOLO ver1 and ver2.

Darknet-53 is a backbone architecture introduced by Redmon et al. in YOLO that harvests feature maps for categorization. Darknet-53, in contrast to Darknet-19, includes residual blocks (short connections) as well as up sampling levels for network concatenation and depth. YOLO makes three predictions for each spatial location in an image at different scales, removing the issue of being unable to detect small objects efficiently. The objectless, boundary box regress, and classification scores are computed for each prediction.

In order to recognize objects in real time, convolutional neural networks are used. It can be done in a single run of an algorithm, because it is a forward propagation method. The COCO dataset is used as the data source. Humans and other moving items (luggage, inanimate objects, automobiles, etc.) are classified using exceedingly comprehensive labels and classifications. We can avoid any errors in the algorithm's execution, because the data set is well-defined. To associate and provide the path to the person in the movie, the object identification prototype is fine-tuned with true and false samples of people's images, as shown in Fig. 2. The surveillance footage is fed to the trained model. For each identified person, the prototype gives a set of leaping boxes.

Pairwise Distance Calculation Using Manhattan Distance

Each detected person has a 3D feature space (x, y, d), in which (x, y) are the centroid coordinates of the bounding box and d represents the depth of the individual as seen by the camera.

$$d = \left((2*3.14*180)/(w+h*360)*1000+3\right)$$

where *w* represents the width of the bounding box and *h* denotes the height of the bounding box. The Manhattan distance between the first person and the second person is calculated as follows. If $x = (a,b)$ and $y = (c,d)$, then the Manhattan distance between *x* and *y* is $|a - c| + |b - d|$.

Closeness Property

When the pairwise distance between two things is greater than 2.0 m (6 ft), they are considered safe. There is a minor chance of transmission and breach of nearby distance protocol if the found distance is less than 2.0 m and greater than or equal to 1.5 m. If the discovered distance is less than 1.5 m, then there is a strong possibility of a collision.

Possibility of the Breach in the Protocol and Transmission

Anyone that meets the closeness property is allocated to an adjacent node or nearby dimensions, which create a cluster that is denoted by various color lines in comparison to different people. The development of collective nodes denotes a breach of the practice of community separation, which can be measured using the following criteria: – *ng* represents the number of identified superclusters, and np represents the closeness of the population detected. The slighter breaches of protocols are represented by orange bounding boxes and connecting lines, the more serious breaches by red bounding boxes and connecting lines, and objects at a safe distance by green bounding boxes and connecting lines.

Object Detection and Distance Calculation Using Proposed Scheme

Input Feed

An input feed is taken for examination using a CCTV live relay. It is determined whether the number of individuals in a room can be kept under safe conditions using this feed, which is then saved as frames per minute. For crowd density estimation, this is employed as an approximation method. This step is critical, because it is the initial stage of our analysis. It is possible to compartmentalize our required info by breaking our feed into frames.

Methods for estimating crowd density can be classified into two categories.

Direct methods: In crowds, some classifiers are employed to segment or detect each individual human body. The bodies are then tallied to determine the human crowd density. These techniques are further separated into two sorts.

Model-based methods: Detection or segmentation is done using human body models or shape contours.

Object Detection

The detection of objects is crucial in this paradigm. The input feeds and detects the required characters in a given frame using this method (in our case, people following social distancing). In YOLO object detection, convolutional neural networks are employed to detect objects in real time. It can be done in a single run of the algorithm, because it is a forward propagation method. The proposed work uses the COCO data set [10] as an input to the object detection process. It has incredibly deep labeling and classifications that allow it to differentiate between humans and other moving things (luggage, inanimate objects, vehicles, etc.). Because it is a well-defined data set, any errors in the algorithm's execution can be avoided.

Decision-Making and Output Formatting

Calculation of Manhattan distance is discovered as an enhancement to existing models. In the event of a pandemic, it is critical not only that a room's threshold is not crossed but also that persons in the room keep a minimum distance of 6 ft (or 2 m) between themselves to minimize contamination. Split the frame into green and red portions to highlight regions where people are obeying the guideline correctly vs badly, accordingly, to make it easier on the eyes. This simplifies the process of analyzing the frame and making it more user-friendly.

People are tallied and numbered from 1 to n, and Manhattan distance is measured in this fashion. The distance between a person and the rest of the world (1–2, 1–3, 1–4 … 1 – n) is now saved. Every measurement that exceeds the 1.5-m limit will be highlighted in red and reported to the appropriate authority, as shown in Figs. 4 and 5.

Performance Evaluation

The total count can be determined by identifying all the objects as people. Table 1 compares the proposed object identification model to faster RCNN and SSD in terms of NoI, mAP, TL, and FPS, whereas Fig. 6 depicts the performance measure.

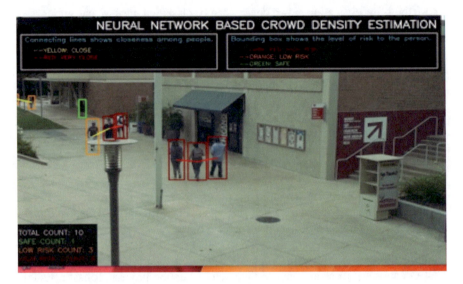

Fig. 4 Person identification in a frame

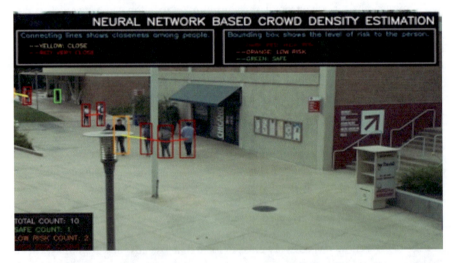

Fig. 5 Manhattan distance calculation between persons

Table 1 Comparison of object detection models

Model	NoI (no. of iteration)	mAP	TL	FPS
Faster RCNN	12,135	0.969	0.02	3
SSD	1200	0.069	0.22	10
YOLO	7560	0.846	0.87	23

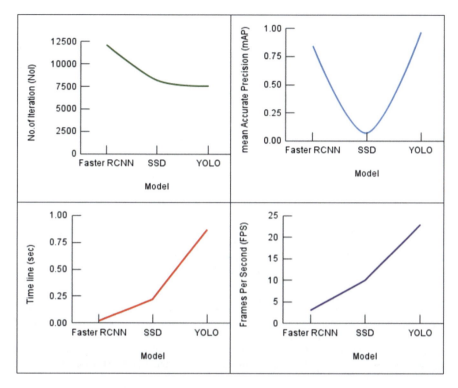

Fig. 6 Comparative analysis of proposed scheme

Conclusion and Future Work

This work develops a real-time deep learning-based system for automating the process of measuring social distance utilizing object recognition and tracking approaches, in which each participant is identified in real time using bounding boxes. The bounding boxes that result can be used to locate clusters or groups of people that satisfy the proximity property of the pairwise vectored approach. Calculating the number of groups established and the violation index term, which is derived as the ratio of persons to groups, validates the number of infractions. Three prominent state-of-the-art object identification models were tested extensively: faster RCNN, SSD, and YOLO, with YOLO displaying efficient performance with balanced FPS and mAP scores. Because it is highly sensitive to the spatial placement of the camera, this technique can be fine-tuned to better adjust with the appropriate field of vision.

Distancing oneself from others is crucial in preventing illness transmission. Using computer vision technology based on OpenCV and YOLO-based deep learning, the social distance of people in video feeds are analyzed, allowing to forecast the number of likely transmissions and so assist in controlling the pandemic.

Precision and accuracy are vital in this application, because it is meant to be employed in a range of operating situations. Additional precautions, such as gaining prior consent for such working settings, concealing a person's identity in general, and preserving transparency about its fair usage among a select group of stakeholders, can address real concerns about privacy and individual rights.

References

1. C.T. Nguyen, Y.M. Saputra, N. Van Huynh, N.T. Nguyen, T.V. Khoa, B.M. Tuan, D.N. Nguyen, D.T. Hoang, T.X. Vu, E. Dutkiewicz, Enabling and emerging technologies for social distancing: a comprehensive survey. IEEE Access **8**, 153479–153507 (Aug. 2020)
2. J. Redmon, A. Farhadi, YOLOv3: an incremental improvement. ArXivabs/1804.02767 (2018)
3. S. Syed Ameer Abbas, M. Anitha, X. Vinith Jaini, Realization of multiple human head detection and direction movement using Raspberry Pi. IEEE **4**, 78–91 (Mar 2018)
4. E.M. Hoeben, W. Bernasco, L.S. Liebst, C. van Baak, M.R. Lindegaard, Social distancing compliance: A video observational analysis. PLOS ONE **2** (Mar 2021). https://doi.org/10.1371/journal.pone.0248221
5. S. Jie, X. He, L. Qing, T. Niu, Y. Cheng, Y. Peng, A novel social distancing analysis in urban public space: a new online spatio-temporal trajectory. Sustain. Cities Soc. **68**, 102765 (2021)
6. A. Al-Sheary, A. Ali, Crowd monitoring system using unmanned aerial vehicle (UAV). J. Civil Eng. Archit. **11** (Nov. 2017). https://doi.org/10.17265/1934-7359/2017.11.004
7. J. Redmon, S. Divvala, R. Girshick, A. Farhadi, You only look once: unified, real-time object detection, in Proceedings of the IEEE conference on computer vision and pattern recognition, 2016, pp. 779–788
8. J. Redmon, A. Farhadi, Yolo9000: better, faster, stronger, in Proceedings of the IEEE conference on computer vision and pattern recognition, 2017, pp. 7263–7271
9. M. Putra, Z. Yussof, K. Lim, S. Salim, Convolutional neural network for person and car detection using yolo framework. J. Telecommun. Electron. Comput. Eng. **10**(1–7), 67–71 (2018)
10. http://cocodataset.org. Accessed on 20 July 2021

Role of Digital Healthcare in Rehabilitation During a Pandemic

Meena Gupta and Ruchika Kalra

Introduction

Rehabilitation is always a very important part of treatment and considered primary. It enhances a person ability to be functional and independent and enriches the natural healing process [1]. Nowadays, the term digitalization has finally entered health care full of zeal with the ability to fulfill the best possible solutions [2]. Digital health is the technological setup created for the health care sectors by the brains of engineers to overcome the inability and inaccessibility regarding social and economic factors [3]. Digital health is the best solution for the organization presenting with absenteeism of employees with health care issues, places where the patient is unable to go to the health care center, or quality health care rehabilitation is not available at their center [4]. Since the development of digital sectors in health care, rehabilitation in digital health sectors has been introduced, where the proper applications are accessible to all smart phones [5]. According to the World Health Organization, digital health is innovating the health care sector providing transparency, accessibility, and availability of health care service everywhere. Digital health increased its efficacy during the pandemic, and it is now available in developing countries where the rehabilitation tool is accessible to the patients in their hands and can connect to their therapist at any moment [6]. The role of digital health on rehabilitation was maximally seen during Covid-19 and allowed patients to access care with their own device [7]. Globally, the pandemic caused by the coronavirus created the situation of unavailability of medical professionals everywhere and the accessibility was limited, thereby creating the need for improving earlier versions of digital rehabilitation, and the pandemic helped created trust on both the medical

---

M. Gupta (✉) · R. Kalra
Amity Institute of Physiotherapy, Amity University, Noida, Uttar Pradesh, India

© The Author(s), under exclusive license to Springer Nature Switzerland AG 2023
G. R. Kanagachidambaresan et al. (eds.), *System Design for Epidemics Using Machine Learning and Deep Learning*, Signals and Communication Technology, https://doi.org/10.1007/978-3-031-19752-9_16

professional and patient's side. The outpatient rehabilitation suffered a lot during the Covid-19 pandemic, including acute to chronic conditions, and the inpatients suffered too, as rehabilitation requires teamwork and the medical professionals were unavailable. It was also difficult to bring the non-covid and covid patients under one roof and treat them with justice, ensuring prevention of spreading infections among them. Therefore, the platform of digital rehabilitation stepped up for not only the medical purpose but with due management of complete data associated with it [8–11]. Digital rehabilitation requires the technology of artificial intelligence to provide the space for the initiation of the robotic, virtual, and smart rehabilitation [12, 13].

Digital health has been introduced in specific areas of practice, such as Telemedicine, M-Health, E-health, and algorithmic medicine [14].

Different Digital Health Platforms in Rehabilitation

Telemedicine

In the 1980s, when personal computers introduced video conferencing, telemedicine emerged and acted in a supportive role to distant health care services, so as to work in places where the specialist was not available. Telemedicine provided teleconsultation in remote areas termed as telecare. In this, the patient and doctor are not in a face-to-face consultation, but the technology on hand created the articulation by involving multifaceted invisible work by medical professional and patient relationship to diagnose the symptoms and improvise the treatment. Digital telemedicine brings the clinic to the home [15–17]. The innovation of telemedicine stood as disaster management in the case of Covid-19 as a part of public health measures.

No telemedicine program can be begun in a short period and earlier constructed telemedicine technology created the sorting of the patients before arriving to the emergency rooms as a central health strategy of central health triage. Technology provides the patient centered environment and allows them to communicate with the doctor 24/7 regarding the symptoms and prevents spreading the infection to the other patients and clinicians [18–20].

Telemedicine had been increasing in rates but questions remained and development was according to countries, but Covid-19 accelerated the speed and questions to be answered in the last 2–3 years. Some of the barriers to trust patients and doctors face include that new physicians cannot be trusted on the telemedicine services compared to a physician that has treated the patient for years; in addition, trust is absent for the illiterate and senior medical professionals with less understanding of how to operate the software on the medical device and whether they can be trusted on the system for confidentiality and the affordance of cost associated with it. These were answered as availability of the telemedicine care, increasing the literacy rate to the extent to understand the software and making it easy to use, as well as making people aware and create trust by them using it in remote places as Covid-19 changing phases have created self-learning to some extent [21, 22]. Telemedicine was used for the non-urgent cases to decrease the outpatient que. An increased use of telemedicine required increasing the government regulations so as to keep the data associated private and confidential, no resistance toward the quality of care on both ends, and infrastructure to be added at a large scale to create better digital data management [23].

Not only did the pandemic disrupt rehabilitation for outpatient patients but inpatients also experienced an unavailability of therapists, which stood to be a disaster, although telemedicine saved it to some extent for both the therapist and patients. The initial barriers were overcome and rehabilitation through telemedicine was the tool to save lives and maintain the quality of life. Telemedicine in rehabilitation in Covid-19 was initially used as a research tool, but when required it expanded to clinical practice [24, 25].

The technology of telemedicine has shown to be functional for rehabilitation in the pandemic period and even post that. The synchronous visit is captured in tele-rehabilitation. This reduced the cost of traveling, inability to travel, and time saved from traveling, especially in remote places. Prior to using telemedicine, there is the requirement of the software program behind it and permission to be granted from the government licensing to prevent malpractices as telemedicine is a part of public health in a few developed countries and yet to be a part in a few. The connect ability and association of telemedicine over the landline telephone is to prevent malpractices by leaking of the confidential personal information. The next step oriented with tele-rehabilitation for conducting a visit is where the staff makes the medical professional understand the software prior to connecting with the patient. Assessment is done on the virtual purpose with the help of the virtual applications allowing a few to many parameters to be assessed, as many are still under research for the assessment. As a part of the delivery, the protocols are suggested and explained to the patient and their family depending on the patient orientation. Documentation is the primary tool to be utilized in the medical practice to work ethically and in a synchronous manner. Telemedicine provides data documentation many ways, from chief complaint to each assessment group, and manage it in a narrative and descriptive manner to prevent mistakes [26–30].

Mobile Health

The World Health Organization defines mobile health as medical and public health operated by mobile devices. In this decade, people have become dependent on mobile technologies for day-to-day activities, which initiated the innovation of the applications related to health inside your phone that are being added to day by day. Mobile devices are in the hands of most of the population of the developed and developing countries, and because they are essential necessities, the addition and programming of the health applications makes it easier for health professionals to monitor and consult. The interest in and awareness of the applications in the mobile devices are also initiating a step ahead in awareness to health with the help of M-health applications [31–33].

The technology associated with M-health is recent and promotes health and motivates people to monitor their daily activities. Sensors associated devices are linked with applications associated with the mobile device having your health records, where the sensors that are worn on the wrist allow the device to read location, walk, sleep, and anxiety according to your vital signs. These sensors monitor the status of the body. These devices not only provide the data for the medical professional or the follow up but also for understanding and adjusting the lifestyle according to the imbalance that is created such as disturbed cycle, sedentary lifestyle with limited number of activities, poor nutrition, and improper intake of water. These can be a self-rehabilitation tool to keep up to date in private life that is documented and presented graphically to show how much it has been improved [34–36].

In the Covid-19 era, M-health had a triple role such as connecting to citizens, digitally relating health issues, and controlling health with the innovation of applications. Traditionally, M-health during the pandemic had advantages such as promoting a heathy lifestyle, awareness and motivation with active participation with technologies, facilitating the doctor–patient communication without a structured work environment setup such as a clinic, monitoring in the remote areas, and ensuring social distancing is properly followed. With the situation of the pandemic, the potential of mobile devices in the health sector is boosted and new boundaries are approached not only for the health benefits but also for contact tracing during the pandemic; in addition to increased memory and better computing capacity, tethering, photoelectric sensors, barometers and many more [37–40].

The role of M-health in rehabilitation is broad spectrum nowadays because mobile devices are in the hands of every age from child to senior citizen and the pandemic made it a more essential tool of life. Mobile health is promoting rehabilitation by making a more comfortable and easier way to adapt and break the absenteeism of young adults who are prevented from meeting the therapist due to the workload but the accessibility of the medical professional is just a touch away on the phone and the control by the applications make the track record easier to document. The treatment sessions are administered by videoconferencing with the help of mobile applications or defined by the mobile applications according to the body type, gender, physical activity, comorbidities, and so many other assessments differ in applications. After looking at this type of technology, the hospital setup has initiated the personal M-health applications that not only works with the therapist and the patient but also the complete hospital, even with the pharmacy, such that all information regarding health data is incoming and so the data is managed and made easier for the patient and medical professional [41–43].

E-health

The world wide web was introduced in the 1990s and created accessibility of the health care information to reach the public and their illness experiences. There are various sites such as health line and many more. The research conducted on E-health introduced the various experiences and helped to access the health information online. There are various sites that support true health consultancy. Simply E-health is the platform for the digital information and communication to be improved and rechecked in health care [44]. During the Covid-19 pandemic, covid-related information was the most explored topic on the electronic platforms, where both true and false statements were presented. Guidelines were provided by the World Health Organization, national and international governments, but on the same link there were also a few fake health care facts that were providing no use treatments. The government and WHO came together to overcome this using E-health and used the platforms such as Facebook, Twitter, Instagram, and YouTube to provide the evidence-based information and increase the E-health literacy rate and for public health measures [45, 46].

E-health in rehabilitation is the knowledge tool used to notify about the disease or condition. E-rehabilitation came to be more common in new patients due to the inability to visit the place for treatment or small difficulties that can be understood and classified by the electronic health and can be discussed with the rehabilitation specialist with the help of the applications provided with mobile health.

E-health can obtain relevant information with the help of E-referral following the assessments, case study, history, and E-diagnosis and establishing the digital information and documenting the pathology. The therapist can easily draft all the information data management and ensure the quality of care, where the E-discharge summaries contain relevant and necessary information and are created quickly. The pros of E-health for rehabilitation specialists is the feedback system is quick and proper according to the session [47–49].

Algorithmic Medicine

Algorithmic medicine involves the increased capacity for storing, sharing, and producing in the era of big data. These algorithms have the capacity to filter and process data. This is the broader area of work aims of medical informatics and decision making, which are creating decision areas of test, assessment, diagnosis, and automatic control [50, 51]. Artificial intelligence plays a role where the neural network created artificially supports clinical decisions and creates the structure and user interface. Errors can be minimized by utilizing an automated algorithm and having the potential to reduce the errors and better score outcomes [52, 53] These algorithms create robotic, virtual, and smart rehabilitation using technology to support clinical decisions and adhere to the evidence-based guidelines. This provides a large aspect for rehabilitation. In various types of devices, using machine learning and sensors creates the environment where the digital computers transfer the current data the patient is carrying without being informed by the patient and assessment and digital diagnosis is taken even at the patient's home. This smart technology with artificial intelligence has moved from just consultation to robotic technology that can conduct robotic surgery even when the specialist surgeon is not with the patient at the hospital [54, 55]. During the pandemic, artificial intelligence with an algorithm interface introduced ease in the ongoing and planned surgeries, ongoing rehabilitation as the interface for the robots or the devices that are inserted in the patient's body, or even the placement over the patient's body depending on the extent of the dependability, can be controlled by the medical professional during the session [56–58]. The algorithm interface is not yet found in the remote areas or even the underdeveloped countries because this interface is very expensive and so this protocol will take a few more years to enter into public health. The challenges so far are being answered with results, but overcoming the challenge to decrease the cost will create the availability for the medical algorithm to be utilized by more countries. This interface is not only to help patients or even the public be aware but also to help the medical professional to understand the significance behind the rehabilitation [59].

Technology such as the robots in rehabilitation, including MIT Manus, mirror image movement enabler, arm assisted rehabilitation measurement, machine learning in the rehabilitation have been mentioned in the research and the medical algorithms for the classification, prediction, and treatment planning. These devices not only have a role to play in the rehabilitation but also the classifier to predict the activity and potential of the patient [60, 61].

Digital Patient Management

Technology improvement stands to be the successful support in assessing and treating patients. The treatment is incomplete if the generation of the data supporting the management and occurrence, improvement, new techniques, and many more things are not analyzed. The role of data patient management is vital and required whether in the private sector or public health sector. It was never thought that this coronavirus would lead to a pandemic as stated in earlier statements, but when we look to the national and international data of patients, it makes us understand how disastrous it has been and will continue to be [62–64].

The digital mode of data management supported and created a lot of technology to resolve the disaster. The extent of this disaster was more easily tracked digitally with the information made public, and made it easy to document by downloading one application on the phone that made us aware of how many people were covid positive in our limited range of meters to kilometers, registering one's number, and becoming covid positive automatically generates the data to the public health sector to be aware of that region and create the zones [65].

Numbers prioritize the criteria defining what is urgent; as the number rose, it set the criteria of whom to admit, depending on how many ICU beds, oxygen beds, or home quarantine facilities are available. The registration of vaccine throughout the world was and still is a challenge, and the patient management supports how many jabs, the ratio, and when the vaccination will be completed according to the population and production of vaccination. This triage of digital patient management was the key to understanding [66–68].

The digital health transformation stood to be greatest in developing and implementing new ideology of care. Digital approaches emerged as a shield for vulnerable patients by creating safety for the staff or patients coming to hospital. For example, software varies from country to country such as EMIS (Egton Medical information systems) in the UK, which keeps the records from primary care, including everything the patient carried, and so on [69].

NHS trusts are rushing to create this kind of setup as soon as possible for the remote areas as much as possible so the patient can be managed according to digital data such as digital methods of rehabilitation. Digital patient management is much needed but it was limited in public health. However, the pandemic led to the understanding of a limited number of working people so the technology can help manage data accurately and provide the data for the extent of how it will proceed such as new variants beginning in different areas, saturation presented by the numbers, ratio of lives saved, death and vaccinated people, the data created awareness of precautions to be followed and motivation by looking for improvement and a sense of winning over the disaster [70, 71].

Discussion

The Covid-19 pandemic made many ongoing research studies a part of clinical practice. Digitalization already existed but had not entered daily practice in the health care sector until it was introduced in clinical practice through a digital platform. The previous challenges and questions were put aside because of the disaster situation and the opportunity was presented to put trust and investment in the digital sector. This digital health care eased the management in patient care with full quality of care. This pandemic made us realize the digital platforms were not only made for office, education, and work but also the health care systems [72–74].

The pandemic created the fear of when and how to access the hospital sector whether with or without covid. However, the emergency was not completely turned off by the digitalization in health care, but ease was created to some extent, especially for non-covid patients [75]. Rehabilitation is the tool to heal completely and a first step to a solution for the discomfort converting to inability to illness, where the rehabilitation was carried out as a team collectively, including doctor, therapist, nurses, and other medical professionals completing the rehabilitation team [76]. The emergency of the disaster disturbed the management cycle created by them in the normal medical profession [77]. The pandemic exposed the limitation of the medical professionals and unlimited patients suffering with covid, non-covid and post covid, where all of them wanted equal attention and rehabilitation. Rehabilitation during the pandemic is a priority not only in the interface of the doctor to the patient but also all the other medical professional requirements [78, 79]. The studies mentioned different measures of the digital health structure, including telemedicine as the rehabilitation tool used, which followed the traditional digital platform followed from years earlier too, and E health as the measure for the awareness tool as the pandemic increased the valuation of life and comorbidities, and the effects of lockdown added the awareness to be careful toward the self and family health [80, 81].

Mobile technology was introduced to daily life years ago as the tool for communication, but the smart phones added the applications, and as the pandemic disoriented the life structure, people became more dependent on the digital devices to survive as an essential aspect [82]. Therefore, this essential aspect can also be used as a health tool creating the accessibility to a healthy life whether ill or just improvement of lifestyle to prevent disorders and a sedentary lifestyle, which have increased a lot during this period apart from Covid-19; rehabilitation awareness helps a person to prevent becoming a patient with the accessibility of the rehabilitation specialist at one touch. The sessions oriented with the mobile phones acted as the structure for the M-health technology and allowed medical professional handheld accessibility without the excuse of unavailability, as this tool was the most bought and appreciated during the pandemic [41, 83].

Algorithmic medicine is the proposal for smart rehabilitation where the rehabilitation is not stuck to the applications but beyond the thought of understanding the digital aspect in health care. According to the studies, these type of intelligent robots play a vital role in improvement of the patient, where return to life is faster. The role of robots and high-end technology is required, but due to the cost of the technology, it is still under research to be accessible to developing and underdeveloped countries. The research is turning into clinical practice in certain countries for this type of rehabilitation. Results oriented with this type of technology are quite promising [84, 85]. There has been an evolution from rehabilitation to digital rehabilitation; according to a study by Jones in 2020, the transformation of medical rehabilitation is evident. Although the benefits of rehabilitation are well established, inefficiencies in the current system of care are also clearly documented. These inefficiencies are influenced by the growing demand for services, continued changes in reimbursement to contain cost, pivoting service delivery models, and increasing provider shortages. Today's priorities in medical rehabilitation are containing costs, improving access, and increasing the amount of time spent on actual rehabilitation. It has been suggested that the transformation toward the greater use of digital health technologies will lead to better outcomes, greater value in care, better patient experiences, and more empowered rehabilitation stakeholders [4, 86, 87]. One of the biggest advantages of digital health care in rehabilitation has been its ability to bring quality care to more people who need it. Add to this the fact that online searches for queries like "physiotherapy," "physical therapy," "back pain exercises," etc., are over 4 million per month. Regarding continuity of care, most patients and providers understand that physical therapy is not restricted to the session at the doctor's clinic. Using digital health, this care can be extended from the clinic to the patient's home. Tools such as tele-rehab or using telehealth for physical rehabilitation allows providers to guide and support their patients to recovery [5, 88]. Rehabilitation requires trust, where the patient is first trusting the software to be opened and then the medical professional doing the consulting because, generally, the medical professional is different on the digital platform [89]. The consultation is not the only part of the health sector to be thought of, where all the management takes place from appointment, visit, billing, session, feedback and reappointment, and so on, depending on the extent of the health sector. This management is carried out by the professionals handling the digital sector and work to be licensed oriented, even in personal practice or public health, as medical data has major importance in the health sector, so the documentation needs to be managed in a similar manner [90, 91]. Data management is not the only task but the patient too, as there are many patients that require rehabilitation management. The introduction of the technology in the health sector did not remove the toughness and emergency mode of the pandemic, but increasing trust in the digital sector is reducing the stress of being surprised by the disaster, as the management is improving in the current situation and varying from country to country, including in their remote areas [92, 93].

Some of the barriers to digital rehabilitation are because health professionals sometimes feel threatened by new technologies. However, the digital transformation should be seen as a tool to complement the professional's service and not as a replacement, as well as helping them to optimize their time. According to Mapfre, only 3 out of 10 public hospitals are adapted to digital transformation while 6 out of 10 private hospitals have a digital transformation plan. At present, only 1% of health expenditure in the autonomous communities is allocated to new technologies and, in order to achieve the necessary standard, health business models should be restructured, and innovation should be a priority. Each technological advance leads to research and development work. This can sometimes be costly, and there is not always a willingness to pay, both on the part of public administrations and on the part of patients [94–96].

Conclusion

This chapter included the aspects of the pandemic on rehabilitation and how the evolution of digital rehabilitation can act as the tool to continue the rehabilitation. Various research studies have been oriented toward efficacy of digital rehabilitation, which has proven to be safe, and the trust aspect, where the studies indicated significant improvement and overcoming the challenges, with many barriers overcome and some needing further attention.

Acknowledgment Gratitude to all authors for their contributions. There are neither conflicts of interests nor funding assistance.

References

1. E. Krug, A. Cieza, Strengthening health systems to provide rehabilitation services. Can. J. Occup. Ther. **84**(2), 72–73 (2017)
2. J. Milward, C. Drummond, S. Fincham-Campbell, P. Deluca, What makes online substance-use interventions engaging? A systematic review and narrative synthesis. Dig. Heal. **4**, 2055207617743354 (2018)
3. P. Dunn, E. Hazzard, Technology approaches to digital health literacy. Int. J. Cardiol. **15**(293), 294–296 (2019)

4. M. Jones, F. DeRuyter, J. Morris, The digital health revolution and people with disabilities: Perspective from the United States. Int. J. Environ. Res. Public Health **17**(2), 381 (2020)
5. M. Falter, M. Scherrenberg, P. Dendale, Digital health in cardiac rehabilitation and secondary prevention: A search for the ideal tool. Sensors **21**(1), 12 (2021)
6. World Health Organization, Is the Eastern Mediterranean Region ready for digitalizing health? implications from the global strategy on digital health (2020–2025)
7. K. Ganapathy, Telemedicine and neurological practice in the COVID-19 era. Neurol. India **68**(3), 555 (2020)
8. M. Bartolo, D. Intiso, C. Lentino, G. Sandrini, S. Paolucci, M. Zampolini, Urgent measures for the containment of the coronavirus (Covid-19) epidemic in the neurorehabilitation/rehabilitation departments in the phase of maximum expansion of the epidemic. Front. Neurol. **11**, 423 (2020)
9. S. De Biase, L. Cook, D.A. Skelton, M. Witham, R. Ten Hove, The COVID-19 rehabilitation pandemic. Age Ageing **49**(5), 696–700 (2020)
10. L.M. Sheehy, Considerations for postacute rehabilitation for survivors of COVID-19. JMIR Public Health Surveill. **6**(2), e19462 (2020)
11. A. Saverino, P. Baiardi, G. Galata, G. Pedemonte, C. Vassallo, C. Pistarini, The challenge of re-organizing rehabilitation services at the time of COVID-19 pandemic: A new digital and artificial intelligence platform to support team work in planning and delivering safe and high quality care. Front. Neurol. **12**, 501 (2021)
12. R. Kalra, Methods of virtual rehabilitation for health care workers-a review. Archivos De Medicina **7**(5), 134 (2021)
13. R. Kalra, M. Gupta, A review on potential of robotic rehabilitation in health care system. Int. J. Med. Sci. Clin. Invent. **8**(05), 5392–5413 (2021)
14. B. Marent, F. Henwood, 21 Digital health, in *Routledge International Handbook of Critical Issues in Health and Illness* (2021).
15. N. Oudshoorn, How places matter: Telecare technologies and the changing spatial dimensions of healthcare. Soc. Stud. Sci. **42**(1), 121–142 (2012)
16. T.L. Finch, M. Mort, F.S. Mair, C.R. May, Future patients? Telehealthcare, roles and responsibilities. Health Soc. Care Community **16**(1), 86–95 (2008)
17. E. Håland, L. Melby, Negotiating technology-mediated interaction in health care. Soc. Theory Health **13**(1), 78–98 (2015)
18. S. Duffy, T.H. Lee, In-person health care as option B. N. Engl. J. Med. **378**(2), 104–106 (2018)
19. N. Lurie, B.G. Carr, The role of telehealth in the medical response to disasters. JAMA Intern. Med. **178**(6), 745–746 (2018)
20. J.E. Hollander, B.G. Carr, Virtually perfect? Telemedicine for COVID-19. N. Engl. J. Med. **382**(18), 1679–1681 (2020)
21. J. Portnoy, M. Waller, T. Elliott, Telemedicine in the era of COVID-19. The journal of allergy and clinical immunology. In Pract. **8**(5), 1489–1491 (2020)
22. American Well, Telehealth index: 2019 consumer survey (2019).
23. R. Bashshur, C.R. Doarn, J.M. Frenk, J.C. Kvedar, J.O. Woolliscroft, Telemedicine and the COVID-19 pandemic, lessons for the future. Telemed. e-Heal. **26**(5), 571–573 (2020)
24. S. Negrini, K. Grabljevec, P. Boldrini, C. Kiekens, S. Moslavac, M. Zampolini, N. Christodoulou, J.F. Kaux, Up to 2.2 million people experiencing disability suffer collateral damage each day of COVID-19 lockdown in Europe. Eur. J. Phys. Rehabil. Med. **56**(3), 361–365 (2020)
25. MEDICA EM, Telemedicine from research to practice during the pandemic. "Instant paper from the field" on rehabilitation answers to the Covid-19 emergency (2020).
26. A.S. Tenforde, M.A. Iaccarino, H. Borgstrom, J.E. Hefner, J. Silver, M. Ahmed, A.N. Babu, C.A. Blauwet, L. Elson, C. Eng, D. Kotler, Telemedicine during COVID-19 for outpatient sports and musculoskeletal medicine physicians. PM&R **12**(9), 926–932 (2020)
27. I.M. Howard, M.S. Kaufman, Telehealth applications for outpatients with neuromuscular or musculoskeletal disorders. Muscle Nerve **58**(4), 475–485 (2018)
28. J. Shih, J. Portnoy, Tips for seeing patients via telemedicine. Curr Allergy Asthma Rep **18**(10), 1–7 (2018)

29. Centers for Medicare & Medicaid Services, Medicare telehealth frequently asked questions (FAQs) (2020).
30. M. Verduzco-Gutierrez, A.C. Bean, A.S. Tenforde, R.N. Tapia, J.K. Silver, How to conduct an outpatient telemedicine rehabilitation or prehabilitation visit. PM&R **12**(7), 714–720 (2020)
31. M. Kay, J. Santos, M. Takane, mHealth: New horizons for health through mobile technologies. World Health Organ. **64**(7), 66–71 (2011)
32. F. Greaves, I. Joshi, M. Campbell, S. Roberts, N. Patel, J. Powell, What is an appropriate level of evidence for a digital health intervention? Lancet **392**(10165), 2665–2667 (2018)
33. M.L. Millenson, J.L. Baldwin, L. Zipperer, H. Singh, Beyond Dr. Google: The evidence on consumer-facing digital tools for diagnosis. Diagnosi **5**(3), 95–105 (2018)
34. S. Pink, V. Fors, Self-tracking and mobile media: New digital materialities. Mobile Media Commun. **5**(3), 219–238 (2017)
35. D. Lupton, The diverse domains of quantified selves: Self-tracking modes and dataveillance. Econ. Soc. **45**(1), 101–122 (2016)
36. J. Pols, D. Willems, M. Aanestad, Making sense with numbers. Unravelling ethico-psychological subjects in practices of self-quantification. Sociol. Health Illn. **41**, 98–115 (2019)
37. A. Gabbiadini, C. Baldissarri, F. Durante, R.R. Valtorta, M. De Rosa, M. Gallucci, Together apart: The mitigating role of digital communication technologies on negative affect during the COVID-19 outbreak in Italy. Front. Psychol., 2763 (2020)
38. S.G. Shah, D. Nogueras, H.C. Van Woerden, V. Kiparoglou, The COVID-19 pandemic: A pandemic of lockdown loneliness and the role of digital technology. J. Med. Internet Res. **22**(11), e22287 (2020)
39. D. Giansanti, G. Maccioni, Health in the palm of your hand – Part 1: The risks from smartphone abuse and the role of telemedicine and e-health. Mhealth, 7 (2021)
40. D. Giansanti, Diagnostics imaging and M-health: Investigations on the prospects of integration in cytological and organ diagnostics. Rapporti ISTISAN **20**(1), 1–66 (2019)
41. C.P. Adans-Dester, S. Bamberg, F.P. Bertacchi, B. Caulfield, K. Chappie, D. Demarchi, M.K. Erb, J. Estrada, E.E. Fabara, M. Freni, K.E. Friedl, Can mHealth technology help mitigate the effects of the COVID-19 pandemic? IEEE Open J. Eng. Med. Biol. **7**(1), 243–248 (2020)
42. P. Bonato, The role of mHealth technology in the COVID-19 pandemic and beyond. Doctoral Dissertation. College of Health and Rehabilitation Science, Boston University, 2020.
43. S.P. Burns, M. Terblanche, J. Perea, H. Lillard, C. DeLaPena, N. Grinage, A. MacKinen, E.E. Cox, mHealth intervention applications for adults living with the effects of stroke: A scoping review. Arch. Rehabil. Res. Clin. Transl. **3**(1), 100095 (2021)
44. R. Harris, P. Spoel, F. Henwood, Integrating the imperatives of healthy living in everyday life, in *Relational Concepts in Medicine* (Brill, 2011), pp. 61–71.
45. G. Brørs, C.D. Norman, T.M. Norekvål, Accelerated importance of eHealth literacy in the COVID-19 outbreak and beyond. Eur. J. Cardiovasc. Nurs. **19**(6), 458–461 (2020)
46. A. Carvalho, M. Moreno, Aging, cognitive rehabilitation and eHealth: Insights from clinical neurosciences to neuropsychology in Portugal. Lusiadas Sci. J. **2**(1), 29–35 (2021)
47. S. ter Stal, M. Tabak, op den Akker H, Beinema T, Hermens H., Who do you prefer? The effect of age, gender and role on users' first impressions of embodied conversational agents in eHealth. Int. J. Hum. Comput. Interact. **36**(9), 881–892 (2020)
48. J.M. Cal, M. Fernández-Sánchez, G.A. Matarán-Peñarrocha, D.A. Hurley, A.M. Castro-Sánchez, I.C. Lara-Palomo, Physical therapists' opinion of E-health treatment of chronic low back pain. Int. J. Environ. Res. Public Health **18**(4), 1889 (2021)
49. T.H. Tebeje, J. Klein, Applications of e-health to support person-centered health care at the time of COVID-19 pandemic. Telemed e-health **27**(2), 150–158 (2021)
50. M. Ruckenstein, N.D. Schüll, The datafication of health. Annu. Rev. Anthropol. **23**(46), 261–278 (2017)
51. Z. Obermeyer, E.J. Emanuel, Predicting the future – big data, machine learning, and clinical medicine. N. Engl. J. Med. **375**(13), 1216 (2016)
52. J. Shabbir, T. Anwer, Artificial intelligence and its role in near future. arXiv preprint arXiv:1804.01396 (2018).

53. E.J. Topol, High-performance medicine: The convergence of human and artificial intelligence. Nat. Med. **25**(1), 44–56 (2019)
54. J. Fong, R. Ocampo, D.P. Gross, M. Tavakoli, Intelligent robotics incorporating machine learning algorithms for improving functional capacity evaluation and occupational rehabilitation. J. Occup. Rehabil. **30**(3), 362–370 (2020)
55. V. Szücs, T. Guzsvinecz, A. Magyar, Movement pattern recognition in physical rehabilitation-cognitive motivation-based IT method and algorithms. Acta Polytechnica Hungarica **17**(2), 211–235 (2020)
56. B. Pradhan, D. Bharti, S. Chakravarty, S.S. Ray, V.V. Voinova, A.P. Bonartsev, K. Pal, Internet of things and robotics in transforming current-day healthcare services. J. Healthc. Eng. **26**, 2021 (2021)
57. M. Kyrarini, F. Lygerakis, A. Rajavenkatanarayanan, C. Sevastopoulos, H.R. Nambiappan, K.K. Chaitanya, A.R. Babu, J. Mathew, F. Makedon, A survey of robots in healthcare. Technologies **9**(1), 8 (2021)
58. D. Khemasuwan, J.S. Sorensen, H.G. Colt, Artificial intelligence in pulmonary medicine: Computer vision, predictive model and COVID-19. Eur. Respir. Rev. **29**(157) (2020)
59. A. Sheikh, M. Anderson, S. Albala, B. Casadei, B.D. Franklin, M. Richards, D. Taylor, H. Tibble, E. Mossialos, Health information technology and digital innovation for national learning health and care systems. Lancet Dig. Heal. **3**(6), e383–e396 (2021)
60. S. Nayak, R.K. Das, Application of artificial intelligence (AI) in prosthetic and orthotic rehabilitation, in *Service Robotics* (IntechOpen, 2020).
61. A. Choudhury, O. Asan, Role of artificial intelligence in patient safety outcomes: Systematic literature review. JMIR Med. Inform. **8**(7), e18599 (2020)
62. L. Ferretti, C. Wymant, M. Kendall, et al., Quantifying SARS-CoV-2 transmission suggests epidemic control with digital contact tracing. Science **368**(6491), eabb6936 (2020). https://doi.org/10.1126/science.abb6936
63. M. Zastrow, South Korea is reporting intimate details of COVID-19 cases: Has it helped? Nature (2020)
64. K. Kupferschmidt, J. Cohen, Can China's COVID-19 strategy work elsewhere?
65. D. Bonsall, C. Fraser, Sustainable containment of COVID-19 using smartphones in China: Scientific and ethical underpinnings for implementation of similar approaches in other settings. GitHub, 16 (2020)
66. Ministry of Health, HaMagen – the Ministry of Health app for fghting the spread of coronavirus. https://govextra.gov.il/ministry-of-health/hamagen-app/download-en/ (2020).
67. Amnesty International, Halt to COVID-19 contact tracing app a major win for privacy. https://www.amnesty.org/en/latest/news/2020/06/norway-covid19-contact-tracing-app-privacy-win/. Accessed 27 July 2020.
68. L. Lai, K.A. Wittbold, F.Z. Dadabhoy, R. Sato, A.B. Landman, L.H. Schwamm, S. He, R. Patel, N. Wei, G. Zuccotti, I.T. Lennes, Digital triage: novel strategies for population health management in response to the COVID-19 pandemic, in *Healthcare* (Elsevier, Vol. 8, No. 4, 2020), p. 100493
69. T. Robbins, S. Hudson, P. Ray, S. Sankar, K. Patel, H. Randeva, T.N. Arvanitis, COVID-19: A new digital dawn? Dig. Heal. **6**, 2055207620920083 (2020)
70. F. Murillo-Cabezas, E. Vigil-Martín, N. Raimondi, J. Pérez-Fernández, Covid-19 pandemic and digital transformation in critical care units. Med. Intensiva **44**(7), 457 (2020)
71. J. Budd, B.S. Miller, E.M. Manning, V. Lampos, M. Zhuang, M. Edelstein, G. Rees, V.C. Emery, M.M. Stevens, N. Keegan, M.J. Short, Digital technologies in the public-health response to COVID-19. Nat. Med. **26**(8), 1183–1192 (2020)
72. J.A. Andrews, M.P. Craven, A.R. Lang, B. Guo, R. Morriss, C. Hollis, The impact of data from remote measurement technology on the clinical practice of healthcare professionals in depression, epilepsy and multiple sclerosis: Survey. BMC Med. Inform. Decis. Mak. **21**(1), 1–7 (2021)

73. S. de Lusignan, N. Jones, J. Dorward, R. Byford, H. Liyanage, J. Briggs, F. Ferreira, O. Akinyemi, G. Amirthalingam, C. Bates, J.L. Bernal, The Oxford Royal College of general practitioners clinical informatics digital hub: Protocol to develop extended COVID-19 surveillance and trial platforms. JMIR Public Health Surveill. **6**(3), e19773 (2020)
74. Z.H. Khan, A. Siddique, C.W. Lee, Robotics utilization for healthcare digitization in global COVID-19 management. Int. J. Environ. Res. Public Health **17**(11), 3819 (2020)
75. M. Shammi, M. Bodrud-Doza, A.R. Islam, M. Rahman, Strategic assessment of COVID-19 pandemic in Bangladesh: Comparative lockdown scenario analysis, public perception, and management for sustainability. Environ. Dev. Sustain. **23**(4), 6148–6191 (2021)
76. M. Sivan, M. Phillips, I. Baguley, M. Nott (eds.), *Oxford Handbook of Rehabilitation Medicine* (Oxford University Press, 2019)
77. M.Z. Nomani, R. Parveen, COVID-19 pandemic and disaster preparedness in the context of public health laws and policies. Bangladesh J. Med. Sci. **5**, 41–48 (2021)
78. D.B. O'Connor, J.P. Aggleton, B. Chakrabarti, C.L. Cooper, C. Creswell, S. Dunsmuir, S.T. Fiske, S. Gathercole, B. Gough, J.L. Ireland, M.V. Jones, Research priorities for the COVID-19 pandemic and beyond: A call to action for psychological science. Br. J. Psychol. **111**(4), 603–629 (2020)
79. A. Akbari, F. Haghverd, S. Behbahani, Robotic home-based rehabilitation systems design: From a literature review to a conceptual framework for community-based remote therapy during COVID-19 pandemic. Front. Robot. AI, 8 (2021)
80. A. McDonnell, C. MacNeill, B. Chapman, N. Gilbertson, M. Reinhardt, S. Carreiro, Leveraging digital tools to support recovery from substance use disorder during the COVID-19 pandemic response. J. Subst. Abus. Treat. **1**(124), 108226 (2021)
81. B.N. Do, T.V. Tran, D.T. Phan, H.C. Nguyen, T.T. Nguyen, H.C. Nguyen, T.H. Ha, H.K. Dao, M.V. Trinh, T.V. Do, H.Q. Nguyen, Health literacy, eHealth literacy, adherence to infection prevention and control procedures, lifestyle changes, and suspected COVID-19 symptoms among health care workers during lockdown: Online survey. J. Med. Internet Res. **22**(11), e22894 (2020)
82. G. Goggin, *Apps: From Mobile Phones to Digital Lives* (Wiley, 2021)
83. J. Bostrom, G. Sweeney, J. Whiteson, J.A. Dodson, Mobile health and cardiac rehabilitation in older adults. Clin. Cardiol. **43**(2), 118–126 (2020)
84. P. Ratta, A. Kaur, S. Sharma, M. Shabaz, G. Dhiman, Application of blockchain and internet of things in healthcare and medical sector: Applications, challenges, and future perspectives. J. Food Qual. **25**, 2021 (2021)
85. P.P. Jayaraman, A.R. Forkan, A. Morshed, P.D. Haghighi, Y.B. Kang, Healthcare 4.0: A review of frontiers in digital health. Wiley interdisciplinary reviews: Data mining and knowledge. Discovery **10**(2), e1350 (2020)
86. A.C. Moller, G. Merchant, D.E. Conroy, R. West, E. Hekler, K.C. Kugler, S. Michie, Applying and advancing behavior change theories and techniques in the context of a digital health revolution: Proposals for more effectively realizing untapped potential. J. Behav. Med. **40**(1), 85–98 (2017)
87. J. Stramm, Responding to the digital health revolution. Rich. JL & Tech **28**, 86 (2021)
88. G.C. Chigbundu, R.C. Emeh, A.O. Ezeukwu, Effect of physiotherapy intervention on low back pain and disability, in *Individuals and Patients with Chronic Low Back Pain: A Systematic Review* (2020).
89. A.G. Ouimet, G. Wagner, L. Raymond, G. Pare, Investigating patients' intention to continue using teleconsultation to anticipate postcrisis momentum: Survey study. J. Med. Internet Res. **22**(11), e22081 (2020)
90. M. Massaro, Digital transformation in the healthcare sector through blockchain technology. Insights from academic research and business developments. Technovation **7**, 102386 (2021)
91. C. Pagliari, Digital health and primary care: Past, pandemic and prospects. J. Glob. Health, 11 (2021)

92. K.K. Stephens, J.L. Jahn, S. Fox, P. Charoensap-Kelly, R. Mitra, J. Sutton, E.D. Waters, B. Xie, R.J. Meisenbach, Collective sensemaking around COVID-19: Experiences, concerns, and agendas for our rapidly changing organizational lives. Manag. Commun. Q. **34**(3), 426–457 (2020)
93. K. Ranasinghe, R. Sabatini, A. Gardi, S. Bijjahalli, R. Kapoor, T. Fahey, K. Thangavel, Advances in integrated system health management for mission-essential and safety-critical aerospace applications. Prog. Aerosp. Sci. **1**(128), 100758 (2022)
94. M. Aapro, P. Bossi, A. Dasari, L. Fallowfield, P. Gascón, M. Geller, K. Jordan, J. Kim, K. Martin, S. Porzig, Digital health for optimal supportive care in oncology: Benefits, limits, and future perspectives. Support. Care Cancer **28**(10), 4589–4612 (2020)
95. L. Desveaux, C. Soobiah, R.S. Bhatia, J. Shaw, Identifying and overcoming policy-level barriers to the implementation of digital health innovation: Qualitative study. J. Med. Internet Res. **21**(12), e14994 (2019)
96. B. Mesko, Z. Győrffy, The rise of the empowered physician in the digital health era. J. Med. Internet Res. **21**(3), e12490 (2019)

An Epidemic of Neurodegenerative Disease Analysis Using Machine Learning Techniques

M. Menagadevi, V. Vivekitha, D. Thiyagarajan, and G. Dhivyasri

Introduction

Neurodegenerative diseases are a collection of neurological disorders in which neurons in the central nervous system die or are harmed, causing significant disabilities and, in the worst-case scenario, death. Figure 1 shows the major neurological disorder, which affects all age groups. Typically, they are stumbled upon in elderly age. However, the development of the disease could occur sooner. Their prevalence has risen dramatically in recent years, and this trend is projected to continue. As the world's population ages, the trend will continue. Neurodegenerative illnesses are difficult to manage and can be costly, since the cause is unknown and there is no recognized cure. Currently, treatments are focused on reducing symptoms.

The use of machine learning algorithms in medical and scientific research has gotten a lot of attention in recent years. New technologies have made it possible to rapidly accumulate patient data, such as ultrasonography and MRI readouts; omics profiles of biological samples; electronically collected clinical, behavioral, and activity data; and social media-derived information in the last decade. The number of characteristics (or variables) recorded in each observation can occasionally surpass the total number of observations in these large health datasets, making them high-dimensional. Machine learning advancements can be of great assistance to diagnosis and monitoring, such as illness onset detection, disease characterization,

---

M. Menagadevi (✉) · V. Vivekitha · G. Dhivyasri
Department of Biomedical Engineering, Dr. N.G.P Institute of Technology, Coimbatore, TN, India

D. Thiyagarajan
Department of Artificial Intelligence and Machine Learning, School of Engineering, Malla Reddy University, Hyderabad, Telangana, India

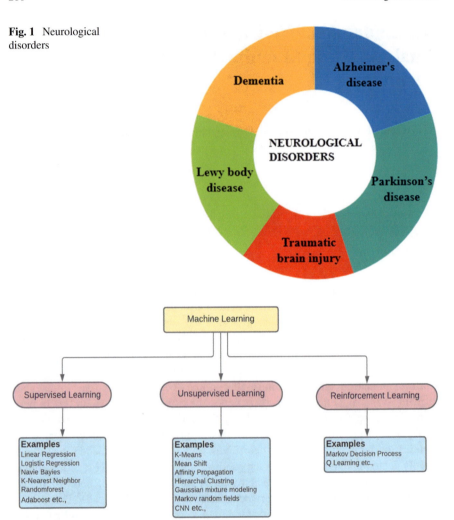

Fig. 1 Neurological disorders

Fig. 2 Divisions of machine learning algorithm

and disease improvement quantification of differential diagnosis. ML approaches have been used to assist physicians with CAD to diagnose the diseases [1, 2].

Classes of machine learning algorithm:

- Supervised learning
- Unsupervised learning
- Reinforcement learning (Fig. 2)

Supervised Learning

These approaches are most typically used to analyze data linked to neurodegenerative diseases. Dataset is required to train the model. Often, these labels necessitate human curation or professional evaluation; for example, a radiologist is required to label a series of radiographs, the size of a brain area on an MRI scan, and the labeling of MRI scan pictures, and a neuropathologist is necessary. The computer may then use this model to predict the label for fresh, unlabeled datasets using the new input characteristics. It can be difficult to collect big enough volumes of correct labels for supervised machine learning. Figure 3 shows the supervised learning model.

Classification is a process that includes finding rules in which new objects are assigned to a predefined category, and it requires two steps. The first step is the building of classification with the help of training dataset that has class attributes. The second step is to analyze the performance of the classification using test dataset. The supervised process is in which prediction is iteratively performed using training data [24, 25]. In supervised learning, some of the commonly used algorithms are decision tree, linear classification, and Naive Bayes.

The dataset must first be preprocessed, which involves a task that transforms the raw data into a finished dataset. It can be fed into the data model. The data cleanup,

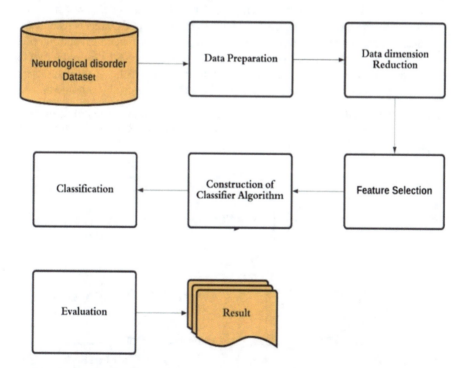

Fig. 3 General block of supervised learning model

data transformation, feature selection, and feature mapping stages in the preprocessing phase all contribute to the classifier's accuracy. Data cleaning is a step that looks upon any missing value in the dataset, and data transformation ensures that the data values fall in a small range. The feature selection is one of the significant steps that limit finite features, which can provide a higher detection rate, and the final step is the feature mapping, which helps in finding a decision region. This can maximize the class separately between the given classes in the newly mapped space. In the training phase, it practically supplies at least 70% of the dataset to create a model that can categorize and predict the right label of the testing set. Using data evaluation is we can analyze the performance of the algorithm in the neurological disorder dataset. Data evaluation includes accuracy sensitivity specificity and error rate. Many literatures suggest that using a supervised algorithm for neurological disorder classification, it was found that it has low specificity, about 0–54%, and the accuracy of the decision was predicted to be nearly 80% only.

Decision Tree

The decision tree (DT) is one of the most well-known and widely used machine learning methods. It is a mimic of the human thinking ability to make a decision. It's a tree-structured decision-making technique. The root, leaf nodes, branches, and internal nodes are the four basic components. The root of a tree connects its classes, with leaf nodes representing classes, branches representing outcomes, and internal leaves representing processes. The classification rules are the paths from the root to the leaves, and the steps involved in predicting the class of the given dataset are given below. Figure 4 shows the basic flow of the decision tree algorithm [31].

Step 1: It starts from the root nodes of the tree which contains the complete dataset.
Step 2: Select the attribute/feature value for the root node. Create a branch for each possible attribute/feature value.

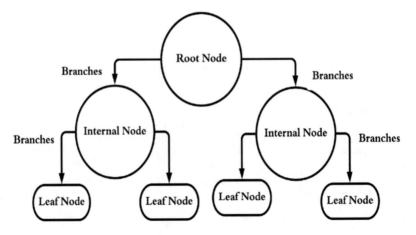

Fig. 4 Basic flow of decision tree algorithm

Step 3: Generate the decision tree which contains the best attribute.
Step 4: Repeat recursively for each branch, and make a new decision tree using the subset of the dataset created in step 2.

The process is continued until a stage where you cannot further classify the nodes and call them as final node/leaf.

Figure 5 explains the use of the decision tree algorithm for the image dataset for analyzing the brain image. Neurological disorder image datasets can be collected from various datasets (e.g., OASIS, TOF-MRA, Allen Brain Atlas, Alzheimer's Disease Neuroimaging Initiative (ADNI), the fMRI Data Center, etc.,). The images were then divided into two groups: testing and training. After collecting the results, the features of the image were extracted using a suitable technique, and the testing was carried out using a decision tree algorithm (C4.5, ID3, CHAID, etc.,). Figure 6 shows the output of lesion detection in the brain MRI image using decision tree algorithm.

Linear Regression

Linear regression was first developed in the discipline of statics to aid in the understanding of the relationship between numerical input and output. A linear model is a linear regression. It assumes that the input variable (x) and output variable (y) have

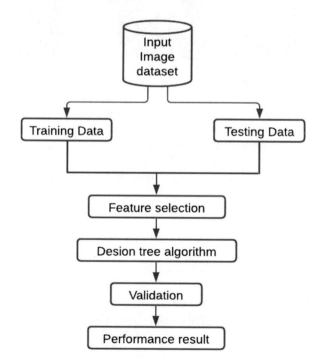

Fig. 5 Decision tree algorithm for image analysis

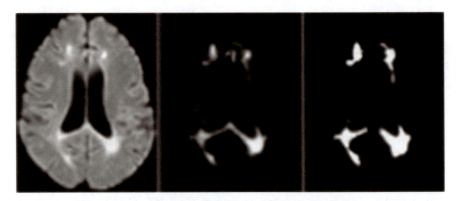

Fig. 6 Decision tree algorithm for lesion detection

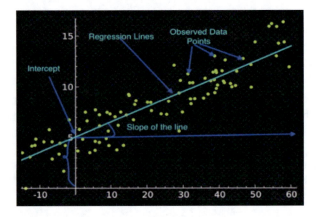

Fig. 7 Plot of linear regression

a linear relationship (y). Simple linear regression and multivariate linear regressions are two separate forms. Simple regression is an approach in which the response prediction is made using a simple feature. The linear regression algorithm's purpose is to discover the optimal values for b0 and b1, such that the best fit line can be found. Figure 7 shows the general plot of the linear regression model [32].

$$y = b_0 + b_1 x_1 \tag{1}$$

When multiple features are used, it is called as multiple linear regression

$$y = b_0 + b_1 x_1 + b_2 x_2 + \ldots + b_n x_n \tag{2}$$

By filtering a linear equation to the observed data, multiple linear regression aims to model the relationship between one or two features and response. Regression analysis formula

$$y = mx + b \tag{3}$$

Regression lines are used to predict the values of "*y*" (dependent variable) for a given value of "*x*" (independent variable). The best-fit regression line times to reduce the sum of squared distance between observed (actual) and forecasted data points. The intercept of regression lines in estimating the value of "*y*" (dependent variable) when "*x*" (independent variable) has no influence.

Figure 8 [34] shows the output of the linear regression model for analyzing the left hippocampus of the functional MRI dataset; Figure 8b shows the linear model analysis of the BOLD signal in the image.

Logistic Regression

One of the supervised machine learning algorithms that may be used to model the probability of an event or class is the logistic regression model. It is used when the data is separable linearly and the outcome is binary. In binary classification, there are primarily two types: one is logistic regression, which is a single independent

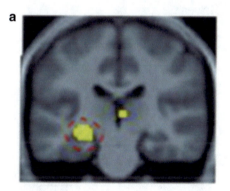
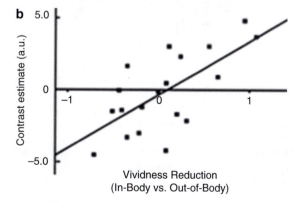

Fig. 8 (a) Linear regression analysis of the fMRI data (b) Linear analysis of BOLD signal

variable to predict the output, and the other one is multiple logistic regression, where multiple independent variables are used to predict the output [33]. Logistic regression models the data using the sigmoid function for single logistic regression which is given as

$$e = 1/\left(1+e^{-(b0+b1x)}\right) \quad (4)$$

Logistic regression models the data using the sigmoid function for multiple logistic regression which is given as

$$e = 1/\left(1+e^{-(b0+b1x+b2x2+...bnxn)}\right) \quad (5)$$

The probability of occurrence of a neurological disorder can be obtained by using this algorithm with high accuracy. The input image is preprocessed, the feature is extracted using a suitable algorithm, and the image is divided into training and testing data. Then, the logistic regression predicts the disorder based on the obtained features. Figure 9 shows the flow diagram of logistic regression [34].

Naive Bayes

The Naive Bayes algorithm is one of the simple and most effective supervised clas-

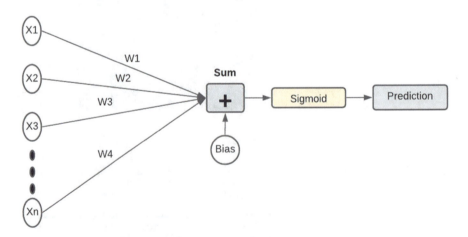

Fig. 9 Flow diagram of logistic regression

sification algorithms. It helps in building fast machine learning that can predict rapidly. It is an object probability-based probabilistic classifier, where naïve assumes the occurrence of a certain feature independent of the occurrence of the other feature and Bayes, as it depends on the Bayes principle: $P(y|X) = \dfrac{P(X|y)P(y)}{P(X)}$, where y is a class variable and x is a dependent feature vector (of size n), which is given as $X = \{x_1, x_2, x_3, \ldots, x_n\}$. Apply Bayes' theorem to the given dataset in the following way: Now, if any two events A and B are independent, then $P(A,B) = P(A)P(B)$. Then; the final result will be given as

$$P(y|x_1 \ldots | x_n) = \frac{P(x_1|y)P(x_2|y)\ldots P(x_n|y)}{P(x_1)P(x_2)\ldots P(x_n)} \qquad (6)$$

It can also be rewritten as

$$P(y|x_1 \ldots | x_n) = \frac{P(y):\Pi(I=i\ldots n)P(x_i|y)}{P(x_1)P(x_2)\ldots P(x_n)} \qquad (7)$$

We can now eliminate that term because the denominator remains constant for every given input:

$$(y|x_1 \ldots | x_n) \alpha \; P(y):\Pi(i=1\ldots n)P(x_i|y) \qquad (8)$$

It was found the best classification results were obtained by mostly using a Naive Bayes classifier for analyzing MRI images from Parkinson's and Alzheimer disease [5].

Support Vector Machine

SVM is abbreviated as support vector machine. It is the most widely used supervised learning method for classification and regression; however, it is more commonly used for classification. The goal of the SVM method is to determine the best line or decision boundary for categorizing n-dimensional space into classes, so that subsequent data points can be easily placed in the relevant category. This ideal decision boundary is referred to as a hyperplane. SVM is used to choose the extreme points/vectors that help build the hyperplane. These extreme points are known as support vectors, and hence, algorithm is called support vector machine. The margin is the difference between two lines on the closest data points of different classes [26]. The perpendicular distance between the line and the support vectors can be used to determine the margin. A wide margin is considered a good margin, whereas a tiny margin is considered a poor margin. The training culminated in the creation of a decision surface that splits the space into two subspaces. Each subspace represents a different training data class. Once the training is complete, the test data is mapped to the feature space. These data are then assigned a class based on which subspace they are mapped to. The fundamental goal of SVM is to divide datasets into classes in order to find the maximum marginal hyperplane (MMH), which can be done in two steps [29]:

1. To begin, SVM will construct hyperplanes that best divide the classes iteratively.
2. The hyperplane that correctly separates the classes will then be chosen.

By applying the above steps, a linear discrimination SVM model, which is a binary classifier, divides the space into two classes of MRI images by predicting the hyperplane.

Unsupervised Learning

Unsupervised machine learning techniques are effective for applications like clustering, since they don't require tagged data. For example, image classification may be studied using clustering methods. Unsupervised clustering, in addition to analyzing existing data, predictions can also be made using algorithms. A model can be trained using the dataset from various data sources.

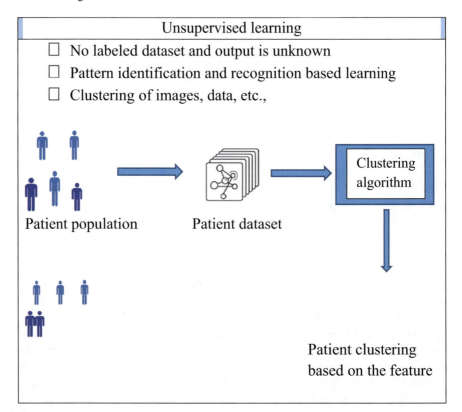

K-Means Algorithm

A popular unsupervised learning approach is the k-means clustering algorithm This approach uses an integer k and n observations. The result is a k-set partition of the n observations, with each observation belonging to the cluster with the closest mean. The operations of k-means are summarized in the stages below.

1. Set up k cluster centers. This can be achieved in practice by selecting k center at random.
2. Points are derived from n observations or k randomly generated center points.
3. Calculate how far each observation is from the cluster centers.
4. Each point should be assigned to the cluster with the smallest distance between its center and the other cluster centers.
5. As the cluster mean, recalculate the placements of the k centers.
6. Once more, compute the distance between each data point and the newly estimated centers.

Steps 3 and 4 should be repeated until all data points have been allocated to the same cluster (data points do not move).

Dataset of individuals with Alzheimer's (AZ) disease having longitudinal evaluations. The National Alzheimer's Coordinating Center database, supplying neuropathological data. The AZ disease in the image was clustered using the means clustering technique. The researchers wanted to look at subgroups of patients with different extrapyramidal sign progression trajectories and their clinical and neuropathological correlates [4]. K-means algorithm to cluster the neurological dataset is based on the disease condition using the above steps [3].

Mean-Shift Clustering Algorithm

The mean-shift clustering method is a centroid-based approach that aids unsupervised learning in a variety of situations. It is one of the most effective image processing and computer vision algorithms. It works by relocating data points to centroids, which then become the mean of other points in the region. The mode searching algorithm is another name for it. The benefit of the method is that it distributes clusters to data without automatically specifying the number of clusters depending on bandwidth.

Unlike the K-means cluster technique, mean-shift does not need a priori cluster number specification. In relation to the data, the algorithm determines the number of clusters [5]. For fMRI (functional magnetic resonance imaging) analysis of neurological disorders the temporal properties of the image is taken. Simulated and actual fMRI data were utilized to compare cluster analysis with mean-shift clustering, which uses a feature space that includes temporal and spatial features [6]. Figure 10 shows the flow of mean-shift algorithm used for clustering medical images.

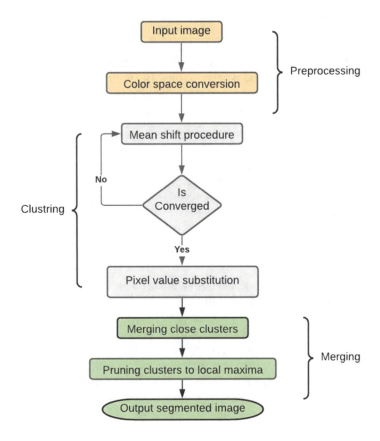

Fig. 10 Flowchart of mean-shift algorithm used for medical image classification

Affinity Propagation and Hierarchical Clustering

To split the brain MRI images into multiple clusters, an affinity propagation approach was used. The affinity propagation method uses tissue-segmented and anatomically parcellated pictures to characterize the similarity between brain images [7]. After clustering, a representative exemplar image is found as the single topic atlas for each clustered, and the MRI images fitting to the same subgroup are recognized. Figure 11 depicts the brain MRI image's tissue segmentation. The algorithm of affinity propagation is:

- Algorithm works based on resemblances among data points.
- All data points are considered as the potential cluster center.
- Cluster centers are identified that represents the dataset.

Affinity propagation requires two data:

- Similarities between data points $s(i,k)$
- Preferences $s(k,k)$

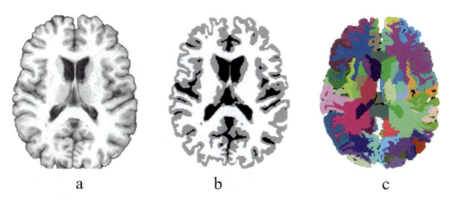

Fig. 11 (**a**) Original image. (**b**) Tissue segmented image using affinity propagation. (**c**) Structure parcellation using affinity propagation

i represents a data point.
k represents the exemplar.

The hierarchical clustering-based segmentation (HCS) is an unsupervised method for separating various sections in image data. The HCS method segments the images by splitting an image into its regions at hierarchical degrees of permitted dissimilarity across the different regions [36]. As the allowable threshold value is increased, the hierarchy represents the uninterrupted merging of similar, adjacent, and disjoint regions [8, 9].

Hierarchical clustering-based segmentation algorithm includes the following.

1. Labeling of each pixel in the image:
   - Label every pixel according to the pre-segmentation if the image has already been segmented.
   - If initial segmentation isn't possible, label every pixel as a separate section.
   - The amount of distinction between areas that can be allowed should be set to zero.

2. Dissimilarity value is calculated among in the given image.
   - The least dissimilarity value should be used as the threshold value.

3. If the threshold and dissimilarity value are equal, then merge all the values close to the dissimilarity value or else move to step 6.

4. If the regions merged in the above step is greater than 0, reclassify the pixels on the boundary of the combined areas with the remaining regions until no further classification is done.

Save the region data for this iteration as an intermediate segmentation among the combined regions after all accessible border pixels have been classed, and move on to step 2.

Otherwise, move to step 5, if the areas merged in step 3 is equal to 0.

Fig. 12 Hierarchical clustering for brain image

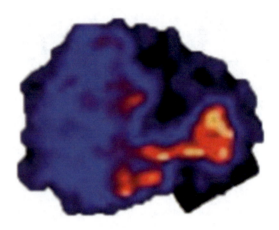

5. Move to step 7 if the number of regions in the image is less than the predetermined value, otherwise go to step 6.
6. If the current dissimilarity permitted value is well below the maximum permissible value, go to step 2 and gradually increase the dissimilarity allowed value. If not, go to step 7.
7. Save the data from the current iteration.

Figure 12 [35] shows the output of the hierarchical clustering algorithm of brain image by applying the abovementioned procedure.

Density-Based Spatial Clustering (DBSC)

Density-based clustering is a term used to describe unsupervised learning approaches for identifying unique groups/clusters in input images. DBSCAN is a density-based clustering base technique. It can detect clusters of various shapes and sizes in a large amount of noisy data including outliers [10].

Two parameters are used in the DBSC algorithm:

minPts: The minimum number of clustered points required for a region to be considered dense (a threshold)
eps (): A distance metric that may be used to find points in the vicinity of a given location

- The algorithm selects a point in the image dataset at random.
- If there are at least "minPoint" points within a radius, we consider it to be part of the same cluster.
- The clusters are then extended, by repeating the neighborhood computation for each nearby point.

Static and dynamic functional connectivity of the fMRI images can be analyzed using the DBSC algorithm by applying the above procedure [11, 12].

Gaussian Mixture Modeling

Histogram thresholding is one of the most often used methods for segmenting pictures, and Gaussian-mixture-based segmentation is based on it. The assumption in histogram thresholding is that an image has two areas or classes: target and background, each with a unimodal gray-level distribution. As a result, the segmentation problem entails selecting an appropriate threshold for partitioning the picture into target and background regions. The probability density function (PDF) of the gray levels in the picture is a combination of two Gaussian density functions with specific means, standard deviations, and proportions in Gaussian-mixing segmentation techniques [12, 13].

$$P(x) = \sum_{a=1}^{b} p_a N\left(x \propto_a, \sigma_a^2\right)$$

where b is the number of regions
$p_a > 0$ -weights, i.e., is $\sum_{a=1}^{b} p_a$

$$N\left(\propto_a, \sigma_a^2\right) = \frac{1}{\sigma\sqrt{2pa}} \exp \frac{-(x-\propto_a)^2}{2\sigma_i^2}$$

where

$\propto_a$ – mean of class a.
σ_a^2 – standard deviation of class a.

Figure 13 [35] shows the input MRI image and Gaussian output image [14]. White and gray matter in the brain MRI image can be classified to analyze neurological disorders, like attention deficit hyperactivity disorder (ADHD).

Convolutional Neural Network (CNN)

CNN stands for convolutional neural network and is a sort of deep learning neural network. In short, consider CNN to be a machine learning system that can take an input image, assign relevance (learnable weights and biases) to various aspects/objects in the image, and distinguish between them. Figure 14 shows the block diagram of CNN [15, 30, 35].

CNN extracts data from images by extracting features.
The following are the components of any CNN:

- A grayscale image serves as the input layer.
- The output is a multi-class labeling system.
- Convolution layers, rectified linear unit layers, pooling layers, and a fully linked neural network are all hidden layers in the CNN architecture.

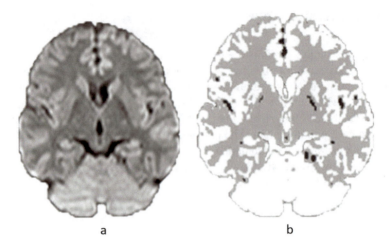

Fig. 13 (**a**) Input MRI image, (**b**) Gaussian image

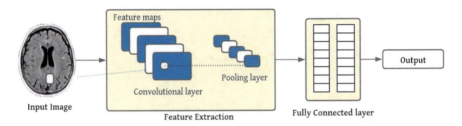

Fig. 14 Block diagram of CNN

Convolutional Layer

It has a convolutional filter of size N*M*D, where D is the image depth. N and M are the image pixel. Kernels are convolved over the image region, and the dot product among the filter entries is computed during the forward pass [16].

Activation Functions

For nonlinear transformation of medical images, the following activation functions are used:

- Sigmoid
- Tan hyperbolic
- Rectified linear unit

Pooling Layer

Convolved features are down sampled in the pooling layer. By dimensionality reduction, it reduces the amount of computing power necessary to process the data. It avoids overfitting and minimizes translation and rotational variance of images by aggregating data over space. It also minimizes spatial size by aggregating data across space or feature types. The input to a pooling process is partitioned into a collection of rectangular patches. Depending on the pooling, each value is replaced with a single value. Maximum pooling and average pooling are the two forms [27, 28].

Fully Connected Layer

The fully connected layer is comparable to a deep neural network in that each node has interconnections to all of the inputs and that each link has weights associated with it. The total of all inputs multiplied by the weights yields the final output. The classifier work is performed by the fully connected layer, which is proceeded by the sigmoid activation function. In Table 1, various types of CNN are used for the classification of neurological disorders. The table highlights some widely used CNN networks used for the analysis of disorders.

S. no.	CNN	Developed by	Neurological disorders
1.	Modified LeNet [17]	R.A. Hazarika, A. Abraham, D. Kandar and A.K. Maji	Mild cognitive impairment (MCI), cognitively normal (CN), Alzheimer's disease (AD)
2.	VGG16 [18]	Jain, R., Jain, N., Aggarwal, A. and Hemanth, D.J.	AD, MCI
3.	AlexNet, GoogLeNet, ResNet50 [19]	Khagi, B., Lee, B., Pyun, J.-Y. and Kwon, G.-R.	AD, healthy control (HC)
4.	ResNet-18 [20]	M. Raza, M. Awais, W. Ellahi, N. Aslam, H.X. Nguyen and H. Le-Minh	CN, significant memory concern (SMC), early mild cognitive impairment (EMCI), mild cognitive impairment (MCI), late mild cognitive impairment (LMCI), and AD
5.	VGG 19 [21]	Bhatele, K.R. and Bhadauria, S.S.	Alzheimer's disease (AD) and Parkinson's disease (PD)
6.	U-Net [22]	Fan, Zhonghao, Li, Johann, Zhang, Liang, Zhu, Guangming, Li, Ping, Lu, Xiaoyuan, Shen, Peiyi, Shah, Syed, Bennamoun, Mohammed, Hua, Tao and Wei, Wei	AD, late MCI, early MCI
7.	3D CNN [23]	Yee, Evangeline, Ma, Da, Popuri, Karteek, Wang, Lei and Beg, Mirza Faisal	Stable dementia, stable normal control

Conclusion

Advanced CNN approaches and models in supervised and unsupervised algorithms, as well as advances in high-speed computing techniques, provide a unique opportunity to predict and manage a variety of neurological illnesses, such as Alzheimer's disease, Parkinson's disease, and schizophrenia, among others. The most popular CNN models were investigated in this article for diagnosing neurological disorders using MRI, fMRI, and CT scan dataset. The use of CNN techniques to classify neurological illnesses identified in the literature has been described.

References

1. A.-M. Tautan et al., Artificial intelligence in neurodegenerative diseases: a review of available tools with a focus on machine learning techniques. Artif. Intell. Med. **117**, 102081 (2021)
2. A. Tagaris, D. Kollias, A. Stafylopatis, G. Tagaris, S. Kollias, Machine learning for neurodegenerative disorder diagnosis—survey of practices and launch of benchmark dataset. Int. J. Artif. Intell. Tools **27**(03), 1850011 (2018)
3. M.B.T. Noor, N.Z. Zenia, M.S. Kaiser, et al., Application of deep learning in detecting neurological disorders from magnetic resonance images: a survey on the detection of Alzheimer's disease, Parkinson's disease and schizophrenia. Brain Inf. **7**, 11 (2020)
4. G. Tosto, S.E. Monsell, S.E. Hawes, G. Bruno, R. Mayeux, Progression of extrapyramidal signs in Alzheimer's disease: clinical and neuropathological correlates. J. Alzheimers Dis. **49**, 1085–1093 (2016)
5. L. Ai, J. Xiong, Temporal–spatial mean-shift clustering analysis to improve functional MRI activation detection. Magn. Reson. Imaging **34**, 1283 (2016)
6. H. Cho, S. Kang, S.I. Cho, Y.H. Kim, Image segmentation using linked mean-shift vectors and its implementation on GPU. IEEE Trans. Consum. Electron. **60**, 719–727 (2014)
7. G. Li et al., Grouping of brain MR images via affinity propagation. The Midwest symposium on circuits and systems conference proceedings: MWSCAS. Midwest symposium on circuits and systems (2009)
8. C. Hejijun, J. Zheng, Y. Guo, Y. Shen, A robust image segmentation method using hierarchical color clustering, pp. 1–6. https://doi.org/10.1145/3028842.3028843 (2016).
9. A. Selvan, L. Cole, L. Spackman, C. Wright, Hierarchical cluster analysis to aid diagnostic image data visualization of MS and Other medical imaging modalities, in *Imaging Mass Spectrometry Methods and Protocols*, Methods in Molecular Biology, ed. by L. Cole, vol. 1, (Humana Press, Totowa, 2017), pp. 95–123
10. https://www.kdnuggets.com/2020/04/dbscan-clustering-algorithm-machine-learning.html
11. D. Rangaprakash, T. Odemuyiwa, D. Narayana Dutt, et al., Density-based clustering of static and dynamic functional MRI connectivity features obtained from subjects with cognitive impairment. Brain Inf. **7**, 19 (2020)
12. H. Bi, H. Tang, G. Yang, et al., Accurate image segmentation using Gaussian mixture model with saliency map. Pattern. Anal. Applic. **21**, 869–878 (2018)
13. J.B. Ashly, S.N. Kumar, F.A. Lenin, K.H. Ajay, V. Suresh, An improved Gaussian mixture model based on prior probability factor for MR brain image segmentation, in *Soft Computing for Problem Solving. Advances in Intelligent Systems and Computing*, ed. by K. Das, J. Bansal, K. Deep, A. Nagar, P. Pathipooranam, R. Naidu, vol. 1057, (Springer, Singapore, 2020)

14. L. Moraru, S. Moldovanu, L.T. Dimitrievici, N. Dey, A.S. Ashour, F. Shi, S.J. Fong, S. Khan, A. Biswas, Gaussian mixture model for texture characterization with application to brain DTI images. J. Adv. Res. **16**, 15–23., issn 2090-1232 (2019)
15. D.R. Sarvamangala, R.V. Kulkarni, Convolutional neural networks in medical image understanding: a survey. Evol. Intel. **15**, 1–22 (2021)
16. R.A. Hazarika, A. Abraham, D. Kandar, A.K. Maji, An improved LeNet-Deep Neural Network Model for Alzheimer's disease classification using brain magnetic resonance images. IEEE Access **9**, 161194–161207 (2021)
17. E. Yagis et al., Effect of data leakage in brain MRI classification using 2D convolutional neural networks. Sci. Rep. **11**(1), 22544 (19 Nov 2021)
18. R. Jain, N. Jain, A. Aggarwal, D.J. Hemanth, Convolutional neural network based Alzheimer's disease classification from magnetic resonance brain images. Cogn. Syst. Res. **57**, 147 (2019)
19. F. Ramzan et al., A deep learning approach for automated diagnosis and multi-class classification of Alzheimer's disease stages using resting-state fMRI and residual neural Networks. J. Med. Syst. **44**(2), 37 (2019)
20. B. Khagi, B. Lee, J.-Y. Pyun, G.-R. Kwon, CNN models performance analysis on MRI images of OASIS dataset for distinction between Healthy and Alzheimer's patient, in *2019 International Conference on Electronics, Information, and Communication (ICEIC)*, (IEEE, Piscataway), pp. 1–4
21. K.R. Bhatele, S.S. Bhadauria, Classification of neurodegenerative diseases based on VGG 19 deep transfer learning architecture: a deep learning approach. Biosci. Biotechnol. Res. Commun. **13**(4), 1972–1980 (2020)
22. Z. Fan, J. Li, L. Zhang, G. Zhu, P. Li, X. Lu, P. Shen, S. Shah, M. Bennamoun, T. Hua, W. Wei, U-net based analysis of MRI for Alzheimer's disease diagnosis. Neural Comput. Applic. **33**, 13587 (2021). https://doi.org/10.1007/s00521-021-05983-y
23. E. Yee, D. Ma, K. Popuri, L. Wang, M.F. Beg, Construction of MRI-based Alzheimer's disease score based on efficient 3D convolutional neural network: comprehensive validation on 7,902 images from a multi-center dataset. J. Alzheimers Dis. **79**, 1–12 (2020). https://doi.org/10.3233/JAD-200830
24. S.A. Mostafa, A. Mustapha, S.H. Khaleefah, M.S. Ahmad, M.A. Mohammed, Evaluating the performance of three classification methods in diagnosis of Parkinson's disease, in *SCDM 2018. AISC*, ed. by R. Ghazali, M. Deris, N. Nawi, J. Abawajy, vol. 700, (Springer, Cham, 2018), pp. 43–52. https://doi.org/10.1007/978-3-319-72550-5_5
25. G.R. Ramani, G. Sivagami, Parkinson disease classification using data mining algorithms. Int. J. Comput. Appl. **32**(9), 17–22 (Oct 2011)
26. D. Gil, M. Johnson, Diagnosing Parkinson by using artificial neural networks and support vector machines. Glob. J. Comput. Sci. Technol. **9**, 63–71 (2009)
27. S. Joshi, D. Shenoy, G.G. Vibhudendra Simha, P.L. Rrashmi, K.R. Venugopal, L.M. Patnaik, Classification of Alzheimer's disease and Parkinson's disease by using machine learning and neural network methods, in *2010 Second International Conference on Machine Learning and Computing*, (2010), pp. 218–222. https://doi.org/10.1109/ICMLC.2010.45
28. S. Sivaranjini, C.M. Sujatha, Deep learning based diagnosis of Parkinson's disease using convolutional neural network. Multimed. Tools Appl. **79**, 15467–15479 (2019). https://doi.org/10.1007/s11042-019-7469-8
29. L. Khedher, I.A. Illan, J.M. Gorriz, J. Ramirez, A. Brahim, A. Meyer-Baese, Independent component analysis-support vector machine-based computer-aided diagnosis system for Alzheimer's with visual support. Int. J. Neural Syst. **27**(03), 1650050 (2017)
30. A. Segato, A. Marzullo, F. Calimeri, E. De Momi, Artificial intelligence for brain diseases: a systematic review. APL Bioeng. **4**(4), Article ID 041503 (2020)
31. J. Maroco et al., Data mining methods in the prediction of dementia: a real-data comparison of the accuracy, sensitivity and specificity of linear discriminant analysis, logistic regression, neural networks, support vector machines, classification trees and random forests. BMC. Res. Notes **4**(1), 299 (2011)

32. A. Mozhdehfarahbakhsh, S. Chitsazian, P. Chakrabarti, T. Chakrabarti, B. Kateb, M. Nami, An MRI-based deep learning model to predict Parkinson's disease stages. J. Critic. Rev. Preprint from medRxiv (Feb 2021). https://doi.org/10.1101/2021.02.19.2125208
33. L. Billeci, A. Badolato, L. Bachi, A. Tonacci, Machine learning for the classification of Alzheimer's disease and its prodromal stage using brain diffusion tensor imaging data: A systematic review. PRO **8**(9), 1071 (2020)
34. L. Bergouignan, L. Nyberg, H.H. Ehrsson, Out-of-body-induced hippocampal amnesia. Proc. Natl. Acad. Sci. U. S. A. **111** (2014). https://doi.org/10.1073/pnas.1318801111
35. G. Li, L. Guo, T. Liu, Grouping of brain MR images via affinity propagation, in *Conference Proceedings (Midwest Symposium Circuits Systems)*, (2009 May 24), pp. 2425–2428. https://doi.org/10.1109/ISCAS.2009.5118290
36. A. Selvan, S. Pettitt, C. Wright, Hierarchical clustering-based segmentation (HCS) aided interpretation of the DCE MR images of the prostate. (2015). https://doi.org/10.13140/RG.2.1.1496.1123

COVID-19 Growth Curve Forecasting for India Using Deep Learning Techniques

V. Vanitha and P. Kumaran

Introduction

The global spread of the COVID-19 pandemic has resulted in considerable number of losses of life. It has been regarded as the world's largest economic and health disaster since World War II. According to the World Health Organization (WHO), the SARS-CoV-2 virus has infected approximately 200 million individuals globally. The virus has been shown to spread between persons via respiratory channels during human movement, enhancing its transmissibility and making the whole population vulnerable. COVID-19 confirmed cases numbered 4,799,266 on May 17th, while 316,520 persons died as a result of the pandemic at global level. Due to the lack of vaccine and drugs at the initial outbreak, different countries have taken varied approaches to contain the outbreak. The most usual responses include strict lockdown, partial lockdown, the closure of all educational institutions, and the cancellation of all sorts of aircraft. Because of the link between human movement and viral transmissibility, governments throughout the world have implemented restrictions, such as mandatory face mask, social distancing, and shutting public transit and restaurants, to avoid crowds. Although the implementation of such regulations has slowed the spread, the emergence of lethal mutations continued to put public health at risk.

V. Vanitha (✉)
Sri Ramachandra Faculty of Engineering and Technology, Sri Ramachandra Institute of Higher Education and Research, Porur, Chennai, Tamil Nadu, India
e-mail: vanikkdi@gmail.com

P. Kumaran
Department of Computer Science and Engineering, National Institute of Technology Puducherry, Karaikal, Puducherry, India
e-mail: kumaran.p@nitpy.ac.in

© The Author(s), under exclusive license to Springer Nature Switzerland AG 2023
G. R. Kanagachidambaresan et al. (eds.), *System Design for Epidemics Using Machine Learning and Deep Learning*, Signals and Communication Technology, https://doi.org/10.1007/978-3-031-19752-9_18

Medical supplies are frequently in low supply due to rising patient numbers, placing a strain on healthcare systems and personnel in many nations. Thus, one of the most important factors to contain and control the spread is understanding the nature of the spread and accurately projecting the patterns. Reliability in forecasting COVID-19 spread trends can aid in the prediction of pandemic outbreaks and boost government readiness to combat the pandemic. Furthermore, precise forecasting can offer feedback on whether the implemented strategy helps reduce the burden on the country's healthcare system.

Such a tumultuous environment of epidemic breakouts sparked numerous broad questions where there is a definite answer: Would coronavirus endure until a vaccine is discovered, or will it be eradicated after a set length of time? How long does it take a medical expert to develop the correct drug or vaccine? What is the estimated number of individuals who will be affected by this epidemic? What is the likelihood of death or recovery among the afflicted patients? Is it different in different age groups and different parts of the world? If that's the case, what may be the reasons? How effective is the lockdown approach at reducing the spread? What are the negative consequences of lockdown, and how long can various countries afford it?

In the last decade, machine learning (ML) has established itself as a distinct academic subject by tackling a slew of extremely complicated and sophisticated real-world challenges. There is extant research that attempts to forecast death daily using the traditional and deep learning methods, like long short-term memory (LSTM) and its variants. The mean squared error (MSE) and absolute error (MAE) score are commonly used to evaluate the prediction capabilities of the models. Recurrent neural network, a type of deep learning, is used in this study to anticipate the pandemic trend for India by forecasting the number of new cases. The reason for choosing India is due to the fact that it is one of the top 10 severely afflicted countries in the world, according to healthcare professionals. Furthermore, the LSTM model built beats several previously published models; therefore, the work utilizes it to anticipate COVID-19 instances a week in advance.

The rest of the paper is organized as follows: section "Literature review" discusses related research in this field, section "Materials and methods" describes the dataset and details the proposed system, section "Results and discussion" discusses the experimental results, and section "Conclusion" concludes the study.

Literature Review

Machine learning models are widely employed to understand the COVID-19 pandemic from various medical perceptives, including understanding the impact of antibodies [1], chest X-rays and chest CT images [2, 3], mutations [4], and forecasting pandemic trends.

The authors of this study [5] focused on predicting the number of COVID-19 cases that will be confirmed, recovered, or died in 60 days in the 16 high-impact nations. They used a seasonal auto-regressive integrated moving average (SARIMA) and an auto-regressive integrated moving average (ARIMA) models. According to their study, the SARIMA model is more realistic than the ARIMA model. Da Silva et al. [6] compared the univariate ARIMA and a proposed hybrid model that examine the number of illnesses in the top 27 afflicted cities in Brazil. Their experiments demonstrated that the ensemble model outperformed the single model by 26.73%.

Researchers have indicated a strong desire to learn more about India's rapid expansion. Swaraj et al. [7] built a model for predicting the COVID-19 epidemic in India that used ARIMA and a nonlinear auto-regressive neural network (NAR). When compared to the single ARIMA model, the hybrid model exhibits a considerable reduction in evaluation metrics. Wadhwa et al. [8] forecast the number of active cases across India 3 months ahead using the linear regression (LR) model. Khan et al. [9] implemented various machine learning models to determine when will the number of cases in India stop growing and to examine policy restrictions. According to their findings, the GPR model surpasses the other models with an accuracy of 95 percent. Using daily fresh confirmed cases in Russia, Peru, and Iran, Wang et al. [9] created an LSTM model to estimate pandemic trends for 150 days. Bayesian model was used on publicly available global data to assess the impact of lockdowns on COVID-19 transmission for five nations with high covid incidence (India, Brazil, Russia, the USA, and the UK). It has been established that if the lockdowns are lifted, the outbreak tempo in Brazil, India, and Russia would considerably rise.

In [10], an auto-regression model was used to predict confirmed and recovered COVID-19 cases in Jakarta. With an MPAE value of less than 20%, the results suggest that this technique delivers adequate forecasting accuracy. When compared to traditional approaches, such as ARIMA, exponential smoothing, BATS, and Prophet, this methodology performed better for pandemic prediction. However, the prediction quality of the Poisson auto-regression technique still has to be improved to achieve good prediction performance. ARIMA, MLP, LSTM, and feedforward neural network (FNN) are four regression models used to forecast COVID-19 spread in [11]. The LSTM model was shown to have the highest forecast accuracy in this investigation.

In [12], a few machine learning models, including susceptible-infected-recovered, linear regression, polynomial regression, and SVR and LSTM, are examined in projecting COVID-19 cases in Saudi Arabia and Bahrain. When utilizing confirmed COVID-19 cases data from Saudi Arabia, the results show that SVR offers the greatest predicting, whereas LR surpasses the other models with Bahrain verified cases data.

Materials and Methods

Description of Dataset

The data for this study was taken from the government of India official website https://www.mohfw.gov.in/. The dataset contains information about the newly confirmed COVID-19 cases, cured cases, and deaths for each day for each state. The confirmed cases, cured cases, new cases, and death are updated by the Ministry of Health and Family Welfare (MoHFW), India, on a regular basis. The website provides state-wise statics of all aforementioned parameters. In the dataset, daily COVID-19 statistics are available for 560 days from January 30, 2020, till August 11, 2021. It contains 18,110 corona records observed for different states at different days. This dataset has been used to analyze the state-wise trend. The data from August 12, 2021 till date of this article was fetched from coronavirus research center of John Hopkins University available at GitHub site and are updated daily. The records are split into 65:35 for training and validation; records of 450 days are used for training, and remaining records are utilized for validation. A time step of seven is considered as the spread of covid is significant from 1 week to another week. COVID-19 statistics plots from data taken from MoHFW are shown in Fig. 1. Figure 2 depicts the total confirmed, recovered, active cases and deaths for each state. Figure 3 shows the top ten states with the highest confirmed cases. Figure 1a–c displays the heatmap plot of confirmed, recovered, and deaths for each state in India.

Forecasting COVID-19 with Recurrent Neural Network

The analysis of underlying patterns in time series data has seen as key way to solve a series of forecasting problems, like stock market forecasting, traffic planning and management, and weather prediction. In healthcare applications, time series

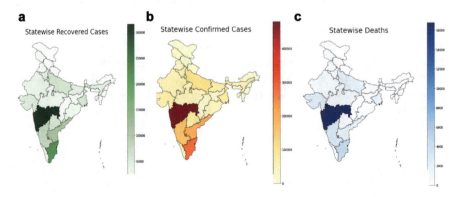

Fig. 1 Plots from dataset. (**a**) State wise recovered cases, (**b**) state wise confirmed cases, (**c**) state wise deaths

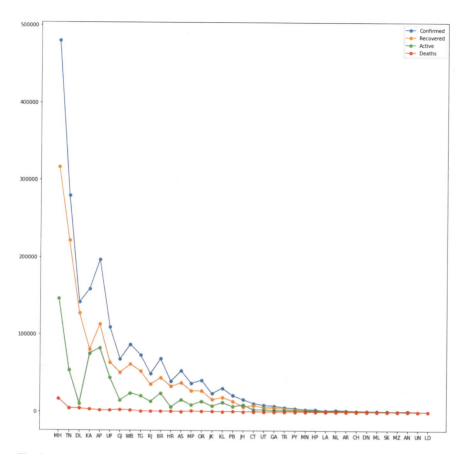

Fig. 2 Total infected cases till August 11, 2021

forecasting model is used to predict the spread of disease, estimate survival and mortality rate, and evaluate the possible risk caused by disease over time.

For short-term forecasting, conventional time series models, e.g., ARIMA and exponential smoothing, are appropriate. Long-term forecasting involves unearthing the underlying trends of the data and the effect of the association among the related parameters to provide estimates for future [13]. As they demand tremendous computations, conventional techniques were limited in their ability in terms of high-dimensional data and complex nature of functions [14].

Currently, deep learning models have been widely employed in forecasting problems [15], owing to its nature to learn the mapping of the input-output pair and support multiple inputs and outputs. Specifically, recurrent neural networks (RNNs) pose the ability to handle the sequence dependency that exists between inputs. However, for any standard RNN, weights on the hidden layers and output layers would either decay or explode. To tackle this gradient problem, long short-term memory (LSTM) has been designed and have been employed successfully in various domains [16].

	State/UnionTerritory	Confirmed	Deaths	Cured	Active
0	Maharashtra	1928603	49463	1824934	54206
1	Karnataka	918544	12081	894834	11629
2	Andhra Pradesh	881948	7104	871588	3256
3	Tamil Nadu	817077	12109	796353	8615
4	Kerala	755718	3042	687104	65572
5	Delhi	624795	10523	608434	5838
6	Uttar Pradesh	584966	8352	562459	14155
7	West Bengal	550893	9683	528829	12381
8	Odisha	329306	1871	325103	2332
9	Rajasthan	307554	2689	295030	9835

Fig. 3 Top ten states with respect to active cases (till August 11, 2021)

```
ADF Statistic: 0.627317
p-value: 0.988270
Critical Values:
        1%: -3.438
        5%: -2.865
        10%: -2.569
Failed to Reject Ho - Time Series is Non-Stationary
```

Fig. 4 ADF statistics for the COVID-19 dataset

ADF (Augmented Dickey-Fuller) Test

The time series forecasting model a stationary time series data for better prediction. So, as the preliminary step, we checked the nature of the dataset used in the study using the augmented Dickey-Fuller (ADF) test. The results of the test are interpreted based on the p-values. The ADF test was performed on the covid dataset and found to be nonstationary as the p-value is over 5% as shown in Fig. 4.

In order to make the dataset stationary, lag 1 difference was performed on the dataset. The ADF statistics after lag difference is shown in Fig. 5.

```
ADF Statistic: -4.160818
p-value: 0.000767
Critical Values:
        1%: -3.438
        5%: -2.865
        10%: -2.569
Reject Ho - Time Series is Stationary
```

Fig. 5 ADF statistics for the COVID-19 dataset after performing lag difference technique

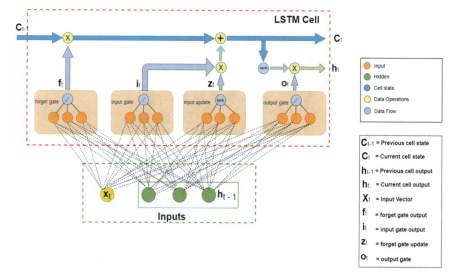

Fig. 6 LSTM cell

LSTM

RNN is the key deep learning technique on time series data to extract temporal correlations hidden in the data [17]. It has one to many hidden states distributed in the temporal way and can forecast the future with good accuracy than traditional methods [18–20]. The major disadvantage with this method is its inability to overcome vanishing gradient problem [21]. To address this shortcoming, LSTM was developed, which regularizes the gradient flow [16]. Long short-term memory is a recent variant of recurrent neural network to resolve exploding and vanishing gradient problems. LSTMs are capable of learning long-range dependencies hidden in the data through memory cells (LSTM cells). The dissection of LSTM cell is shown in Fig. 6.

These dependencies and temporal correlation of the input are captured in the LSTM cell through the series of gates, viz., forget gate, input gate, and output gate, along with the sigmoid and tangent activation function. The computation at each gate in LSTM cell is shown in the equations below [22].

$$\text{Input gate } i_t = \sigma\left(W_{xi}x_t + W_{hi}h_{t-1} + W_{Ci}C_{t-1} + b_i\right) \quad (1)$$

$$\text{Forget gate } f_t = \sigma\left(W_{xf}x_t + W_{hf}h_{t-1} + W_{Cf}C_{t-1} + b_f\right) \quad (2)$$

$$\text{Output gate } o_t = \sigma\left(W_{xo}x_t + W_{ho}h_{t-1} + W_{Co}C_t + b_o\right) \quad (3)$$

$$\text{Cell state } c_t = \sigma(f_t c_{t-1} + i_t \tanh\left(W_{xc}x_t + W_{hc}h_{t-1} + b_c\right) \quad (4)$$

$$\text{Hidden state } h_t = o_t \tanh(c_t) \quad (5)$$

where σ represents sigmoid function and $\tanh$ is tangent function. In this paper, variants of LSTM are implemented and are discussed in the following sections.

Stacked LSTM

In stacked LSTM, multiple LSTM layers stacked together as depicted in Fig. 7. Each intermediate LSTM output layer provides a sequence of outputs which is fed to the next LSTM layer. Also, it provides output for each time step rather than a one

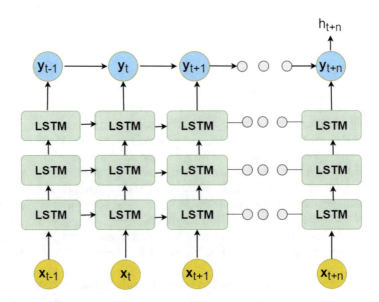

Fig. 7 Stacked LSTM

output for all input time steps. The computation at each stage is given in Eqs. (6), (7), (8), (9) and (10) [22].

$$\text{Input gate } i_t^L = \sigma\left(W_{ih}^L h_{t-1}^L + W_{ix}^L h_t^{L-1} + b_i^L\right) \quad (6)$$

$$\text{Forget gate } f_t^L = \sigma\left(W_{fh}^L h_{t-1}^L + W_{fx}^L h_t^{L-1} + b_f^L\right) \quad (7)$$

$$\text{Output gate } o_t^L = \sigma\left(W_{oh}^L h_{t-1}^L + W_{ox}^L h_t^{L-1} + b_o^L\right) \quad (8)$$

$$\text{Cell-state } c_t^L = (f_t^L W c_{t-1}^L + i_t^L c_t^{L-1}) \quad (9)$$

$$\text{Hidden state } h_t^L = o_t^L \tanh\left(c_t^L\right) \quad (10)$$

Bidirectional LSTM

Unlike LSTM, which can process inputs only in the forward direction, bidirectional LSTM uses information from both directions (from future to past and from past to future) as shown in Fig. 8.

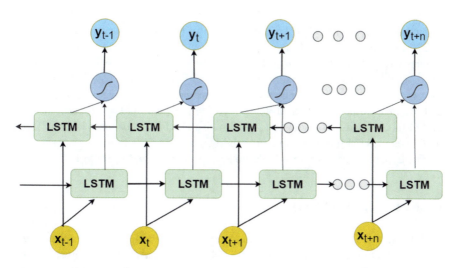

Fig. 8 Bidirectional LSTM

The computation at each stage for producing output is given below [22].

$$\text{Input gate } i_t^{\leftarrow L} = \sigma\left(W_{\leftarrow ih}^L h_{t-1}^L + W_{\leftarrow ix}^L h_t^{L-1} + b_{\leftarrow i}^L\right) \tag{11}$$

$$\text{Forget gate } f_t^{\leftarrow L} = \sigma\left(W_{\leftarrow fh}^L h_{t-1}^L + W_{\leftarrow fx}^L h_t^{L-1} + b_{\leftarrow f}^L\right) \tag{12}$$

$$\text{Output gate } o_t^{\leftarrow L} = \sigma\left(W_{\leftarrow oh}^L h_{t-1}^L + W_{\leftarrow ox}^L h_t^{L-1} + b_{\leftarrow o}^L\right) \tag{13}$$

$$\text{Cell-state } c_t^{\leftarrow L} = (f_t^{\leftarrow L} W c_{t-1}^{\leftarrow L} + i_t^{\leftarrow L} c_t^{\leftarrow L-1}) \tag{14}$$

$$\text{Hidden state } h_t^{\leftarrow L} = o_t^{\leftarrow L} \tanh\left(c \leftarrow_t^L\right) \tag{15}$$

The output of the network is the cumulative outputs from both directions and is given by

$$\text{Output } y_t = W_{hy}^{\leftarrow} h_t^{\leftarrow} + W_{hy}^{\rightarrow} h_t^{\rightarrow} + b_y \tag{16}$$

The Proposed Models

LSTM Model

Three LSTM models are built for this study and experimented on the dataset. The first model based on stacked LSTM is shown in Fig. 9. It has an input layer, two LSTM hidden layers, a fully connected layer, and an output layer. The input time sequence is set to 7, considering the significance of a week of COVID-19 data. Both the first and second LSTM hidden layers have 150 units and a rectified linear unit (ReLU) activation function. The fully connected layer is designed with 64 neurons, and the final output layer has a dense layer with 1 neuron. The proposed second LSTM model is similar to the first model with an additional dropout layer after the first hidden LSTM layer (dropout probability 0.5).

The hyperparameters set for both models are summarized in Table 1.

Bidirectional LSTM Model

A bidirectional STM model with architecture as shown in Fig. 10 was implemented. It has an input layer, two bidirectional LSTM hidden layers, a fully connected layer, and an output layer. The input time sequence is set to 7 as that of stacked LSTM model. Both the first and second LSTM hidden layers are an LSTM layer with 300 units and a rectified linear unit (ReLU) activation function. The fully connected layer is designed with 150 neurons, and the final output layer had a dense layer with 1 neuron.

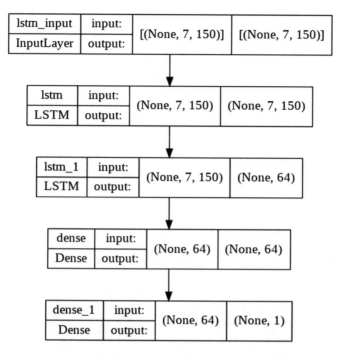

Fig. 9 Proposed stacked LSTM model

Table 1 Hyperparameters of the proposed model

Parameters	Value
Time step	7
Activation function	ReLU
Batch size	32
Epochs	150
Optimizer	Adam
Loss function	Squared error loss
No. of fully connected layers	1 (64 neurons)
Dropout probability (stacked LSTM+ dropout model)	0.5

Results and Discussion

In this section, the performance of three proposed models on Indian covid dataset is discussed. Three variants of LSTM models, namely, stacked LSTM, stacked LSTM + dropout, and bidirectional LSTM, are built and experimented on the dataset. Each model has been trained using the same dataset and evaluated by the same validation dataset. The forecasting for all proposed models is based on the attribute confirmed

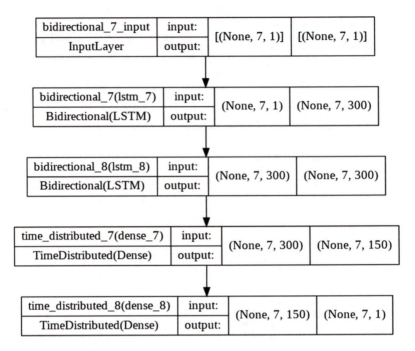

Fig. 10 Proposed bidirectional LSTM model

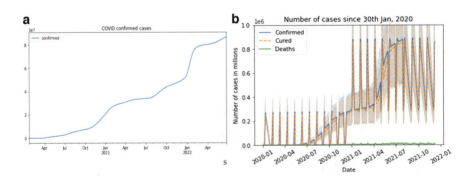

Fig. 11 Confirmed cases (**a**) for 1 year period, (**b**) for 2 years period

cases in the dataset. The confirmed covid cases plotted for 1 year period (2021–2022) and 2 years period (2020–2022) are shown in Fig. 11a, b, respectively.

From Fig. 11a, rise is event at two periods: January 2021 peaking in March 2021 and January 2022 peaking in February 2022. These two peaks indicate the second and third wave in India, respectively. The second wave in India started in January 2021, peaked in March 2021, and declined in June 2021. The third wave driven by the Omicron variant started in January 2022, peaked in February 2022, and declined in March 2022. The start of the first wave (January 2020) and its trend for 2 years period of 2020–2022 can be interpreted in Fig. 11b.

The trend of active, cured, and death for top three states, namely Maharashtra, Karnataka, and Tamil Nādu for the period of 2 years from 2020 to 2022 are shown in Fig. 12. These three states top the list of severely affected states. Though the number of active, cured, and death cases vary for each state, they exhibit more or less same trend throughout the 2-year period.

The proposed three models, namely, stacked LSTM model, LSTM with dropout layer, and bidirectional model, are built on training dataset and checked against the validation dataset. All the experiments are conducted using a 16GB graphics processing unit and Keras framework with TensorFlow back end.

The proposed models are trained on the dataset for different epoch sizes of 50,100,150 and 500. The training loss and validation loss for three models at epoch size = 150 are given in Figs. 13a, b and 14, respectively. The loss plot curve can used to interpret the performance of the model whether are underfit, overfit, or perfectly fit the data. Underfitting models have high bias, meaning that training loss will not decrease with increase in data. It indicates that the model is not able learn from the training data. On the other hand, overfitting indicates high variance. The model can perform well on the training data, but poor on the unseen data. It means that model cannot generalize well.

The training-validation loss plot of stacked LSTM revealed that both training loss and validation loss are high with smaller training samples. As the samples are increased, both the losses came down. More to that, both the losses follow the same path, and distance between them is less. It indicated that the proposed stacked LSTM model shows good fit on data and can generalize well on the unseen data.

The training-validation loss plot of bidirectional LSTM revealed that validation loss is very high than training loss and shoots up at several batches of datapoints. This indicate that the proposed bisectional model has overfitting problem and not able to generalize on new data.

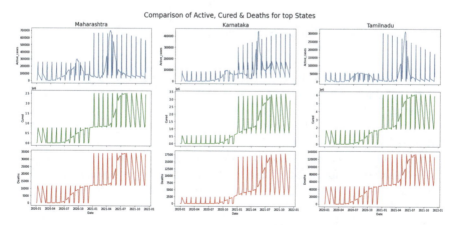

Fig. 12 Trend of active, cured, and death in top three states

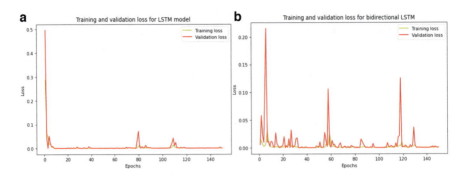

Fig. 13 (**a**). Plot of training/validation loss for LSTM, (**b**) training/validation loss for bidirectional LSTM

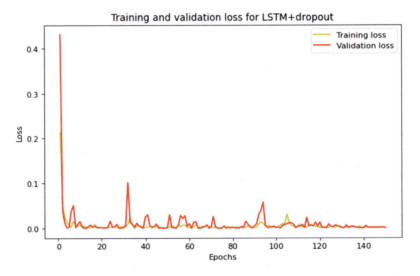

Fig. 14 Training/validation loss for LSTM + dropout

The training-validation loss plot of stacked LSTM + dropout model has shown a similar behavior of the first model, but with the validation loss greater than the first model.

Error measures of the proposed models are calculated using the metrics RMSE and MAPE and are tabulated in Table 2.

As the LSTM and bidirectional LSTM models have shown better, these two models are used for forecasting. These models forecast the confirm cases for 7 days from June 21, 2022, to June 28, 2022, and are shown in Fig. 15a, b, respectively.

Table 2 Performance measure

Model	RMSE	MAPE
LSTM	0.1504	0.1077
LSTM+ dropout	95.20	0.1568
Bidirectional LSTM	131.24	0.2924

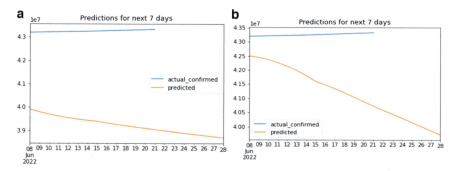

Fig. 15 Forecasting using (**a**) LSTM model, (**b**) LSTM + dropout model

Conclusion

This study proposed three LSTM variant models to forecast confirmed cases of COVID-19 in India. The data was collected through the government of India website and Johns Hopkins University. The necessary preprocessing techniques on data were carried out and was normalized. The data was split into training and testing dataset. The first model is LSTM model with input layer, two hidden layers, a dense layer, and an output layer. In the second model, dropout layer was added to the first model. The third model is bidirectional LSTM model. The performance of the proposed models has been evaluated using MAPE, and RMSE, on test dataset. The findings revealed that the proposed stacked LSTM outperforms other models and is best suited for Indian covid dataset.

References

1. R. Magar, P. Yadav, A. Barati Farimani, Potential neutralizing antibodies discovered for novel corona virus using machine learning. Sci. Rep. **11**, 5261 (2021). https://doi.org/10.1038/s41598-021-84637-4
2. N. Zhu, D. Zhang, W. Wang, A novel coronavirus from patients with pneumonia in china, 2019, 9.22.21, NEJM, 2020 [WWW Document]. URL https://www.nejm.org/doi/full/10.1056/nejmoa2001017

3. M. Toğaçar, B. Ergen, Z. Cömert, COVID-19 detection using deep learning models to exploit social mimic optimization and structured chest X-ray images using fuzzy color and stacking approaches. Comput. Biol. Med. **121**, 103805 (2020). https://doi.org/10.1016/j.compbiomed.2020.103805
4. B. Mullick, R. Magar, A. Jhunjhunwala, A. Barati Farimani, Understanding mutation hotspots for the SARS-CoV-2 spike protein using Shannon entropy and K-means clustering. Comput. Biol. Med. **138**, 104915 (2021). https://doi.org/10.1016/j.compbiomed.2021.104915
5. K. Arun Kumar et al., Forecasting the dynamics of cumulative covid-19 cases (confirmed, recovered and deaths) for top-16 countries using statistical machine learning models: Auto-regressive integrated moving average (arima) and seasonal auto-regressive integrated moving average (sarima). Appl. Soft Comput. **103**, 107161 (2021)
6. T.T. da Silva, R. Francisquini, M.C.V. Nascimento, Meteorological and human mobility data on predicting COVID-19 cases by a novel hybrid decomposition method with anomaly detection analysis: a case study in the capitals of Brazil. Expert Syst. Appl. **182**, 115190 (2021). https://doi.org/10.1016/j.eswa.2021.115190
7. A. Swaraj, K. Verma, A. Kaur, G. Singh, A. Kumar, L. Melo de Sales, Implementation of stacking based ARIMA model for prediction of Covid-19 cases in India. J. Biomed. Inf. **121**, 103887 (2021). https://doi.org/10.1016/j.jbi.2021.103887
8. P. Wadhwa, Aishwarya, A. Tripathi, P. Singh, M. Diwakar, N. Kumar, Predicting the time period of extension of lockdown due to increase in rate of COVID-19 cases in India using machine learning. Mater. Today Proc.., International Conference on Newer Trends and Innovation in Mechanical Engineering: Materials Science **37**, 2617–2622 (2021). https://doi.org/10.1016/j.matpr.2020.08.509
9. P. Wang, X. Zheng, G. Ai, D. Liu, B. Zhu, Time series prediction for the epidemic trends of COVID-19 using the improved LSTM deep learning method: case studies in Russia, Peru and Iran. Chaos Solit. Fractals **140**, 110214 (2020). https://doi.org/10.1016/j.chaos.2020.110214
10. B.I. Nasution, Y. Nugraha, J.I. Kanggrawan, A.L. Suherman, Forecasting of covid-19 cases in Jakarta using Poisson autoregression, in *2021 9th International Conference on Information and Communication Technology (ICoICT)*, (IEEE, Piscataway, 2021), pp. 594–599
11. C.-S. Yu et al., A covid-19 pandemic artificial intelligence-based system with deep learning forecasting and automatic statistical data acquisition: development and implementation study. J. Med. Internet Res. **23**, e27806 (2021)
12. H. Khaloofi, J. Hussain, Z. Azhar, H.F. Ahmad, Performance evaluation of machine learning approaches for covid-19 forecasting by infectious disease modeling, in *2021 International Conference of Women in Data Science at Taif University (WiDSTaif)*, (2021), pp. 1–6. https://doi.org/10.1109/WiDSTaif52235.2021.9430192
13. J.S. Armstrong, *Long-Range Forecasting* (Wiley, New York, etc, 1985)
14. Y. Bengio, Y. LeCun, Scaling learning algorithms towards AI. Largescale Kernel Mach. **34**(5), 1–41 (2007)
15. I.H. Witten et al., *Data Mining: Practical Machine Learning Tools and Techniques*, 4th edn. (Morgan Kaufmann, Burlington, 2016) https://www.amazon.com/exec/obidos/ASIN/0128042915/departmofcompute. Accessed on 30 Nov 2018
16. S. Hochreiter, J. Schmidhuber, Long short-term memory. Neural Comput. **9**(8), 1735–1780 (1997). https://doi.org/10.1162/neco.1997.9.8.1735
17. A. Sherstinsky, Fundamentals of recurrent neural network (RNN) and long short-term memory (LSTM) network. Phys D (2020). https://doi.org/10.1016/j.physd.2019.132306
18. K. Singh, S. Shastri, A.S. Bhadwal, P. Kour, et al., Implementation of exponential smoothing for forecasting time series data. Int. J. Sci. Res. Comput. Sci. Appl. Manage. Stud. (2019) issn: 2319-1953
19. Z. Zhao, K. Nehil-Puleoa, Y. Zhao, How well can we forecast the COVID-19 pandemic with curve fitting and recurrent neural networks? medRxiv preprint 2020. https://doi.org/10.1101/2020.05.14.20102541

20. S. Shastri, A. Sharma, V. Mansotra, A model for forecasting tourists arrival in J & K. India. Int. J. Comput. Appl. **129**(15), 32–36 (2015) issn: 0975-8887
21. M. Fakhfakh, B. Bouaziz, F. Gargouri, L. Chaari, ProgNet: Covid-19 prognosis using recurrent and convolutional neural networks. medRxiv preprint 2020. https://doi.org/10.1101/2020.05.06.20092874
22. Y. Yu, S. Xi, C. Hu, J. Zhang, A review of recurrent neural networks: LSTM cells and network architectures. Neural Comput. **31**, 1235–1270 (2019). https://doi.org/10.1162/neco_a_01199

Index

A
Algorithmic medicine, 272, 275–276
Artificial intelligence (AI), 27, 28, 38, 49–61,
  89, 101, 102, 105, 108, 110, 112–120,
  125–149, 179, 180, 207, 210, 213, 215,
  219, 221–228, 272, 275
Audio classification, 191

B
Billing, 22, 222, 278
Blockchain, 63–80

C
Cardiovascular diseases, 10, 221, 223–225
Circular economy, 50
Clinics, 111, 208, 216, 223, 227, 238, 272,
  274, 278
CNN architecture, 39, 40, 115, 191
Computer-aided diagnostic (CAD),
  38, 85, 286
Convolutional neural network (CNN), 38–40,
  44, 45, 85, 89–92, 94, 138, 140, 141,
  146, 148, 192, 194, 196, 208, 217,
  218, 299–302
COVID-19, 1–16, 37–45, 99–120, 125, 129,
  134, 137, 143–148, 167–175,
  177–180, 185–204, 207, 209–212,
  216, 218, 221, 223, 226–228,
  231–253, 257–270, 305–319
CT images, 115, 148, 185–204, 306

D
Data transparency and COVID, 68
Deep convolutional generative adversarial
  network (DCGAN), 153–165
Deep learning, 38, 39, 44, 52, 85, 89, 91, 94,
  95, 101, 120, 141–142, 144, 148, 155,
  165, 185–204, 207, 208, 210, 211, 213,
  215, 219, 221, 223, 224, 269,
  299, 305–319
Digital rehabilitation, 271, 272, 278, 279

E
Edge computing for good, 207–219
Effective, 4, 12, 45, 50, 60, 86, 89, 91, 101,
  103, 104, 111, 116, 127, 134, 138, 144,
  168, 177, 180, 201, 219, 223, 232, 233,
  235, 236, 243, 246, 248, 251–253, 292,
  294, 295, 306
E-health, 83, 143, 275, 277
Epidemic, 3, 5, 12, 16, 52, 58, 120, 129,
  131–138, 141–143, 148, 186, 189,
  207–219, 231, 257, 285–302,
  306, 307

Epidemic solutions, 207–219
E-prescription, 26
Expert systems, 102, 111, 113, 120, 135, 136, 143, 144

F

Features, 13, 21, 33, 34, 39, 40, 42–45, 85–88, 91, 101, 103, 112, 115, 140, 144, 146, 148, 149, 154, 171, 180, 191–199, 201–204, 210, 258–260, 262–265, 288–290, 292, 293, 295, 299, 301
Forecasting, 12, 54, 111, 138, 305–319
Frechet Inception Distance (FID), 161, 164, 165

G

Graphics processing unit (GPU), 155–157, 159, 162, 163, 208, 213–215, 219

H

Health, 2, 3, 7, 10, 11, 14, 16, 19–35, 37, 51–52, 58–60, 66, 77–79, 83, 85, 99–120, 126, 128, 129, 134, 141, 143, 178, 186, 207–210, 212, 213, 219, 221, 223–225, 227, 228, 231–253, 271–279, 285, 305, 308
Health sector, 52, 167–180, 271, 274, 276, 278, 279

I

India, 2–4, 9, 22–23, 32, 55, 100, 110, 186–188, 246, 247, 249, 305–319
Indian Internet of Medical Things (IIoMT), 207–210, 212–215
Internet of Things (IoT), 22, 49, 63–80, 100, 102, 108, 139, 142, 144, 207, 209, 214

L

Long short-term memory (LSTM), 144, 146, 197, 199, 201, 204, 306, 307, 309, 311–319

M

Machine learning, 12, 19, 20, 22, 26–28, 31, 33, 38, 52, 53, 58, 89, 101, 104, 105, 107, 115, 119, 135, 137–142, 144–149, 155, 180, 201, 204, 210, 221–228, 275, 276, 285–302, 306, 307
Machine learning model, 1–16, 28, 29, 34

Magnetic resonance image, 295
m-health, 114
Multiclass classification, 40, 190, 201

N

Neural networks, 49, 52, 88–91, 139, 140, 142, 144, 146, 148, 149, 153, 210, 222, 257–270, 275, 299, 301, 307–309
Neurodegenerative, 285–302

O

Object detection, 258–259, 264–268
Object tracking, 257, 258, 260–262
Optical character recognition (OCR), 30–32

P

Pandemic, 1–16, 19–35, 37, 99–120, 129–144, 148, 149, 167–180, 185–187, 189, 207–219, 221, 223, 226, 227, 231–233, 236, 244, 245, 249, 251, 253, 257–279, 305–307
PatchCamelyon (PCam), 155–160, 165
Photonics devices, 167–180
Policy, 60, 69, 186, 307

R

Radiograph images, 38, 41, 42, 45
Random forest, 91, 92, 94, 95, 138, 144, 199
Remote health monitoring, 100–103, 108, 110, 113, 118
Remote monitoring, 100, 101, 103–107, 113, 114, 119
Role of edge computing, 207–219
RT-PCR test, 218, 234, 235, 238

S

SARS and MARS, 4
Screening, 4, 11, 56, 109–111, 115, 135, 139, 142–143, 175, 201, 221, 222, 231–253
Security, 27, 32, 33, 60, 61, 68, 80, 107, 119, 210, 219, 249
Sensors, 52, 54, 58, 60, 66–80, 90, 100, 101, 103–113, 119, 142, 168, 172, 174, 175, 180, 208, 209, 213–215, 227, 274, 275
Severe acute respiratory syndrome coronavirus 2 (SARS-CoV-2), 3, 4, 11, 12, 37, 99, 102, 104–107, 131, 133, 143, 169, 175, 176, 190, 191, 231, 232, 236–238, 240–242, 244, 246, 247, 249, 305

Smart city, 50
Sustainable Development Goals (SDGs), 49–61

T
Telemedicine, 24, 25, 27, 35, 107, 110, 117, 227, 272–273, 277
Transfer learning, 40–42, 115

V
Vaccination, 58, 99, 134, 168, 231–253, 276
VGG16, 38–40, 42, 45, 46, 301
VGG19, 46, 162–165

W
Wireless body area networks (WBAN), 100, 104–107, 119, 120

X
X-ray, 19, 37–39, 41, 44, 45, 84, 115, 144, 146, 148

Y
You just Look once (YoLo), 216, 264–265, 267, 268

Printed in the United States
by Baker & Taylor Publisher Services